Practical Pharmacognosy

Fourth Edition

Practical Pharmacognosy

Fourth Edition

T. E. Wallis

B.Sc. (Lond.), F.I.C., Ph.C., F.L.S.

Reader in Pharmacognosy, University of London

Member of the Society of Public Analysts

PharmaMed Press

An imprint of BSP Books Pvt. Ltd.

4-4-309/316, Giriraj Lane,

Sultan Bazar, Hyderabad - 500 095.

Practical Pharmacognosy
by **T. E. Wallis**

This Reprint is published in arrangement with legal heirs of Author.

Nineth Reprint 2024

Published by:

PharmaMed Press
An imprint of BSP Book Pvt. Ltd.
4-4-309/316, Giriraj Lane, Sultan Bazar, Hyderabad - 500 095.
Phone: 040-23445688 Fax: 91+40-23445611
E-mail: info@pharmamedpress.com
www.pharmamedpress.com/pharmamedpress.net

Printed at
Repro India Limited.

Price: Rs. 295.00
ISBN: 978-93-81075-02-9 (Paperback)

PREFACE TO THE FOURTH EDITION

In preparing this fourth edition, the text has been revised throughout and some slight rearrangement of the contents has been made, so that the course of instruction may follow a more rational order of development. For example, belladonna, stramonium and henbane have been put with the herbs, because they now consist of stems, leaves, flowers and fruits as do other herbs, such as lobelia. It seems better to take them later in the course after a study of leaves, fruits and seeds which occur separately. The insects, cantharides, mylabris and cochineal have been put immediately after the herbs, because they are whole insect organisms just as the herbs are whole plant organisms. Instructions for determining stomatal number and index have been added to the histological schedules and also the flowers of belladonna, henbane and stramonium.

Under quantitative analysis six new exercises have been introduced including analysis of herbal mixtures, ash and volatile oil determinations, yield of extractive to solvents and the testing of strophanthus.

A second appendix has been added, summarising those pharmacognostical numerical data which are now available.

I am indebted to Mr. J. W. Fairbairn, B.Sc., for assistance with the reading of proofs. I also take the opportunity of thanking my publishers, Messrs. J. & A. Churchill, for the excellence of the workmanship put into the book and for their courtesy and helpfulness in overcoming any difficulties which have arisen.

T. E. WALLIS.

CONTENTS

Part II

DRUG DESCRIPTION AND HABITATS

Part III

HISTOLOGICAL SCHEDULES

Part IV

QUANTITATIVE ANALYSIS

Part V

THE EXAMINATION OF POWDERED DRUGS

INTRODUCTION

THE study of materia medica during a long period of time has resulted in the accumulation of much detailed knowledge of individual drugs, some of which concerns the behaviour of animal organisms to which the drug is administered, and is now separately treated under the designation of Pharmacology or Pharmacodynamics, while a further section is separately treated as Pharmacy, which studies the manufacture of galenical preparations of the drugs and the different ways of combining them for administration according to the wishes of the physician or of members of the public. The remaining part of this general body of information relates to the physical, sensory and chemical characteristics of the actual materials, characteristics which are used to determine their identity and quality ; with this section is also associated the study of their cultivation and preparation for purposes of commerce. The whole of this third section has been systematised and treated scientifically and is now distinguished as the *science* of *Pharmacognosy.* The study of the constitution of the constituents of the drugs belongs to the subject of pharmaceutical chemistry.

The present work aims at directing the student in making a practical study of the drugs he daily handles, and consists of a number of schedules of instructions, detailing the observations of greatest importance in the case of a number of typical drugs. Each schedule provides sufficient work for a period of about three hours, and, if carefully followed as a supplement to the reading of general text-books, will enable the student to understand more clearly the statements, and the reasons for the statements, that are made in the description of the drugs. Each schedule is followed by a few short notes, which explain the significance of some of the observations and experiments suggested in the schedule ; illustrative sketches are added in several instances, so as to suggest the kind of drawing which students may make for themselves when writing up the results of their experiments and observations.

A certain amount of microscopical work has been included in the schedules of Part I because there are several drugs, such as starches, hairs and glands, and broken leaves, whose characters can only be studied by this means. There are also numerous instances where drugs can only be identified with certainty when the naked-eye characters have been supplemented by the observation of certain additional microscopical details. One has to remember that, although it is often a comparatively easy matter to distinguish good commercial samples of entirely different drugs, the question which more often arises in practice is to ascertain that the specimen under examination has been derived from the correct botanical source and not from a nearly related species or genus, which might yield material having a general external resemblance to the genuine drug and yet possessing quite different medicinal properties ; it is under such circumstances that microscopical details frequently assume a critical importance.

APPARATUS

The apparatus needed for the practical study of pharmacognosy will include a microscope, dissecting instruments, bottles of reagents, and a few miscellaneous articles.

The microscope should be a substantially built student's instrument, which will allow of the addition of such further accessories as may become necessary for more advanced work later on. There should be two objectives—a $\frac{2}{3}$ in. (16 mm.) and a $\frac{1}{6}$ in. (4 mm.). These are the most generally useful powers, and, together with an eyepiece magnifying about eight diameters, would be a good selection. This is all that would be needed at first. An instrument of this type is shown in Fig. 1.

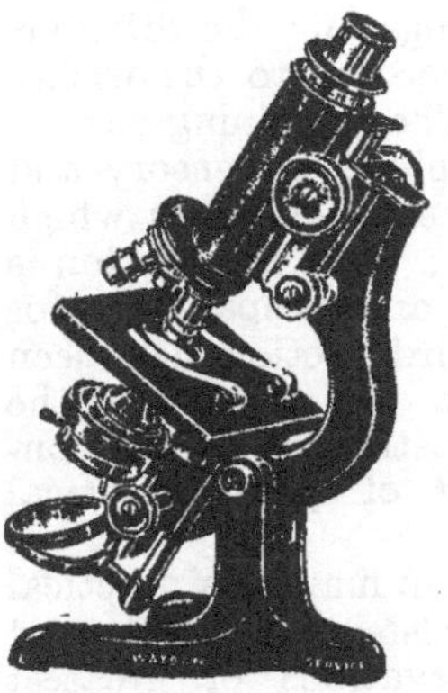

FIG. 1.—The "Service" Microscope, made by W. Watson & Sons, 313, High Holborn, W.C.1. A form of microscope suitable for the study of pharmacognosy.

The instrument is fitted with an eyepiece and a rotating triple objective-changer with three objectives, 16 mm., 4 mm., and 2 mm., the focussing substage is provided with an Abbe condenser. An attachable mechanical stage can be added at any time, if desired.

Daylight is a satisfactory illuminant for this work ; but, if it is necessary to work by artificial light, a paraffin lamp with a $\frac{1}{2}$ or $\frac{3}{4}$ in. flat wick is the most generally useful source of light.

If electricity is available, the most convenient source of artificial illumination is a metal-filament lamp with an opal bulb (such as the "Fullolite" lamp), which should be attached to a simple wooden base and covered by a black-japanned tin, constructed so as to screen the light from the observer's eyes (see Fig. 2).

The dissecting instruments should include a scalpel, a razor, which should be either ground flat on one side or very slightly hollowed, a pair of forceps, or two pairs (a light, fine-pointed pair, and a stronger and more heavily constructed pair), a pocket lens, a camel-hair brush, one or more hollowed glass blocks with covers, a spirit lamp, some 3×1 in. microscopic slides, a supply of $\frac{3}{4}$ in. (19 mm.) square or circular cover-glasses, and some needles fixed in handles. The most useful forms of needle are an ordinary sewing needle, a triangular glover's needle, and a bent needle, which can easily be made by heating a sewing needle in the flame until red-hot, bending it to the required shape, and tempering it by heating it red-hot a second time and dipping it into cold water. See illustrations in Fig. 3.[1]

[1] A set of instruments, made to this specification, is sold by Messrs. Britton, Malcolm and Waymark Ltd., of 38 Southwark Bridge Road, S.E.1, and can be obtained from the makers, post free, for about 12*s*. 6*d*., and a suitable strop costs an additional 2*s*.

The reagents that will be needed at the outset are water, alcohol, dilute glycerin, and iodine water. The alcohol should be about 90 per

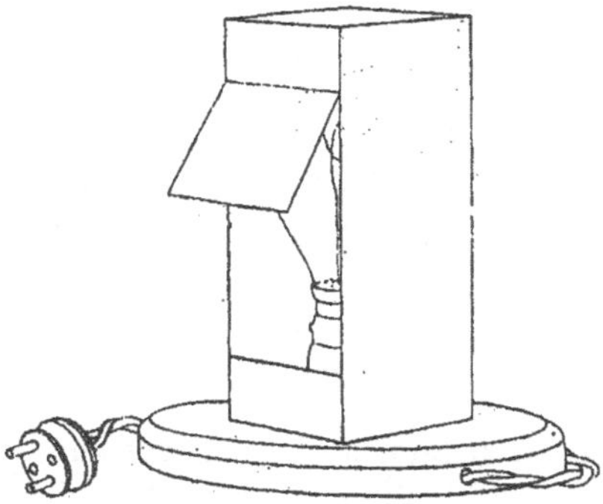

FIG. 2.—Simple electric lamp with cover, designed for use with the microscope.

cent., the dilute glycerin is made by mixing one volume of glycerin with two volumes of water, and the iodine water by mixing one volume

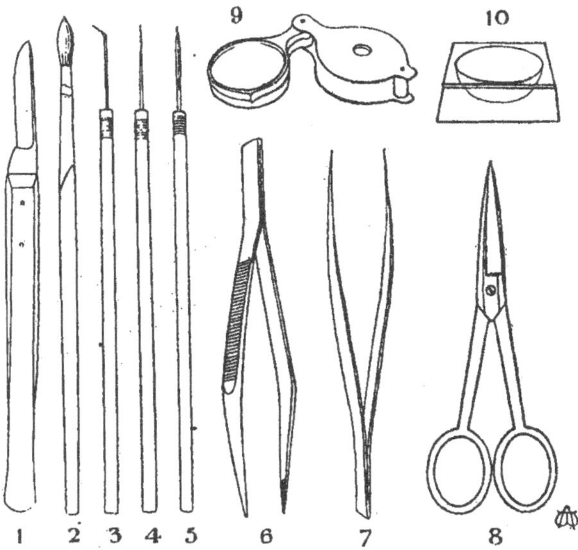

FIG. 3.—Dissecting instruments. 1. Scalpel. 2. Camel-hair brush. 3. Bent needle. 4. Straight needle. 5. Glover's needle. 6. Heavy forceps. 7. Fine-pointed forceps. 8. Dissecting scissors. 9 Pocket lens. 10. Hollowed glass block. All one-third actual size.

of decinormal iodine with four volumes of water, or by diluting the weak tincture of iodine of the Pharmacopœia to ten times its volume with water. The composition of other reagents will be described when the occasion for their use arises. These liquids are conveniently stored in small stoppered bottles of about 23 ml. capacity, and the whole of the bottles may be kept in a box with a lid and of sufficient depth to just take the bottles. Such an arrangement is very convenient, as it protects the bottles from dust and enables one to move the reagents as a whole with a minimum of trouble and risk.

The miscellaneous articles required will include several thin glass rods with rounded ends for removing drops of reagents from the bottles, some microscope slides (3 × 1 in.) and cover-glasses, slide labels, elder pith, a dipping tube (see Schedule XL), a one- or two-pound earthenware pot to hold water, into which slides or other dirty apparatus may be dropped, a duster, some plotting-paper, a razor-strop, a pencil (H or HB) and a note-book, which should be exercise-book size and have paper without lines.

There will be needed, in addition, test-tubes and a test-tube stand, a tripod, a micro-burner and tubing, some flasks, beakers, funnels, etc.

PRACTICAL PHARMACOGNOSY

PART I

SCHEDULES OF INSTRUCTIONS FOR THE EXAMINATION OF DRUGS

SCHEDULE OF INSTRUCTIONS—I

COMMERCIAL STARCHES

Starch of Potato. 1. Measure 8 ml. of distilled water and pour it into a test-tube, add 3 drops of a universal indicator.[1] Divide the tinted water between two test-tubes, noting that the colour is the same in both tubes. From the label on the indicator,[2] read off the corresponding approximate *p*H. To one tube add 0·2 gm. of potato starch, shake and observe the change of *p*H as shown by the alteration of the tint of the indicator. Record your *p*H readings and state your conclusion as to the reaction of the starch.

2. Take up a little commercial potato starch on the point of a needle, place it on a slide, moisten it with alcohol, stir up with a drop of water, and apply a cover-glass. Examine first with the 16-mm. objective and then with the 4-mm. objective. Observe that it consists almost entirely of single granules, the larger of which are ovoid or irregularly ovoid, while the smaller are sub-spherical or rounded. In each granule, usually nearer the smaller end of those which are ovoid, one may find a point—the hilum—which appears light or dark according to the focus, and is surrounded by a number of fine concentric lines—the striations. A very few granules show 2 or 3 hila, each with its concentric rings ; these are compound granules with two or three components, which may become separated during the preparation of the commercial starch, giving rise to granules having one or two flat surfaces and a curved surface. Sketch a few granules as seen with a 4-mm. objective, making the larger ones about 2 to 3 cm. in length, which corresponds to a magnification of about 300 diameters.

3. Mount a little potato starch in a small drop of water ; place one drop of solution of iodine in contact with the edge of the cover-slip,

[1] The B.D.H. universal indicator shows the following colour changes :—

*p*H up to 3·0 . .	Red.	*p*H 8·0 .	Green.
,, 4·0 . .	Deeper Red.	,, 8·5 .	Bluish Green.
,, 5·0 . .	Orange Red.	,, 9·0 .	Greenish Blue.
,, 5·5 . .	Orange.	,, 9·5 .	Blue.
,, 6·0 . .	Orange Yellow.	,, 10·0 .	Violet.
,, 6·5 . .	Yellow.	,, 10·5 .	Reddish Violet.
,, 7·0–7·5. .	Greenish Yellow.	,, 11·0 .	Deeper Reddish Violet.

[2] A suitable universal indicator is that made by the British Drug Houses, Graham Street, City Road, London, N.1.

and examine under the low power; note the gradual change from colourless to blue.

4. *Mucilage of Starch*, preparation of. Heat 45 ml. of distilled water

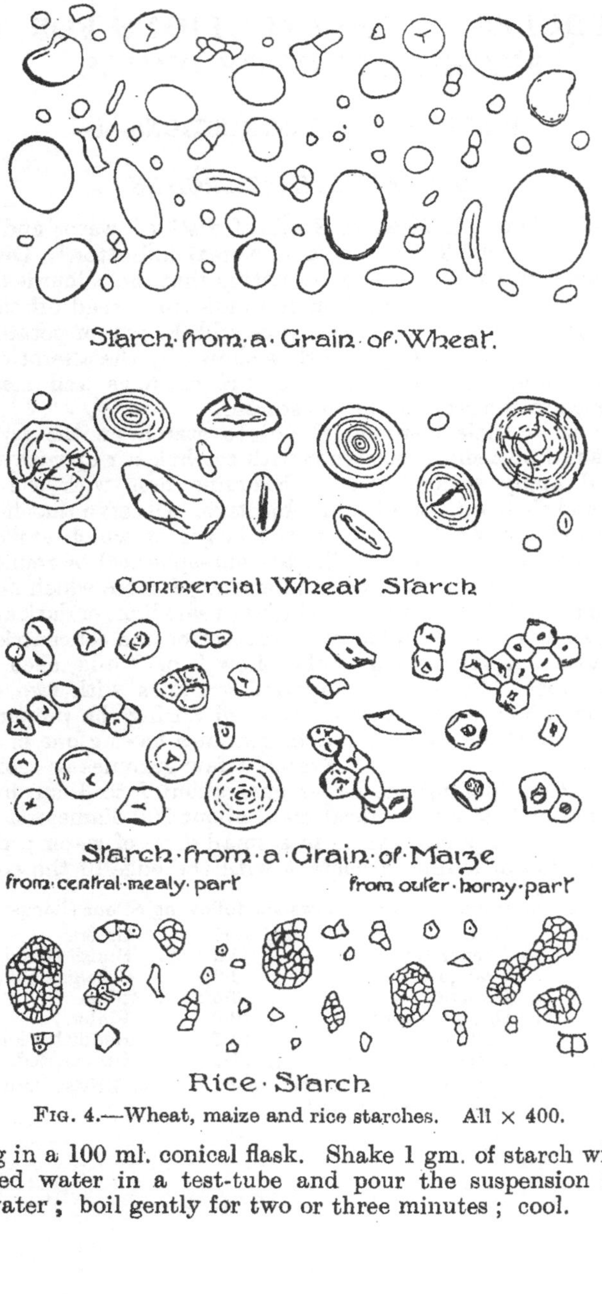

FIG. 4.—Wheat, maize and rice starches. All × 400.

to boiling in a 100 ml. conical flask. Shake 1 gm. of starch with 5 ml. of distilled water in a test-tube and pour the suspension into the boiling water; boil gently for two or three minutes; cool.

5. Put 4 ml. of the mucilage into a test-tube and heat it by immersing the tube in the water of a water-bath for a few minutes. Into a separate test-tube put 3 ml. of Fehling's reagent and heat on the water-bath. Add the starch mucilage to the Fehling's reagent and note the absence of reduction, even after a further heating on the water-bath.

6. *Hydrolysis of Starch.* To 4 ml. of the starch mucilage add 0·5 ml. of hydrochloric acid (sp. gr. 1·16) and heat for half an hour on a water-bath. Add 1·0 ml. of 20 per cent. aqueous solution of caustic soda, test the alkalinity with litmus paper and replace it in the water-bath for a few minutes. Put 3 ml. of Fehling's reagent in a separate test-

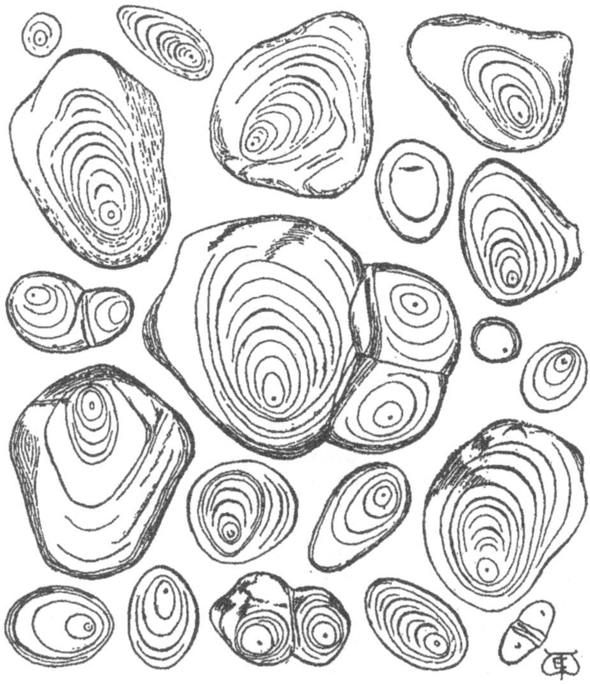

FIG. 5.—Potato starch. × 400.

tube and heat it on the water-bath. Pour the alkaline solution into the Fehling's reagent and note the abundant reduction.

Note. 1 ml. of 5 per cent. *v/v* sulphuric acid may be used in place of the hydrochloric acid.

7. To 4 ml. of the starch mucilage add 0·1 ml. of N/50 solution of iodine. Note the deep blue colour; heat the liquid and the colour disappears, cool it and the blue colour returns.

Starches of Maize, Rice and Wheat. 1. Determine the reaction of each starch to the universal indicator as for potato starch. Note your conclusions.

2. Examine the starches microscopically and observe their characteristic shapes. Sketch a few grains of each, being careful to make

the size proportional to that of the potato starch sketches. Maize grains should be drawn approximately 0·5 cm. in diameter, rice grains about 1 to 2 mm., and wheat 1 cm. long. Notice in wheat starch the concentric striations.

3. Test each starch with iodine water as directed for potato starch.

NOTES ON SCHEDULE I

Wheat starch is prepared by making wheat flour into a dough with water, washing the starch out by kneading the dough enclosed in a piece of closely woven material, in a current of water, and allowing the turbid liquid to deposit the starch grains suspended in it. In *rice* the starch grains are compacted together with a film of protoplasm, from which they are released by maceration with a very dilute solution of caustic soda ; they are subsequently washed and dried. Hence wheat starch is faintly acid from the fermentation of the traces of protein mixed with it, while rice starch is faintly alkaline, owing to the difficulty of completely removing the alkali used during its manufacture. Maize starch is neutral or, in some samples, faintly alkaline. Potato starch is neutral.

Starch is best identified by the iodine reaction. The starches from different sources may be distinguished from one another by the size and shape of the component granules. Note that commercial wheat starch shows distinct concentric striations in most of the larger grains, and that a few of these are split from the rough handling received during manufacture. Wheat starch taken from a corn of wheat does not usually show these striations. Commercial potato starch and starch taken directly from a potato tuber show somewhat similar differences, but less strongly marked.

The points referred to above are illustrated in Figs. 4 and 5, which also serve to indicate the kind of drawing which the student should strive to make. Each grain depicted should be a careful representation of some particular grain of starch viewed through the microscope and the details should be filled in to correspond as nearly as possible with the original. Do not copy the drawings in the book, and avoid making diagrammatic representations sketched in hastily from memory after a rapid glance at the actual preparation.

N.B. *For further details of the starches, see the table on pp.* 196 and 197.

To understand the processes of preparation of maize and potato starches the structure of the fruit of maize and the tuber of potato need to be studied :-

Caryopsis of Maize (*Zea Mays* Linn.).

1. Examine the maize cob with its double rows of fruits attached to the pithy axis. Note that each fruit is partially embedded in a pit which has several chaffy scales, the pales and glumes, at its base.

2. Soak some grains of maize for seven days in water ; examine and compare them with unsoaked grains. Externally note the short broad chaffy stalk at the narrower end and, at the broader end at the centre of one side, find a small point-like scar, produced by the fall of the stigma. Note also on the same side as the scar, the large oval paler coloured area, somewhat shrivelled in the dry grain, but swollen in the soaked grain and extending to the stalk ; this area covers the embryo and its outline corresponds with the margin of the scutellum of the embryo.

Make sketches to show these features and state, with reasons, why the grain is a fruit and whether it is superior or inferior.

3. Cut a soaked fruit by a median vertical section, which will divide the embryo longitudinally. Sketch the cut surface and mark the following structures : pericarp and seed coat, remains of stigma, endosperm (aleurone layer, horny part and mealy part), scutellum, plumule and plumule-sheath or coleoptile, primary root and root-sheath or coleorhiza.

4. Remove some starch from a grain of maize and make separate mounts for the microscope from the horny and mealy parts of the endosperm respectively ; compare with the appearance of the commercial starch.

Tuber of Potato (*Solanum tuberosum* Linn.).

1. At one end of the potato note the scar of attachment to the cord-like branch of the potato plant and at the other end, find the growing-point about which are grouped the majority of the eyes or buds. Sketch the tuber to show these features and also the structure of the eyes, each of which consists of a scale leaf with an axillary bud.

2. Cut a potato longitudinally by a median section and sketch the cut surface to show the skin (cork), cambium line, buds, growing-point, etc.

3. Gently scrape the cut surface with a scapel and examine the turbid fluid with the microscope. Compare the starch granules with those of commercial potato starch.

SCHEDULE OF INSTRUCTIONS—II

SOLUBLE STARCH AND DEXTRIN

Soluble Starch. Prepared from starch of *Solanum tuberosum* Linn.

1. Mount a little in alcohol and examine it under the microscope ; irrigate with water and note that the striations become visible, but the granules do not dissolve.

2. Irrigate a preparation with iodine and observe the blue stain.

3. Into a conical flask put 1 gram of the starch and 5 ml. of cold distilled water ; mix by agitation. Boil 45 ml. of water in a separate flask and pour it quickly into the soluble starch suspension. Boil for two minutes, cool and made the following tests :–

(*a*) To 4 ml. of solution add 0·1 ml. of $\frac{N}{50}$ iodine ; note the blue colour which disappears on heating and reappears on cooling.

(*b*) To 10 ml. of the solution add 0·1 ml. of Fehling's reagent and heat the test-tube on a water-bath for ten minutes. Allow to stand so that any precipitate may settle, and notice that the supernatant liquid remains permanently blue. Compare with the result of the next experiment.

(*c*) To 4 ml. of the solution add 0·5 ml. of hydrochloric acid (sp. gr. 1·16), heat on a water-bath for thirty minutes and add 1·0 ml. of 20 per cent. solution of sodium hydroxide and 3 ml. of Fehling's reagent which has been heated to about 100° C. on a water-bath ; observe and record the result.

N.B. 1 ml. of 5 per cent. *v/v* sulphuric acid may be used in place of the hydrochloric acid.

Dextrin. 1. Make experiments with yellow and with white dextrin as directed for soluble starch and record your results.

2. To a 2 per cent. solution of dextrin add solution of lead subacetate. Note the absence of any precipitate.

3. To a 2 per cent. mucilage of starch add solution of lead subacetate and note the formation of a white precipitate.

NOTES ON SCHEDULE II

Soluble starch is the first stage in the degradation of the starch molecule in the process of hydrolysis. It is usually prepared by the prolonged action upon starch of a dilute solution of hydrochloric acid (about 7·5 per cent.); potato starch is the kind that is generally used.

Dextrin is made by roasting starch, either alone at a temperature of 150° to 250° C., or with a small quantity of very dilute acid, hydrochloric or nitric acid being most commonly used, and the temperature being about 100° to 125° C. Yellow dextrin is more completely dextrinised than white dextrin; it is almost entirely soluble in cold water, whereas white dextrin varies in solubility from 20 to 75 per cent. The starch most commonly used for making dextrin is potato starch.

SCHEDULE OF INSTRUCTIONS—III

CHALK AND MATERIALS USED FOR FILTERING

Prepared Chalk. A native form of calcium carbonate, freed from most of its impurities by elutriation.

1. Take up a little prepared chalk on a needle, transfer it to a slide, mix it with cresol, apply a cover-glass and warm gently if necessary. Examine the preparation with the 16-mm. objective, and, having found a shell, examine it with the 4-mm. objective and sketch it; select in a similar way other shells of different types and sketch them. Note also and sketch some morpholites and the detritus of shells.

2. Irrigate aqueous mounts of chalk with acetic acid and with hydrochloric acid, and watch the action under the microscope, using the 16 mm. objective. Make a similar experiment with sulphuric acid (20 per cent. by volume). Record the changes observed by sketches and notes.

3. Note and record the feel of the powder when rubbed on the back of the hand. Make the experiments with acids in test-tubes and identify the gas evolved.

4. Compare precipitated chalk with prepared chalk and record the differences observed.

Diatomaceous Earth. 1. Mount some diatomaceous earth, often known as kieselguhr, in the manner described for prepared chalk. Notice that it is composed almost entirely of diatomaceous skeletons; sketch a few typical forms as seen with the 4-mm. objective. Sketch also one or two sponge spicules.

2. Determine the action of acetic and of hydrochloric acid upon diatomaceous earth both by microscopical methods and in test-tubes as directed for prepared chalk.

Glass Wool. 1. From a piece of glass wool cut some clippings about 1 mm. long and mount them in cresol on a microscope slide. Examine them with the 4-mm. objective and note their solid, structureless appearance. Sketch some pieces.

2. Examine the same preparation by polarised light and notice that the threads are invisible with crossed Nicols.

3. Mount portions of glass wool separately in strong hydrochloric acid, 66 per cent. by volume sulphuric acid, and in 5 per cent. caustic potash. Record the solubilities. Experiments with the acids should also be made in test-tubes.

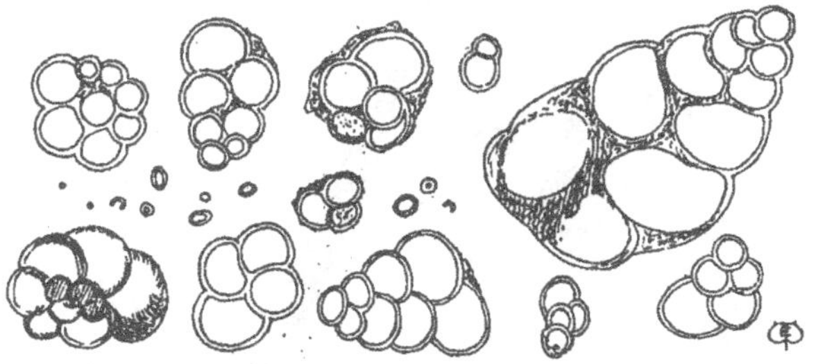

FIG. 6.—Foraminiferous shells and morpholites from prepared chalk. All × 200.

4. Heat a thread of glass-wool in the bunsen flame and note that it fuses and forms a droplet of molten glass.

Asbestos and Talc. Asbestos is a fibrous mineral, consisting chiefly of silicates of magnesium and calcium; talc is a foliated mineral, consisting of magnesium silicate.

1. Examine asbestos and talc as directed for glass wool. Sketch typical pieces of each.

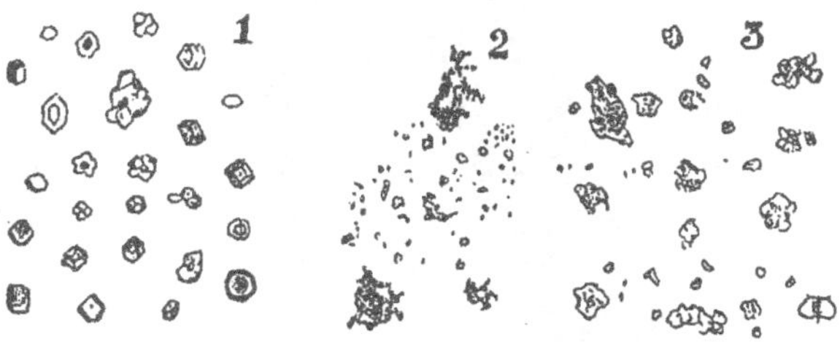

FIG. 7.—Commercial samples of precipitated chalk. 1. A "heavy" chalk showing a micro-crystalline structure. 2. A "very light" specimen, amorphous in structure. 3. A "heavy" chalk of a more commonly occurring type than that shown in 1. All × 200.

2. Heat a strand of asbestos in the bunsen flame and note that it glows brightly, but is otherwise unaffected.

NOTES ON SCHEDULE III

Prepared Chalk. This native calcium carbonate consists of the accumulated calcareous shells of Foraminifera, such as *Globigerina* and *Textularia.* These are unicellular animal organisms each encased in a chalky shell; when the animals die, the shells fall to the bottom of the sea, where they accumulate in enormous numbers and have given rise in geological times to the great masses of limestone which form ranges of hills, such as the North and South Downs. Powdered commercial prepared chalk always shows, in each field of the microscope, a few well-formed shells scattered here and there amongst a large number of very fine particles, some of which are irregular and are the *débris* of crushed foraminiferous shells and the remainder have the form of small closed rings or discs, or portions of such, and are known as morpholites.

Precipitated Chalk. The heavier varieties of precipitated chalk show a crystalline or semi-crystalline structure (see Fig. 7 (1) and (3)); the

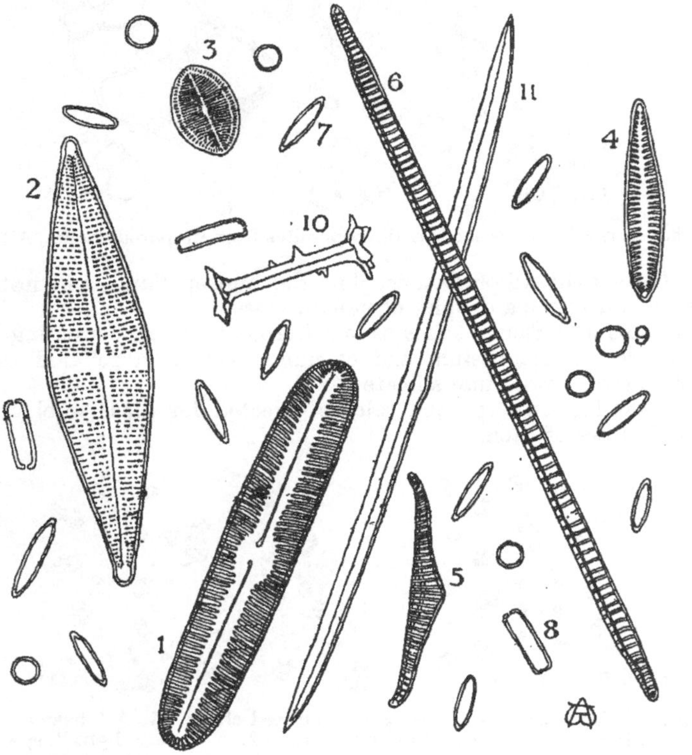

Fig. 8.—Diatoms (1–9) and sponge spicules (10 and 11) from a specimen of Diatomaceous earth. × 400.

lightest forms are not crystalline, but consist of minute amorphous particles which often adhere to form larger masses (see Fig. 7 (2)).

Precipitated chalk mounted in cresol is nearly invisible; it is clearly visible if mounted in solution of chloral hydrate (see diatomaceous earth, below).

Diatomaceous earth is an earth composed almost entirely of the siliceous skeletons of diatoms, which are unicellular plants that secrete a skeleton of silica. These earths are often known as "kieselguhr." When the plants die the skeletons fall to the bottom of the water in which they were living, and have accumulated in vast numbers during geological times, thus forming the diatomaceous earth. Each diatomaceous skeleton consists of two portions which fit together like the lid and bottom of a box, and they vary greatly in size and in shape. The flat upper and under surfaces of the box-like structure are called the valves, and a valve-view of a diatom shows the intricate sculpturings with which many of the valves are adorned. A side view of a diatom shows the two overlapping flanges, and is called the girdle-view.

Diatomaceous earth is very clearly visible if mounted in cresol; it is nearly invisible if mounted in solution of chloral hydrate (see precipitated chalk, above).

Both *asbestos* and *talc* show brightly in polarised light, with crossed Nicols, showing their crystalline nature, while *glass* is amorphous. In appearance asbestos resembles glass wool in being formed of solid threads, but the threads are much finer. Talc consists of particles of many sizes and shapes, many of them showing evidence of having been formed by the crushing of crystals (note the sharp edges, jagged ends and laminated appearance).

SCHEDULE OF INSTRUCTIONS—IV

HAIRS AND FIBRES

Cotton. The hairs covering the seeds of various species of *Gossypium* (Fam. Malvaceæ).

1. Moisten a few threads of cotton-wool with alcohol and mount in water. Examine first with the low and then with the high power; observe the shape of the hairs, the thickened edges, and the twisted appearance. Sketch a few hairs.

2. Irrigate with cuoxam or ammoniacal solution of copper oxide (for method of preparation, see below). Observe and sketch the swollen and dissolving hairs.

3. Compare raw cotton-wool with the absorbent wool, especially noting the action upon it of ammoniacal copper oxide. Sketch a swollen hair to show the peculiar behaviour of the cuticle.

4. Mount some cotton hairs in 5 per cent. caustic alkali and warm the preparation; note that they are not dissolved. Mount some cotton hairs in sulphuric acid (66 per cent. by volume) and note their rapid solution.

5. Soak a few cotton hairs in iodine water for a few minutes; remove excess of iodine by blotting paper, add 66 per cent. *v/v* sulphuric acid and note the blue colour, indicating cellulose.

6. Moisten some cotton hairs on a microscope slide with a 1 per cent. solution of phloroglucin in alcohol, allow to become nearly dry and add a drop of strong hydrochloric acid (s.g. 1·16) and apply a cover-glass. Record the observed effect.

7. Make experiments with Kapok or Vegetable Down in the same way as for cotton and record the observed differences.

Flax. The pericyclic fibres separated from the stem of *Linum usitatissimum* Linné (Fam. Linaceæ).

1. Cut some raw flax into short lengths (about 1 cm.) and boil it for half an hour with 10 per cent. solution of sodium carbonate under a reflux condenser. Tease out a little of the prepared flax in dilute glycerin and sketch a few of the isolated fibres to show the relative

width of the wall and the cavity, and also the fine transverse lines produced by injuries received during the beating.

2. Mount some flax in the same reagents as were used for cotton and record your observations.

Jute. The strands of phloem fibres removed from the bark of the stem of *Corchorus spp.* (Fam. Tiliaceæ).

1. Cut some jute into short lengths (about 5 mm.) and mount a

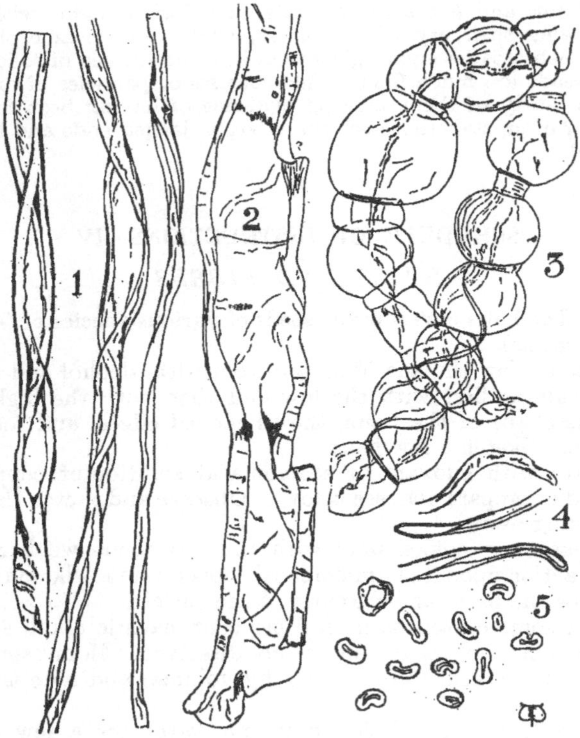

FIG. 9.—Cotton. Hairs from the seeds of *Gossypium sp.* 1. Hairs mounted in dilute glycerin. 2. Absorbent cotton treated with ammoniacal copper oxide. 3. Raw cotton treated with ammoniacal copper oxide. 4. Tips of cotton hairs. 5. Transverse sections of cotton hairs. All × 200.

little in chloral hydrate solution. Sketch a piece to show the bundles of fibres.

2. Mount other pieces of jute separately in ammoniacal copper oxide and in iodine water followed by sulphuric acid (66 per cent. *v/v*). Note the results and state what conclusion you draw.

3. Make further mounts in solution of aniline hydrochloride and in hloroglucin and hydrochloric acid. Record the results and your conclusions.

4. Cut pieces about 1 cm. long from some strands of jute and place them in a hollowed glass block. Cover the jute with a little solution

containing 10 per cent. of chromic anhydride and 10 per cent. of nitric acid (s.g. 1·42). Allow the jute to soak for about 15 minutes, then remove a piece and try to tease it with needles in a drop of water on a slide. When the jute readily breaks down into its constituent cells (phloem fibres), wash away the chromic acid mixture and make preparations from the jute to show the characters of the fibres. Apply a cover-glass and sketch some of the isolated phloem fibres, noting especially the form of the lumen and the shape of the tips of the fibres.

5. Measure the width and length of individual phloem fibres.

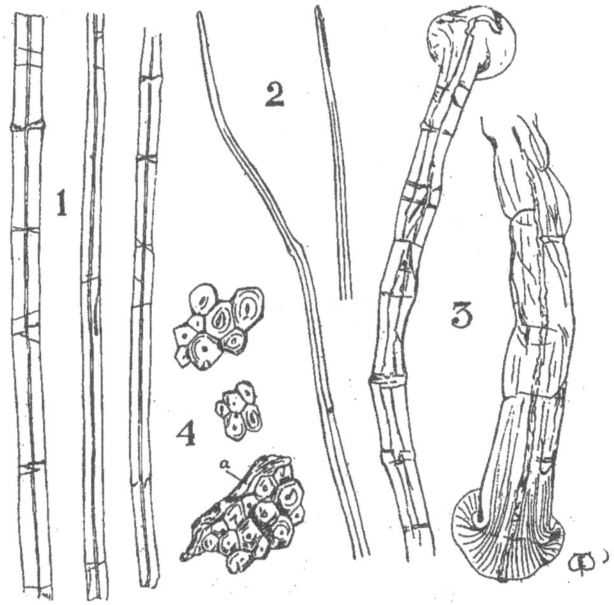

FIG. 10.—Flax. Fibres from *Linum usitatissimum*. 1. Isolated fibres. 2. Apices of fibres. 3. Fibres swelling under the action of ammoniacal copper oxide. 4. Transverse sections of flax fibres. (*a*) Soft tissue adhering to the fibres. All × 200.

Cellulose Wadding. The fibres of delignified and disintegrated timber, usually pine.

1. Examine some cellulose wadding fibres mounted in lactophenol and in water. Sketch individual elements to show the type of timber used for its preparation.

2. Subject some of the material to the reagents and tests as used for cotton and record its behaviour, noting especially the characters which distinguish this material from other fibres.

NOTES ON SCHEDULE IV

Cotton-wool consists of the hairs covering the seed of various species of *Gossypium* (family Malvaceæ). These hairs, in their natural state, are covered with a cuticle in which fatty or waxy matter is present. They may be freed from this waxy matter by boiling under pressure in a dilute solution of caustic soda, washing and drying. The cotton-wool is then readily wetted by water, and is known as absorbent wool (*Gossypium absorbens*, B.P.C.).

Cuoxam or *ammoniacal solution of copper oxide* is prepared by rubbing down 0·5 gm. of commercial copper carbonate with 10 ml. of water and gradually adding 10 ml. of strong solution of ammonia (s.g. 0·880) with continued stirring.

Ammoniacal copper oxide swells absorbent cotton-wool uniformly, and ultimately dissolves it entirely. Many samples of raw cotton (but not all samples, nor all the hairs of certain samples) when treated with the copper reagent show balloon-like swellings separated by ring-shaped, constricting bands formed from the cuticle (see Fig. 9 (3)).

Kapok or *vegetable down* consists of the hairs lining the capsule wall of the fruit of the white-cotton tree, *Eriodendron anfractuosum* (= *Ceiba pentandra*), family Bombacaceæ. The hairs are cylindrical and the wall is lignified ; they are used for stuffing cushions.

Flax. The fibres are loosened by allowing the plants to rot in water, and are then separated from the other tissues by mechanical means. One often finds brown fungal spores adhering to raw flax, and also occasional fragments of the softer tissues (see Fig. 10 (4) (*a*)).

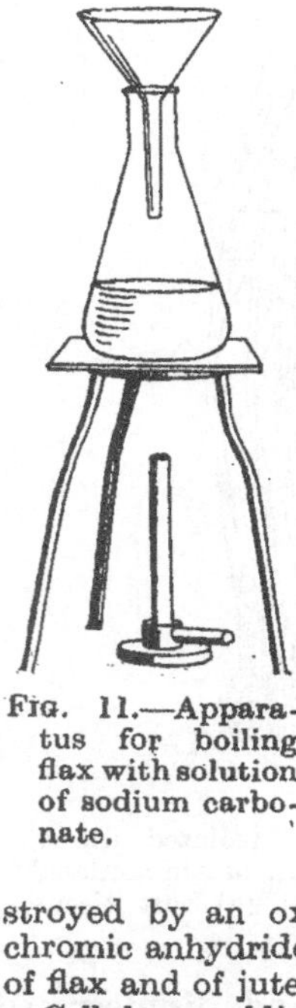

FIG. 11.—Apparatus for boiling flax with solution of sodium carbonate.

A convenient arrangement, giving sufficient reflux action for boiling the flax with the solution of sodium carbonate, is to stand a funnel in the mouth of the boiling flask, as shown in the sketch (Fig. 11).

The middle lamella of the cellulose-walled fibres of flax is pectosic in nature and is therefore converted into soluble substances by an alkali such as solution of sodium carbonate, consequently the fibres fall apart.

Linen cloth, which is made from flax, is used for certain filtering operations.

Jute consists of lignified fibres, the middle lamellæ of which are even more strongly lignified than the walls. This middle lamella is therefore easily destroyed by an oxidising agent such as a mixture of nitric acid and chromic anhydride ; hence different methods are used to isolate the fibres of flax and of jute.

Cellulose wadding or wood cellulose gives all the chemical reactions for cotton and must therefore be identified by its structural differences as seen microscopically. The large circular bordered pits, often in single rows on the tracheids, are characteristic of pine wood, as also is the absence of vessels.

SCHEDULE OF INSTRUCTIONS—V

WOOL, SILK AND FILTER PAPERS

Wool consists of the hairs from the fleece of the sheep, *Ovis aries* Linn.

1. With sharp scissors, cut from the end of a piece of white knitting wool some short pieces about 4 mm. long and let them fall on to a glass slide ; moisten them with alcohol and mount in dilute glycerin.

Examine the preparation with the 16-mm. objective and note the variation of the fibres in thickness and in the possession of a central medulla. Choose some typical fibres and sketch them in detail under the 4-mm. objective.

2. Mount some small pieces of animal wool in a saturated aqueous solution of picric acid and note whether staining is produced. If necessary, allow the preparation to stand for half an hour or more until staining takes place.

3. Mount some animal wool in 5 per cent. caustic alkali and warm gently—what action do you observe ? Mount some more in cuoxam and observe the result. Mount a third quantity in strong sulphuric acid (66 per cent. by volume)—does solution take place ?

4. Warm some wool on a slide with Millon's reagent ; note the coloration produced.

Silk. The fibre from the cocoons of various species of *Bombyx* and of *Antheræa.*

1. Remove some silk from a cocoon, or use some genuine silk thread, cut the filaments into short lengths (about 5 mm.) and mount in lactophenol. Observe and sketch the structureless, nearly cylindrical, yellowish threads.

2. Burn a few threads ; note the odour of the smoke and determine its action upon moistened litmus paper.

3. Mount some silk threads in strong hydrochloric acid and describe the observed effect. Compare with animal wool.

4. Boil a little silk in a test-tube with solution of caustic potash (5 per cent.) for some time and note that it dissolves slowly. Compare with animal wool.

5. Test silk with Millon's reagent, with cuoxam, with sulphuric acid (66 per cent. by volume) and with saturated solution of picric acid (trinitrophenol) as for wool.

6. Mount some silk in iodine water and record the effect.

Filter Papers. 1. Cut a square inch from a white filter paper, tear it up into very small pieces and put them into a test-tube one-third filled with water. Shake vigorously until the paper is completely disintegrated and reduced to a pulp. Remove a few fibres upon the point of a needle and mount them in dilute glycerin ; identify the fibres present.

2. Treat similarly a square inch cut from a grey filter paper and mount a little of the pulp in a saturated solution of picric acid in water (soluble 1 in 95). Certain of the fibres stain yellow ; these fibres are animal hair, search amongst them for wool fibres.

N.B. Some animal hairs stain rather slowly, and, if no immediate staining is visible, allow the preparation to stand for half an hour or more and examine it again.

3. Test a piece of white filter paper with iodine water. If it stains blue, search for starch grains.

NOTES ON SCHEDULE V

Sheep's wool consists of fibres which show a number of irregular transverse lines joined by others at right angles to them (see Fig. 12). These lines are the edges of the overlapping flattened cells of which the outer surface of the hairs is composed. Some of the hairs show a central granular-looking pith, which consists of polydehral or rounded cells, containing nuclei and globules of fat. Air is often present between these cells and produces the dark appearance of the medulla. Between the outer surface, or cuticle, and the medulla, is the cortex, which consists of closely arranged, flattened, spindle-shaped, nucleated cells or fibres, and constitutes the bulk of the hair. Animal wool is dissolved by warm 5 per cent. solution of caustic soda or potash, but is insoluble in strong sulphuric acid; whereas cotton-wool is insoluble in the dilute caustic alkali, but is rapidly dissolved by strong sulphuric acid. Animal wool is insoluble in hydrochloric acid.

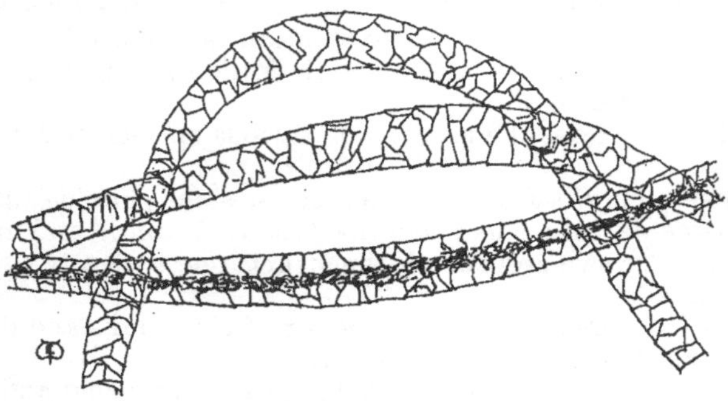

FIG. 12.—Fibres of sheep's wool. × 200. Note that the lowermost hair shows a well-marked medulla.

Silk threads are quite solid and structureless, being non-cellular. They are completely and easily soluble in hydrochloric acid which is the best reagent to separate silk from wool and other fibres. The smoke from burning silk is alkaline. Silk, like wool, is coloured red by Millon's reagent, pale yellow by iodine and deep yellow by picric acid; it is dissolved by cuoxam and by cold sulphuric acid.

Ordinary *white filter paper* is made from white rags, and frequently consists almost entirely of cotton fibres; some white filter papers are made of wood cellulose. The grey filter papers are strengthened by the addition of wool or other animal hair, and these fibres become clearly evident in the pulp when the preparation is stained with picric acid.

The fibres of white filter paper frequently give a blue coloration with iodine; this is due to their partial conversion into hydroxy-cellulose, which gives a reaction similar to that of starch.

SCHEDULE OF INSTRUCTIONS—VI

LINEN TESTER, SURGICAL DRESSINGS

Linen Tester. Note that the metal linen tester consists of three parts, viz. (1) a lens in a metal mount; (2) a square metal frame; and (3) a metal plate, to opposite sides of which the other two parts are hinged. Unfold the tester and turn the lens and square frame as far back as they will go. The instrument now forms a stand having the square frame for its base, and the lens held rigidly above it at a distance approximately equal to its focal length. On now placing the eye close to the lens, a magnified view is obtained of an object placed in the plane of the square metal frame (see Fig. 13).

To Make Counts with the Linen Tester. 1. Measure exactly the length of the inner edge of the square metal frame.

2. Stand the tester with the frame upon the material to be counted, and with its edges parallel to the warp and weft respectively.

3. Look through the lens and count the number of threads in the warp and in the weft of the portion of bandage enclosed by the square frame. If the edge of the square is ½ in., make counts in at least ten different places on the material. Take the average of the results and multiply by two.

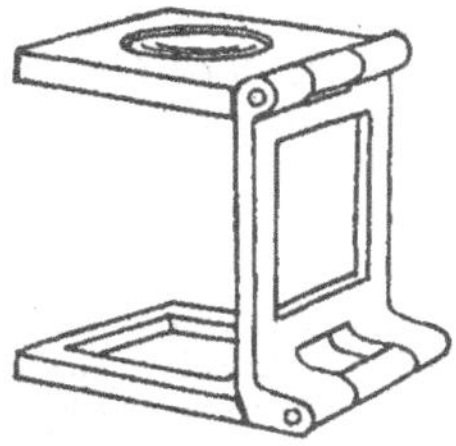

FIG. 13.—Linen tester.

Surgical Dressings. 1. Examine a specimen of *absorbent gauze* and report upon its compliance with the following requirements, " Absorbent gauze consists of cotton cloth of plain weave. It is free from foreign matter. Average number of threads per inch, not less than 19 in the warp, and not less than 15 in the weft " (*cf.* British Pharmaceutical Codex). To determine the number of threads per inch of a *gauze*, count the number in a length of 10 inches and calculate for 1 inch.

2. *Lint.* From a piece of lint separate a thread from the warp (the threads from which a nap has been raised), cut off a piece about ¼ in. long, and tease it out with needles in water. Treat similarly a thread from the weft. Examine each separately and identify the fibres.

3. Examine the specimens of *flannel bandage* and ascertain whether they conform to the following requirements: " Flannel bandage consists of a raised fabric of plain weave, made entirely of wool. . . . Weight of the bandage, not less than 900 grains per 2 inches by 6 yards " (*cf.* British Pharmaceutical Codex).

4. Take a small piece of *domette bandage*, remove a thread from the warp and one from the weft and examine each separately as directed for lint (see 2, above). What is the nature of the fibres present in each case ? Determine the number of threads per inch.

5. Determine the nature of the fibres present in a *crepe bandage :* ascertain whether the arrangement of threads conforms to the following requirements : " The warp threads are arranged as follows : 1 two-fold cotton thread (right twist), 2 wool threads, 1 two-fold cotton thread (reverse twist), 2 wool threads. . . . The weft consists of cotton.

There are 2 two-fold cotton binding threads at each edge." Before counting the number of threads per inch, stain the bandage by soaking in solution of picric acid, washing with water and drying.

6. Examine the *gauze and cotton tissue.* Test the gauze as directed under 1, above, except that " the weft has not fewer than 12 threads per inch." Determine the nature of the fibre of the cotton-wool and test its absorbency thus : " 1 gramme compressed to a volume of about 20 millilitres, and placed lightly by means of a forceps on the surface of water at about 20°, sinks or becomes saturated within ten

seconds." Check the superficial area, which should be "not less than 1,800 square inches per pound."

7. *Cellulose Tissue.* Determine the nature of the fibres in the gauze and in the cellulose wadding. Find also the superficial area, which is "not less than 1,350 square inches per pound."

8. *Bleached Calico Bandage.* Determine the number of threads per inch, using the special linen tester described below.

NOTES ON SCHEDULE VI

Linen Tester. For more accurate work and for counting the threads per inch in closely woven materials, a more precise counting-glass is used, such as that made by Messrs. Casartelli and Sons, of Manchester, and shown in Fig. 14. In this instrument, the magnifying-glass and a pointer are moved together by means of a screw over a standard scale, so that each thread can be numbered as the pointer passes it.

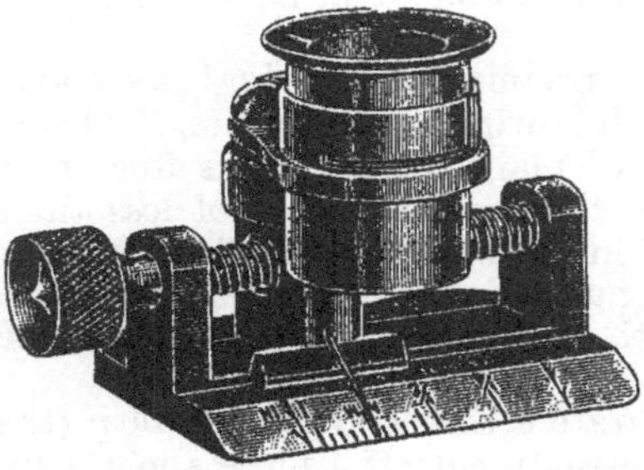

FIG. 14.—A form of linen tester which gives more accurate counts than can be made by the instrument described above.

Lint, as its name implies, was originally made from linen, and consisted of flax fibres. The lint most commonly sold at the present time consists wholly of cotton, and the variety known as "flax lint," which does not now appear to be manufactured, has the warp composed of flax and the woof or weft of cotton fibres.

Domette bandage of the quality required by the British Pharmaceutical Codex has a weft consisting entirely of wool and a warp composed of cotton. The thin threads which run through the whole length of the bandage are the warp, and the thicker threads crossing them are the weft.

Bandages and Dressings. Full details of the specifications for bandages and surgical dressings will be found in the British Pharmaceutical Codex.

SCHEDULE OF INSTRUCTIONS—VII

CALCIUM OXALATE

1. Prepare some microcrystals of calcium oxalate by slowly adding a boiling 0·5 per cent. solution of calcium chloride to an equal volume of a boiling 0·5 per cent. solution of oxalic acid (the mixing of 500 ml. of each should take about an hour). Allow to stand till cold, filter and wash with precipitate. Examine and sketch some of the crystals as seen with a 16 mm. objective, using a mount in solution of chloral hydrate.

2. Mount separate small quantities of the crystals in acetic acid and in caustic alkali (5 per cent.) respectively; record the effects as seen with the 16 mm. objective.

3. Mount further quantities of the crystals in hydrochloric acid (s.g. 1·16) and in sulphuric acid (20 per cent. by volume). Record the changes observed by sketches and notes.

4. Carry out similar tests upon the crystals of Quillaia bark and record your observations and conclusions (see Schedule X, p. 27).

N.B. Compare the results of these experiments with those made with calcium carbonate—see Schedule III., p. 10.

NOTES ON SCHEDULE VII

Although it will be found that calcium oxalate is insoluble in solution of chloral hydrate and in caustic alkali, both these reagents will completely destroy the crystals in the course of time. Chloral hydrate solution gradually attacks calcium oxalate and the crystals dissolve completely

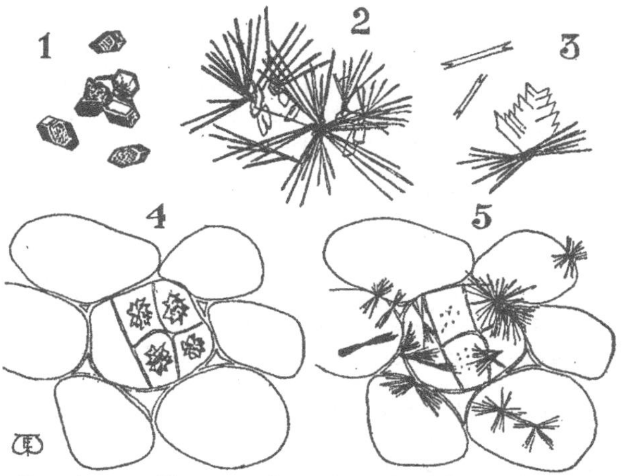

FIG. 15.—Drawings to illustrate the action of sulphuric acid upon calcium oxalate. All × 200. 1. Crystals of calcium oxalate prepared as explained in the text. 2. Needle-shaped crystals of calcium sulphate, formed by the action of sulphuric acid (20) per cent. *v/v*) upon artificial calcium oxalate. 3. Calcium sulphate crystals formed by irrigating a solution of calcium carbonate in acetic acid with sulphuric acid (10 per cent. *v/v*). 4. Part of a section of a petiole in ivy (*Hedera helix*), showing four cluster crystals of calcium oxalate. 5. The same section ten minutes after treatment with 20 per cent. *v/v* sulphuric acid. A few dots represent two of the rapidly disappearing cluster crystals. It will be noticed that the needles of calcium sulphate do not necessarily form in the position previously occupied by the oxalate.

in about three weeks. Both calcium oxalate and calcium tartrate crystals are insoluble in acetic acid, but they can be distinguished by caustic alkali which dissolves calcium tartrate very rapidly, whereas calcium oxalate crystals are apparently unaffected. The calcium oxalate is, however, gradually attacked and disappears after a few weeks, being replaced by crystals of a different form, probably consisting of calcium sodium (or potassium) carbonate.

Hydrochloric acid and sulphuric acid both dissolve the calcium oxalate without effervescence. With hydrochloric acid nothing further is observed, but with sulphuric acid new crystals make their appearance in the vicinity of the original calcium oxalate. These new crystals are mostly needle shaped and in bunches accompanied by a few lamellæ, showing the characteristic angles of calcium sulphate crystals.

SCHEDULE OF INSTRUCTIONS—VIII

QUASSIA, GUAIACUM, LOGWOOD, SAPPAN AND RED SANDERS

Quassia. The dried stem-wood of *Picræna excelsa* (Sw.) Lindl., known in commerce as Jamaica quassia.

1. Take a small piece of quassia wood and smooth a transverse surface with a sharp knife ; examine it with a pocket lens and notice the narrow pale coloured lines running radially across the wood ; these are the medullary rays. Determine the number of rays per millimetre of arc.

2. At right angles to the medullary rays notice some narrow bands and short lines of light coloured tissue, somewhat irregularly outlined and showing small pores at intervals. The bands and lines are the wood parenchyma ; the pores are the vessels ; the remainder of the wood which is darker in colour consists of fibres. Sketch a piece of the transverse surface.

3. Split a piece of the wood longitudinally by a plane at right angles to the medullary rays ; observe the nature of the split surface, smooth a part of it with a sharp knife and examine it with a lens. Notice the transverse rows of small vertical dashes, each about 0·3 mm. high and rather darker or paler (according to the illumination) than the remainder of the wood ; these are the medullary rays seen in a tangential longitudinal section of the wood. Make a sketch to show these characters.

4. Examine a radial surface of the wood and note the very narrow rectangular darker patches crossing the grain at right angles ; these are the medullary rays. Note also the narrow, dark, longitudinal cavities, which are the pores or vessels and can be similarly seen in the tangential surface examined above (No. 3). Sketch these details.

5. Take a shaving of the wood, moisten it with alcoholic solution of phloroglucin, allow it to soak in and then add a drop or two of concentrated hydrochloric acid and note the bright red colour produced (reaction of lignin).

6. Note the odour and taste, and write a description of the wood (see p. 122) and compare it with that of the British Pharmacopœia.

7. From a piece of the wood, scrape some fine powder with a scalpel ; mount a small quantity in solution of chloral hydrate and find the prisms of calcium oxalate ; sketch some crystals. Mount a further quantity of the powder in water on a microscope slide and irrigate it with solution of iodine ; note and sketch any starch which is present.

Guaiacum. The heart-wood of the stem of *Guaiacum officinale* Linn., or of *Guaiacum sanctum* Linn., family Zygophyllaceæ.

1. Note the greenish-brown colour of the heart-wood. Try to split a piece of wood longitudinally and record your conclusion. Observe what happens when the wood is put into water.

2. *Reaction for Guaiaconic acid.* Extract about 0·5 gm. of fine raspings or powder by shaking with 5 ml. of 90 per cent. alcohol, filter and to the filtrate add one-fifth of its volume of a 0·05 per cent. aqueous ferric chloride solution. Note the deep blue colour produced.

Logwood. The heart-wood of *Hæmatoxylon campechianum* Linn., family Leguminosæ.

Reaction for Hæmatoxylin. Cut a number of very small chips from a piece of logwood and weigh out 0·1 gm.; boil them in a test-tube with 5 ml. of distilled water, filter, and add lime water to the filtrate; a fine purplish-blue colour is produced.

Note. Lime water gives a better blue than caustic soda.

Sappan. The heart-wood of *Cæsalpinia sappan* Linn., family Leguminosæ.

Reaction for Brasilin. Carry out a test as directed for logwood; a crimson-red colour is produced.

Red Sanders Wood. The heart-wood of *Pterocarpus santalinus* Linn., family Leguminosæ.

1. Boil chips of red sanders wood with water, as directed for logwood, and note that whereas logwood and sappan impart a colour to the water, red sanders wood does not colour the water.

2. Warm chips of red sanders wood with alcohol, filter, and note that the alcohol acquires a deep red colour.

NOTES ON SCHEDULE VIII

Quassia. It is best to saw a disc of wood, about 3 cm. thick, from the end of a log of quassia and to cut up the disc by splitting it vertically into pieces of a convenient size for examination. The number of medullary rays per millimetre of arc is about six to eight. The crystals of calcium oxalate are an important character distinguishing Jamaica quassia from Surinam quassia, obtained from *Quassia amara*. There are always a few rounded starch granules in quassia.

Guaiacum wood contains from 20 to 25 per cent. of a resin, one of the constituents of which is guaiaconic acid.

SCHEDULE OF INSTRUCTIONS—IX

BARKS; CASCARA, CINNAMON, WILD CHERRY

Cascara Bark. The bark of *Rhamnus Purshiana* DC., family Rhamnaceæ.

1. Examine a piece of the dry bark and note, on the outer surface of some pieces, the presence of epiphytic bryophytes and the whitish patches of lichen with occasional black apothecia. Scrape the surface and observe the purplish colour of the exposed layer—this colour is not so pronounced as the somewhat similar crimson-red colour given by frangula bark. Note the colour of the smooth inner surface (it varies from pale yellow to reddish-brown and sometimes nearly black). Break a piece of the bark transversely and note the very short fracture. The taste is bitter. Make sketches to show the characters of the outer and inner surfaces.

2. Soak some of the bark in water for eighteen to twenty-four hours and cut a piece transversely with a sharp scalpel. Examine the cut surface with a pocket lens and sketch it to show the secondary phloem or inner bark with numerous pale-coloured medullary rays, which are often curved and wavy towards the outside, where they approach one another, and form irregular triangular groups. On the outside is a dark brown line of cork, between which and the phloem is an irregular

yellowish-grey band—the cortex—in which darker, oval groups of sclerenchymatous cells are visible. In the secondary phloem small groups of sclerenchymatous fibres are visible as narrow, dark patches running in irregular, broken lines at right angles to the medullary rays.

3. Test for *anthraquinone derivatives*. Boil 0·1 g. of the drug, in powder or in small pieces, with 5 ml. of sulphuric acid (10 per cent.) for at least 2 minutes. Filter while hot; cool the filtrate and shake gently for a minute with an equal volume of benzene. Allow the benzene layer to separate completely from the lower aqueous layer and, by means of a teat-pipette, transfer the benzene layer to a clean test-tube. Add about half its volume of solution of ammonia, 10 per cent., shake gently and allow the layers to separate. If anthraquinone derivatives were present in the drug, the lower ammoniacal layer will have acquired a delicate rose-pink colour.

Note. If a separator is used in place of a test-tube, carbon tetrachloride is a more suitable solvent than benzene.

4. Scrape some powder from a radial longitudinal surface, mount in solution of chloral hydrate, boil and examine for crystals of calcium oxalate.

Alder Buckthorn Bark. Frangula bark. The stem bark of *Rhamnus Frangula* Linn., family Rhamnaceæ.

Compare frangula with cascara; note that the quills are smaller, the lenticels are more strongly marked, lichens and other epiphytes are generally absent, the outer surface in the younger pieces is covered by a smooth, glossy cork and, if this is removed by scraping, the exposed inner cork shows a deep crimson colour.

Cinnamon. The dried inner bark of the shoots of coppiced trees of *Cinnamomum zeylanicum* Nees.

1. Examine pieces of commercial bark; describe their form and the external surface, noting especially the longitudinal, yellowish, parallel lines (bundles of pericyclic fibres), which may become spirally curved near the scars of the lateral branches. Make sketches to show the features observed.

2. Measure the thickness of the bark; note the nature of the fracture and examine and describe the inner surface of the bark.

3. Examine the smoothed transversely cut surface of a piece of soaked bark with a pocket lens and observe the pale, buff-coloured outer region (the pericycle) and the wider and darker inner region (the secondary phloem) through which run the medullary rays. Stain the cut surface with phloroglucin and hydrochloric acid and note that the pale region becomes deep red.

4. *Test for Tannin.* Prepare a 2 per cent. decoction of broken cinnamon, using about 1 gm. of the bark; filter and to 3 ml. of the filtrate add 2 or 3 drops of a 5 per cent. solution of ferric chloride. Record the result and state your conclusion.

5. Record the odour and taste and describe the bark, using the scheme on p. 122.

Wild Cherry Bark. The bark of *Prunus serotina* Ehrh., collected in autumn.

1. Find the thin, brown layer of cork, the coloured cortex, the lenticels and their scars and record the peculiarities of each. Record

also the average size, thickness and form of the pieces of bark. Sketch a piece to show the characters of the outer surface.

2. Sketch a piece of the inner surface as seen with a lens, name the various structures present and record any characteristic appearances.

3. Observe the nature of the fracture. Cut a piece of soaked bark transversely; examine and sketch the cut surface as seen with a lens; name all evident structures.

4. Is there any characteristic taste when the bark is chewed?

5. Into a test-tube put 1·0 ml. of distilled water and add 1·0 gm. of the bark broken into small pieces. Close the tube with a cork between which and the side of the tube a piece of moist sodium picrate paper is

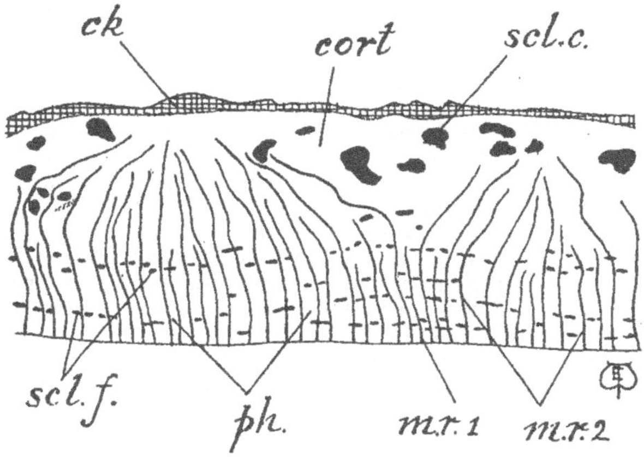

FIG. 16.—Bark of *Rhamnus Purshiana.* Transverse section. × 8. *Ck.*, cork; *cort.*, cortex; *m.r.*1, primary medullary ray; *m.r.*2, secondary medullary ray; *ph.*, phloem; *scl.c.*, group of sclerenchymatous cells; *scl.f.*, group of sclerenchymatous fibres.

held. Allow the tube to stand for half an hour or more, if necessary, and note any change in the colour of the paper. What conclusion do you draw?

NOTES ON SCHEDULE IX

To obtain good sections, soak the barks in water until they are thoroughly softened. Lay the softened bark upon the bench or upon a piece of board and section it transversely by a single, steady cut with a sharp scalpel. In this way an even, smooth surface is obtained and will clearly exhibit all the features when examined with a good pocket lens.

Commercial barks include all the tissues of the stem or root from the outside down to the cambium line, which is the place where separation from the stem or root takes place most easily, because the cells are here very soft, having been only recently formed by cell division. A commercial bark may therefore consist of some or all of the following tissues, commencing from the inside: Secondary phloem, cortex, phelloderm, phellogen, cork, and dead tissues cut off by the cork and forming the rhytidoma. The limit of the secondary phloem is marked by the width of bark traversed by the medullary rays and, in some barks, such as quillaia, this is the only tissue present. Between the outer ends of the medullary rays and the brown outermost part of the bark, the cork and rhytidoma, lies the cortex, when present. In a few barks there is found, at the inner limit of the cortex, a line of pale-coloured sclerenchyma which belongs to the pericycle, and marks, therefore, the outer limit of the stelar tissues in those cases where it occurs. Such a pericyclic band of sclerenchyma is found in wild cherry and cinnamon barks. If preferred, a section may be cut, not necessarily very thin, and stained with phloroglucin and hydrochloric acid, which assists in distinguishing details.

In barks such as cascara and canella, where the cortex is present, the medullary rays commonly fall into groups, each consisting of rays bending towards the central line of the group as they approach the outside. There are thus left between the groups areas of an inverted triangular shape, which mark the position of the primary medullary rays, the other rays being secondary ones. In quillaia and canella barks, and also in some other barks, the innermost, youngest portion of the secondary phloem, being formed of much softer cells than the remainder, dries up, to form an extremely hard layer, which gives the bark a very hard, smooth surface on the inner side. It is this hard surface which produces the metallic sound when sharply struck with a knife handle or some similar object.

A scheme of marking of the tissues has been adopted in constructing the diagrammatic drawings which accompany these descriptions. The cork and dead tissues are represented by two sets of lines crossing each other vertically and horizontally; phelloderm by vertical lines; sclerenchymatous tissues by dead black areas; the medullary rays by lines, and, in the inner, paler part of the bark, the medullary rays are dotted, because they are not so clearly visible in this region.

Cascara Sagrada. Calcium oxalate occurs in two forms, as cluster crystals in the cortex and as prisms associated with the strands of phloem fibres and with the ovoid masses of sclereids.

Wild cherry bark contains a cyanophoric glycoside, prunasin, which in the presence of water is decomposed by an enzyme with the evolution of hydrocyanic acid. Sodium picrate paper is made by dipping narrow strips of filter paper in solution of picric acid and drying them; when required for use, moisten a strip with 10 per cent. solution of sodium carbonate and expose it, while damp, to the vapour. Hydrocyanic acid reacts with the yellow sodium picrate to give brick-red sodium iso-purpurate.

SCHEDULE OF INSTRUCTIONS—X

QUILLAIA, CINCHONA

Quillaia Bark. The bark of *Quillaia Saponaria* Molina, family Rosaceæ.

1. Take a piece of the dry bark and note the slight, brownish patches of dead tissue and cork—rhytidoma—on the outside; strike the inside surface with a knife handle and note the hard metallic sound of the rap. Break a piece of bark across and note the splintery fracture, with numerous sparkling points sprinkled freely over it—due to the presence of large calcium oxalate crystals—and observe the sternutatory character of the dust that arises when the bark is broken. Make sketches to illustrate these features.

2. Soak a piece of quillaia bark for two or three days in water and then cut it across transversely by a single cut with a sharp scalpel. Examine the cut-surface with a pocket lens, and sketch it at a magnifica-

tion of ten diameters. Show in your drawing the medullary rays, which appear as fine radial lines traversing the bark from the inner to the outer surface, and the parallel alternating groups of parenchyma and bast fibres, which appear as tangential lines crossing the medullary rays at right angles and having a pale and dark colour respectively. Observe the semi-translucent inner part of the secondary phloem.

3. From a piece of dry bark scrape a little fine powder and allow it to fall on to a slide; moisten it with alcohol and mount it in chloral hydrate solution. Examine the preparation with the 4 mm. objective, and sketch a few of the large, prismatic crystals of calcium oxalate. Mount a further quantity in iodine water and observe the starch granules.

4. Soak some of the powder in a little water in a test-tube, shake violently and note the abundant and persistent froth, indicating the presence of a saponin.

Red Cinchona Bark. The dried bark of the stem and branches of cultivated plants of *Cinchona succirubra* Pav., family Rubiaceæ.

1. Examine the inner and outer surface of a piece of red cinchona bark and record the colour, surface condition, etc., of each and make sketches.

2. Remove a portion of the white material from the outside, mount it in chloral hydrate and examine it microscopically. Sketch a piece and record your conclusion as to its nature.

3. Break a piece of bark transversely and describe the fracture; is it alike all through? If not, what differences are observable in different parts?

4. Break a piece of bark longitudinally and with a lens observe especially the numerous fine yellow dashes and minute white points. With the point of a needle pick off some of the white specks and boil them in chloral hydrate on a slide; examine with the microscope and determine their nature. Similarly, pick off and mount one or two of the yellow dashes and determine their nature.

5. Cut a piece of soaked bark transversely and sketch the exposed surface, marking the cortex, cork, secondary phloem, medullary rays, etc.

6. Test cinchona bark for tannin as directed for cinnamon.

7. In a porcelain dish mix together 2 gm. of powdered cinchona, 1 gm. of quicklime and 5 ml. of water; set aside for five minutes and evaporate to dryness on a water-bath. To the residue add 20 ml. of alcohol, 95 per cent., and warm on a water-bath for about five minutes, keeping the dish covered by a watch-glass and stirring three or four times during the five minutes. Filter, wash with two quantities of 5 ml. of alcohol and evaporate the filtrate and washings; take up the residue with 5 ml. of sulphuric acid (5 per cent. *v/v*) and filter. To 1 ml. of the clear filtrate add a few drops of Mayer's reagent; record the result and your conclusion. *Thalleioquin reaction.* To 2 ml. of the same clear filtrate add solution of ammonia, 10 per cent., till just faintly cloudy; boil to expel excess of ammonia, cool and adjust the volume to 4 ml. with water. Take 1 ml. and add 1 ml. of freshly prepared 20 per cent. solution of saturated bromine water and 2 ml. of solution of ammonia, 10 per cent. An emerald green colour results.

NOTES ON SCHEDULE X

Quillaia Bark. The groups of bast fibres can be made to stand out very clearly by treating the transversely cut surface of the bark with phloroglucin and hydrochloric acid, when the masses of fibres appear as elongated red spots.

Cinchona Bark. It is difficult to obtain authentic red cinchona bark; much of the cinchona of commerce is now obtained from hybrid trees. The

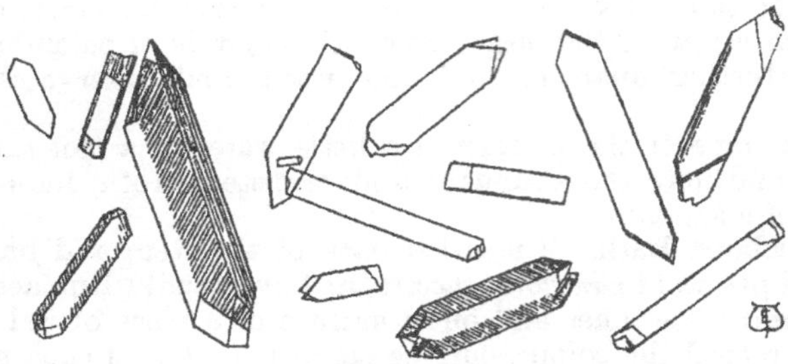

FIG. 17.—Prismatic crystals of calcium oxalate from the bark of *Quillaia saponaria.* × 200.

hybrid barks may be examined as described in the schedule, but will not show clearly the longitudinally wrinkled outer surface, the red colour of the inner bark or the soft texture. The white specks will be found to consist of cells filled with microcrystals of calcium oxalate and the yellow dashes to be due to the large phloem fibres. Treatment of the cinchona with lime decomposes the tannates of the alkaloids which are set free for solution in the alcohol, while the tannin is removed with the lime during the filtration.

SCHEDULE OF INSTRUCTIONS—XI

BARKS; CANELLA, BLACK HAW, EUONYMUS, CASCARILLA, WITCH-HAZEL

Canella Bark. The bark of *Canella alba* Murray, family Canellaceæ.

1. Examine the dry bark and note its pale buff colour and the hard nature of both the inner and outer surfaces. Break a piece across and note the short fracture and the aromatic odour.

2. Soak a piece of a quill in water for eighteen to twenty-four hours and cut it transversely with a sharp scalpel. Examine the cut surface with a pocket lens and sketch it at a magnification of ten diameters. On your drawing mark the pale, yellowish-white, wavy medullary rays arranged in somewhat triangular groups. On the outer edge observe a narrow, semi-transparent, irregular, brownish band of sclerenchyma—the phelloderm; between this and the phloem, the limits of which are marked by the medullary rays, is the whitish cortex extending downwards at intervals as wide primary medullary rays. The whole section is marked by the presence of numerous yellowish oil-ceils, which are largest and most abundant in the cortex and primary medullary rays. Note also the paler coloured innermost layer, which is the youngest part of the secondary phloem. Mark all these details in your drawing.

Cascarilla Bark. The dried bark of *Croton Eluteria* J. J. Benn., family Euphorbiaceæ.

1. Examine pieces of the commercial bark; describe their form and the character of the outer surface, the inner surface and the fracture.
2. Carefully scrape off some of the chalky-looking surface; mount the dust in chloral hydrate and determine its nature with the microscope. Sketch the structures visible.
3. Treat some of the chalky dust with dilute sulphuric acid (1 volume of acid s.g. 1·843 and 5 volumes of water); observe the action under the 16 mm. objective and sketch any new structures produced. In a similar way observe the action of hydrochloric acid (s.g. gr. 1·16) and of 33 per cent. acetic acid separately upon the dust. Record your conclusion.
4. With a sharp scalpel, cut a piece of soaked bark transversely. Examine the cut surface with a pocket lens. Make a sketch and mark the pale cork, the narrow cortex, the pale-coloured medullary rays (primary and secondary), the secretion cells and the secondary phloem.
5. Make a note of the odour and taste.

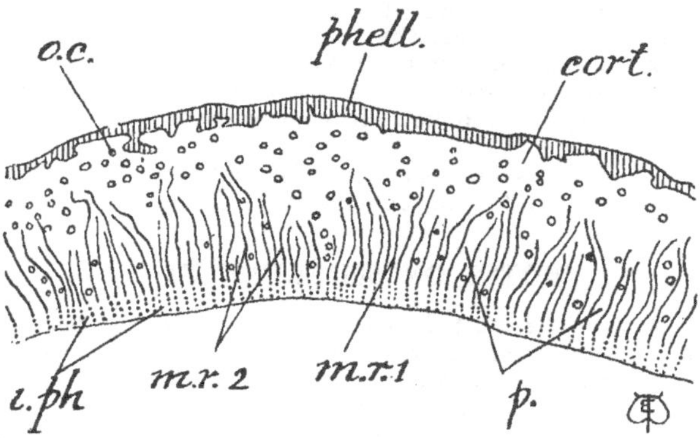

FIG. 18.—Bark of *Canella alba*. Transverse section. × 8. *Cort.*, cortex; *i.ph.*, inner part of the secondary phloem; *m.r.*1, primary medullary ray; *m.r.*2, secondary medullary ray; *o.c.*, oil-cell; *p.*, phloem; *phell.*, phelloderm.

Black Haw Bark. The dried bark of *Viburnum prunifolium* Linn., family Caprifoliaceæ.

1. Record the colour and surface condition of the outside and inside of the pieces of bark. Are there any lenticels? If so, in what pieces do you find them? What is the shape of the pieces? What is the nature of the fracture?
2. With a pocket lens note especially the minute, glittering points scattered over the surface of the dry bark. The points are seen to sparkle as the bark is moved in a strong light. Cut a transverse section of the soaked bark to discover the nature of these small specks.
3. Cut a soaked piece transversely. Sketch the exposed surface to show the dark outline of cork, the medullary rays and the scattered yellowish groups of stone-cells.
4. Note the odour of the bark as perceived by smelling a quantity of bark in a box, what does the odour resemble?

Euonymus Bark. The dried root-bark of *Euonymus atropurpureus* Jacq.

1. Examine pieces of commercial bark and describe the usual form and size of the pieces. Note the external cork and record its colour and any markings present. Observe the colour and condition of the inner surface

and the occurrence of adhering pieces of wood (what colour ?). Record the taste.

2. Remove some of the dark matter from the outside of a piece of bark and examine it microscopically. State its nature.

3. Observe the fracture and find out whether the silky threads have any structure when examined microscopically.

4. Prepare a smooth transverse surface as for canella bark and examine it with a lens. Is there any cortex ? Are there any lignified structures present ? Sketch the cut surface and make a description of the bark.

Witch-hazel Bark. The dried bark of *Hammamelis virginiana* Linn.

1. Examine a piece of commercial bark and make notes of the colour of the external and internal surfaces, the presence or absence of lenticels or striations and the characters of the fracture. Does the inner surface show any special features ?

2. Measure the thickness of several pieces of bark and record the maximum and most common thicknesses.

3. Record the taste and odour (if any) of the bark.

4. With a sharp scalpel, cut the bark transversely as directed under canella bark, and sketch the cut surface as seen with a pocket lens. Mark on your drawing the pale-coloured band of sclerenchyma, marking the position of the pericycle, and key all other structures of the cortex and secondary phloem.

5. Test the cut transverse surface with solution of ferric chloride. Record the result and state your conclusion.

NOTES ON SCHEDULE XI

Cascarilla Bark. The whitish material is seen to consist of tabular, polygonal cells containing small crystal prisms. There is no effervescence with acid, but with sulphuric acid the crystals dissolve, and are later replaced by bunches of needles, indicating the presence of a calcium salt other than carbonate. The insolubility in acetic acid and solubility in hydrochloric acid indicate oxalic acid combined with the calcium (see Schedule VII., p. 20).

Black Haw Bark. The presence of lenticels indicates stem bark. The glittering points will be found to be due to the presence of numerous cluster crystals of calcium oxalate. The bark has a faint odour, resembling valerian.

Euonymus Bark. The dark matter on the outer surface will be found to resemble clay ; it is earthy matter and indicates a root bark. Lignified structures may be detected by staining the cut transverse surface with phloroglucin and hydrochloric acid.

Witch-hazel Bark. The pale-coloured band of sclerenchyma seen in the transverse section consists partly of fibres and partly of stone-cells ; it marks the position of the pericycle. Ferric chloride shows the presence of tannin, which explains the astringent taste.

SCHEDULE OF INSTRUCTIONS—XII

LEAVES ; BUCHU, EUCALYPTUS, JABORANDI

Buchu Leaves. The leaves of *Barosma betulina* Bartling and Wendland, family Rutaceæ.

1. Measure a leaf and draw it six times the natural size ; make a separate drawing of the recurved apex. Indicate carefully the indenta-

tions of the margin and the distribution of the veins and of the oil-glands. Key your drawings.

2. Make similar sketches at a magnification of six diameters of the leaves of *Barosma crenulata* Hooker, and of *Barosma serratifolia* Wildenow, to show how they differ from the leaf of *B. betulina* in the characters of the outline, margin, and distribution of the oil-glands.

3. Examine the stem of buchu and note that it is brownish-red, with opposite and decussate leaf-scars. Two lines or ridges extend longitudinally down each internode from each leaf-scar. Note also the glands which appear as small elevations on the surface. Sketch to show these features; sketch also the transversely cut surface.

4. Examine a commercial specimen of buchu for the presence of stems, flowers, fruits, seeds and foreign leaves. If any are present, make sketches of the structures found and determine the amounts of stem and of other organic matter.

Eucalyptus Leaf. The ensiform leaves of *Eucalyptus globulus* Labill., family Myrtaceæ.

1. Measure the length and the greatest breadth of a leaf. Make a sketch to scale of the leaf to show the ensiform shape, the twisted petiole, the venation and the corky points.

2. Hold a leaf to the light and examine it with a pocket lens. Observe the punctate appearance, due to the presence of the oil-glands.

3. Write a description of the leaf.

Jaborandi Leaves. The dried leaflets of *Pilocarpus microphyllus* Stapf., family Rutaceæ.

1. Trace the outline of some typical leaflets, indicating the venation, the apex and the symmetry. How many differently shaped leaflets can be found and how can their occurrence be explained?

2. Hold a leaflet to the light and examine it with a pocket lens; what peculiarity does it show? Note the texture of the leaflet.

3. Cut a small square from a leaflet, mount it in chloral hydrate solution, apply a cover-glass, and boil it till transparent. Sketch the preparation to show the veinlets and the distribution of the glands. What explanation of the appearance by transmitted light does this preparation supply?

4. Make a brief statement of the important diagnostic characters you have observed.

NOTES ON SCHEDULE XII

The illustrations of buchu leaves are given to indicate how keyed drawings may be made. The actual drawings should be at least twice the size of those in the figures, and the degree of magnification or of reduction should be marked upon them as in the illustrations. The lettering should be kept in horizontal lines, which are more easily read and make a neater drawing than any other arrangement.

Buchu Leaves. To see the oil-glands, hold the leaf up to the light and examine it with a pocket lens; note the presence of an oil-gland in the apex of the leaves. The margin of the leaf of *Barosma betulina* is dentate in the upper two-thirds, and becomes serrate towards the base.

Eucalyptus Leaf. The glands of this leaf discharge their contents through the epidermis when the leaf is strongly bent; the emptied gland then becomes lined by a layer of cork, thus producing a minute corky point upon the leaf blade.

Jaborandi Leaves. Three differently shaped leaflets are present in the drug. A few leaflets are symmetrical, and have a short petiole into which the lamina gradually tapers; these are terminal leaflets. The remaining leaflets are all asymmetric—*i.e.*, the margin of the lamina forms a much

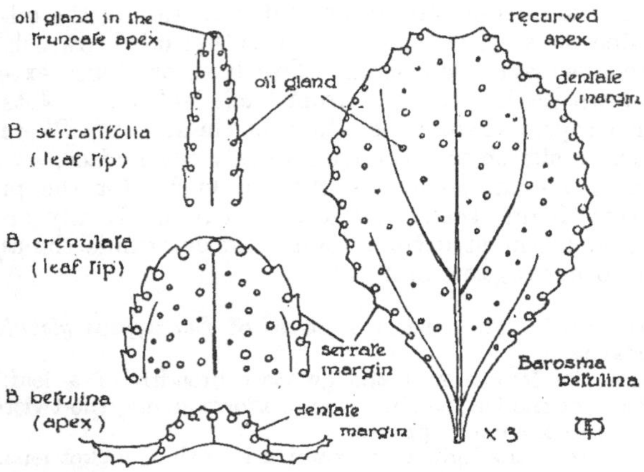

FIG. 19.—Buchu leaves, to show how enlarged keyed drawings of these leaves should be made.

more acute angle with the midrib on one side than on the other. If a large number of the asymmetric leaflets is examined, it will be found that half of them have the more acute angle on the left and the other half on the right. This acute-angled side of the lamina is the side directed towards the apex of the compound leaf. The asymmetric leaflets are

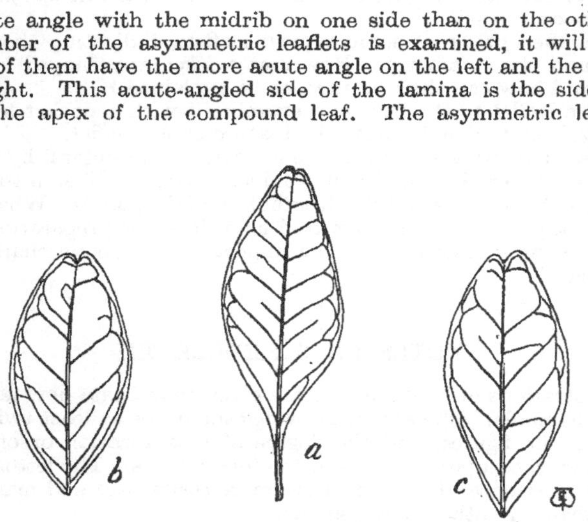

FIG. 20.—Leaflets of *Pilocarpus microphyllus* Stapf. *a.* Terminal leaflet. *b* and *c.* Leaflets from the left-hand and right-hand sides respectively of the imparipinnate leaf. All natural size.

sessile. One may conclude from the presence of these three forms of leaflet in a drug that it has been derived from imparipinnately compound leaves. Compare with Senna leaflets, which are of two shapes only, indicating a paripinnate leaf. In the case of an imparipinnate leaf, it is possible to determine the average number of leaflets in the leaf by taking a considerable quantity of the drug. The number of symmetrical leaflets gives the number of leaves present, and the number of asymmetric leaflets divided by two gives the average number of pairs of leaflets in the imparipinnate leaf.

A chloral hydrate preparation of a leaflet shows large oil-glands sparsely scattered throughout the mesophyll, thus explaining the translucent points seen by transmitted light when the lamina is examined with a lens. Such leaves are termed punctate, a feature which is characteristic of the family Rutaceæ.

SCHEDULE OF INSTRUCTIONS—XIII

LEAVES: COCA, WITCH-HAZEL, SENNA

Coca Leaf. The leaf of *Erythroxylum Coca* Lamarck, family Erythroxylaceæ, Bolivian coca.

1. Make drawings natural size. Trace off the outline and fill in the veins, etc. Make a second sketch of the lower surface to show the characteristic longitudinal lines on either side of the midrib. Mark all other features of importance, and make a note of the colour and texture of the leaf.

2. Measure some leaves and determine the average ratio of the length to the breadth of the lamina.

3. Compare with a commercial specimen of Peruvian coca, the leaves of *E. truxillense* Rusby, and record the differences in colour, condition, texture and prominence of the smaller veinlets as seen on the under surface.

Witch-hazel Leaves. The dried leaves of *Hamamelis virginiana* L., family Hamamelidaceæ.

1. Sketch a leaf to show the type of venation, the apex and the margin. What are the peculiarities of the venation ?

2. With a pocket lens, search for hairs, especially upon the lower surface and record their colour and position.

3. Cut out a small square of leaf with hairs upon it, place it under side uppermost on a microscope slide, mount it in chloral hydrate solution, apply a cover-glass and boil till transparent. Examine the preparation with the 16 mm. objective, and sketch a hair in detail.

4. *Test for Tannin.* Make a 5 per cent. decoction of the roughly powdered leaf, cool, filter and to 3 ml. of the filtrate add a few drops of solution of ferric chloride. Note the colour produced.

5. Write a description in technical language, see p. 122.

6. Examine leaves of sweet chestnut (*Castanea sp.*) and of *Hamamelis japonica* and compare with Hamamelis, noting points of difference.

Senna Leaves. The leaflets of *Cassia acutifolia* Delile (Alexandrian senna), and of *Cassia augustifolia* Vahl (Tinnevelly or Indian senna), family Leguminosæ.

1. Draw leaflets of both kinds of senna natural size, tracing the outlines. Key the drawings and make notes of the colour, distribution of hairs, etc.

2. Examine a number of leaflets and find whether or no all the leaflets are asymmetric. Draw any different types you find and state,

with reasons, any conclusion that may be made as to the type of leaf characteristic of the senna plant.

3. Test for anthraquinone derivatives as directed under Cascara Sagrada (p. 24). The colour may take 5 minutes to develop.

4. With a pair of scissors, cut out from a Tinnevelly senna leaf a small piece about 2 mm. square, so as to include a piece of the midrib. Place the piece of leaf upon a slide, moisten it with alcohol, mount in chloral hydrate and boil gently over a very small spirit-lamp or gas-flame. As soon as bubbles appear remove it from the flame, and when bubbles cease to leave the leaf heat it again, and so on, until the leaf is sufficiently transparent. During the boiling replace any liquid evaporated by running in more chloral hydrate solution until the space under the cover-glass is completely filled.

Cool and examine the preparation under the 16 mm. objective, and sketch a piece diagrammatically to show the general distribution of the veinlets and of the prismatic and cluster crystals of calcium oxalate. Sketch a few crystals in detail under the 4 mm. objective. Now focus carefully the epidermis of the leaf and sketch it to show the shape of the epidermal cells and the unicellular, pointed and warty hairs.

5. Examine a sample of senna for the presence of stalk. Note that a few pieces are rather thicker (stem), while the majority are very slender (leaf rachis). The rachis is characterised by the presence on the upper surface of a longitudinal groove and by four to six pairs of scars of leaflets, all towards the upper surface and the last pair at the apical extremity of the rachis. Sketch a rachis.

6. Determine the percentage amount of stalks present in a sample of leaf.

NOTES ON SCHEDULE XIII

Coca Leaves. When in bud, the leaves of coca are rolled longitudinally, the two margins being rolled inwards to meet one another on the upper surface above the midrib. This type of vernation (*i.e.*, the arrangement of the leaves in the bud) is termed involute. In the case of coca leaves, a longitudinal ridge of tissue is developed on either side of the midrib in the position where the two inrolled halves of the leaf come into contact. These two ridges meet and close the gap which would otherwise exist between the curved surfaces, thus affording additional protection to the young leaves.

The *chloral hydrate solution* to be used for treating the leaves is prepared by dissolving 5 parts by weight of chloral hydrate in 2 parts by volume of distilled water. This solution dissolves many of the cell contents, such as starch and protein matters; it also expands the walls of collapsed cells. Boiling the preparations ensures the complete removal of air, so that the combined action of chloral hydrate and boiling results in "clearing" the pieces of leaf and so rendering them transparent.

Witch-hazel Leaves. The leaf of the sweet chestnut has a coarsely serrate margin with very acute teeth; the lamina is oblong-lanceolate, the apex very acute and the secondary veins rather close together. The leaf of *H. japonica* is obovate with a cordate base and the secondary veins are more closely arranged than in *H. virginiana*.

Senna Leaves. It will be found that all the leaflets are asymmetric, and that there are two types present in equal numbers. For half the leaflets, the left-hand portion of the lamina has a more acute basal angle, while, for the remainder, the right-hand portion is more acute at the base. These facts indicate that the senna plant bears paripinnate leaves. Compare with jaborandi (p. 32).

Notice that the veinlets are of two kinds—viz., larger ones, which are accompanied by numerous prismatic crystals and, within the meshes of

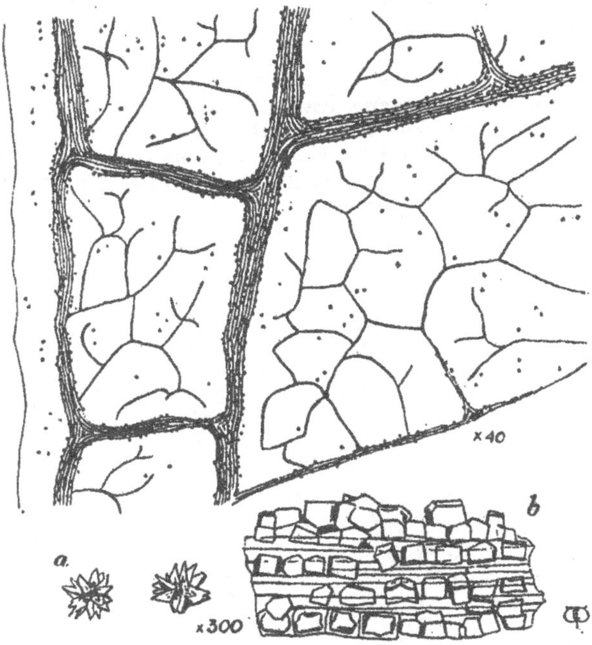

Fig. 21.—Diagram of a portion of a leaflet of *Cassia angustifolia* Vahl. as seen in surface view, after clearing with chloral hydrate, × 40. The left-hand side shows part of the margin of the leaflet. The dots represent prismatic crystals and the crosses cluster crystals of calcium oxalate. *a*. Two clutser crystals drawn in detail, × 300. *b*. Portion of a vein showing rows of prismatic crystals associated with its fibres, × 300.

these larger veinlets, a network of much smaller veinlets, which are not accompanied by crystals. The cluster crystals are rarely found near the veins; they generally occupy positions scattered sparsely throughout the interneural mesophyll. These features are shown in the figure, Fig. 21, where prismatic crystals are represented by dots, and cluster crystals by crosses. The student should make his drawings at least twice the size of those shown here.

SCHEDULE OF INSTRUCTIONS—XIV

LEAVES: FOXGLOVE, CHERRYLAUREL, BEARBERRY

Foxglove Leaves. The leaves of *Digitalis purpurea* L., collected from plants commencing to flower.

1. From a sample of commercial foxglove leaves select some that are as perfect as possible or choose some pieces including the petiole and others showing the margin. Expose the leaves for eighteen to twenty-four hours to a moist atmosphere, after which they are sufficiently softened to be spread out by hand. Sketch a leaf or portions of leaves to show the characters of the margin, venation and petiole. Make notes of the distribution and nature of the hairs, the prominence of the veins, and the variations in outline and indentation of the margin.

2. Prepare foxglove leaves by boiling with chloral hydrate solution, as described above for senna leaves. Make two preparations, one having the upper surface and the other the lower surface towards the cover-glass. Examine with the microscope and note the absence of crystals. Find the long, pluricellular, uniseriate, protective hairs,

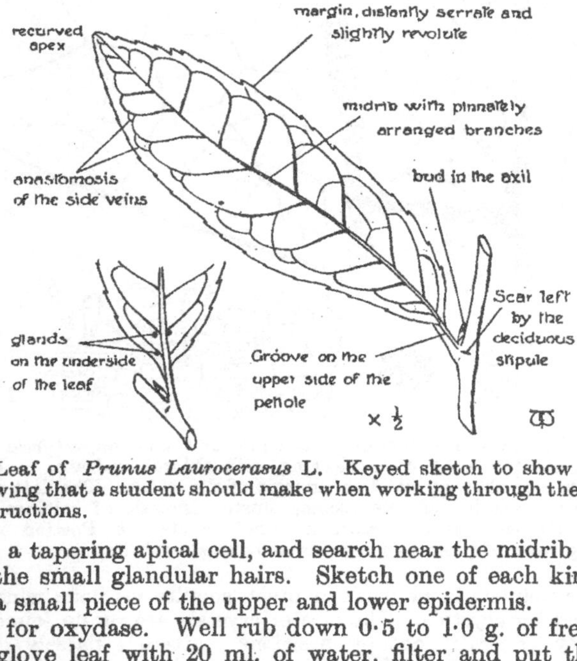

Fig. 22.—Leaf of *Prunus Laurocerasus* L. Keyed sketch to show the kind of drawing that a student should make when working through the schedule of instructions.

each with a tapering apical cell, and search near the midrib or a large vein for the small glandular hairs. Sketch one of each kind of hair and also a small piece of the upper and lower epidermis.

3. Test for oxydase. Well rub down 0·5 to 1·0 g. of fresh or air-dried foxglove leaf with 20 ml. of water, filter and put the filtrate into a small burette. Into each of two test-tubes put 3 ml. of water and add to each 3 drops of the digitalis extract. Boil the contents of one tube and then cool it. Add from burettes 0·3 ml. of solution of hydrogen peroxide and 0·3 ml. of a 1 per cent. solution of benzidine in alcohol (90 per cent.). A blue colour is formed with the unboiled liquid, no colour with the boiled one.

4. Compare foxglove leaves with those of comfrey, mullein and primrose. Make sketches to show the differences.

Cherrylaurel Leaf. The fresh leaf of *Prunus Laurocerasus* L., family Rosaceæ.

Make a drawing natural size, and mark upon it the recurved apex, the slightly revolute and distantly serrate margin, and the marked anastomosis of the side veins. Note the groove down the upper side of the petiole and the scars left upon the twig after the fall of the fugaceous stipules; mark these features upon the drawing, and make a note of the coriaceous

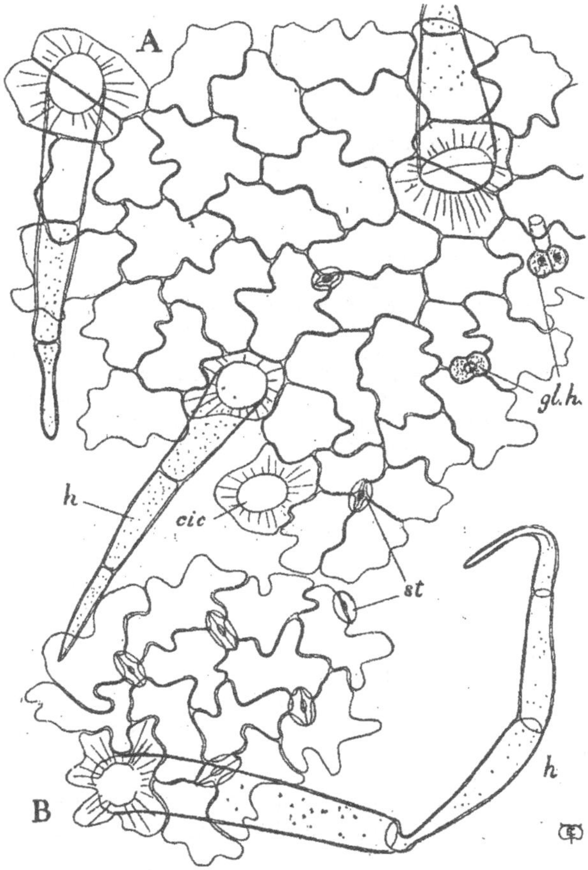

FIG. 23.—Epidermis of the leaf of *Digitalis purpurea* Linn., as seen in surface view, in a preparation made by clearing with chloral hydrate solution, × 200. A. Upper epidermis. B. Lower epidermis. *cic.*, scar left by the fall of a hair; *gl h*, glandular hair; *h*, protective hair; *st*, stoma.

texture, evergreen habit, and any other points worthy of notice, but not evident in the drawing. Upon a separate drawing of the under surface of the basal part of a leaf mark the nectaries on either side of the midrib near its base.

Bearberry Leaf. The leaf of *Arctostaphylos Uva-ursi* Sprengel, family Ericaceæ.

1. Sketch two or three leaves natural size to show the outline and

characters of the apex, margin, etc. Make notes of the texture, presence or absence of hairs, prominence of the veins, taste, etc.

2. *Reaction for Tannin.* Break a few leaves into small pieces and boil them in a test-tube one-third filled with water for a minute. Filter off the decoction into a clean test-tube and add to it a drop or two of solution of ferric chloride; note the bluish- or greenish-black colour, indicating the presence of tannin.

NOTES ON SCHEDULE XIV

Foxglove Leaves. The most convenient way of exposing leaves to a moist atmosphere is to put them into an ordinary desiccator containing water in place of a desiccating agent, and to allow them to stand at room temperature until sufficiently softened. Note the very great variation in the margin of foxglove leaves. It is sometimes typically crenate, but one may find all stages of transition from crenate to serrate or dentate.

The leaves do not show calcium oxalate crystals, but have numerous characteristic hairs. The drawing in Fig. 23 shows how to make a sketch of the epidermis of a leaf. In this instance it will be noticed that the protective hairs of the upper epidermis frequently arise from two (more rarely from one or three) epidermal cells, which cells have straighter walls than the surrounding cells. The similar hairs of the lower epidermis arise nearly always from single cells. The glandular hairs are quite small and most numerous near the veins. Each one consists of a short cylindrical stalk cell carrying a glandular head composed of two rounded cells having dense contents. The stomata are much more numerous in the lower than in the upper epidermis.

SCHEDULE OF INSTRUCTIONS—XV

FLOWERS OF CLOVE AND CHAMOMILE

Cloves. The dried flower-buds of *Eugenia aromatica* (Linn.) Baill. family Myrtaceæ.

1. Measure the length of a clove and also the length and width of the head and of the stalk. Sketch a clove at a magnification of four or five times and mark the calyx, corolla and hypanthium (so-called gynophore or calyx tube). Count the sepals and petals and observe their æstivation.

2. Cut a vertical section of a clove and make a drawing to show the position of the ovary, calyx, corolla, stamens, style, nectary, oil-glands, etc.

3. Cut a transverse section through the ovary and sketch it to show the number of loculi, the placentation and the oil-glands. Make a floral diagram and write the floral formula.

4. Examine specimens of clove stalks and of "mother cloves" and make sketches of each.

Chamomile Flowers. The flower-heads of *Anthemis nobilis* Linn., family Compositæ.

1. Cut a vertical section of a relaxed flower-head from below upwards and determine the following points: How many rows of involucral bracts do you find? How long are the bracts compared with the height of the receptacle? How many florets can you count in passing

from the base to the apex of the receptacle? How many tubular florets, if any, are there at the summit of the receptacle? Are the florets subtended by paleæ? Note the relative height of the tubular florets and the relative length of the recurved straps of the ligulate florets as compared with the height of the receptacle Measure the actual height of the receptacle. Make a drawing to show all these features, making the receptacle 2·5 cm. (1 in.) high and drawing the other structures in proportion.

2. With a finely-pointed pair of forceps remove some of the tubular florets, mount in chloral hydrate solution, apply a cover-glass and boil gently until cleared. Sketch one to show the five petals, five syngenesious anthers, bifid stigma and the inferior ovary. Mark the glands scattered on the surface of the ovary and corolla.

3. Take a ligulate floret and spread the corolla upon a microscope slide with a camel-hair brush dipped in water. Mount in chloral hydrate solution and examine the preparation with a pocket lens. Sketch a floret to show the number of teeth at the apex of the strap-shaped corolla and the number of veins. Note also the bifid stigma, the style, and the inferior ovary. Observe and mark on your drawing the glands, which are dotted over the ovary, the corolla tube and strap. These glands are more easily seen with a 16 mm. objective.

4. Remove a few of the involucral bracts and mount them in chloral hydrate solution, boiling if necessary. Sketch one of them to show the outer surface and mark the position of the hairs and glands found upon it.

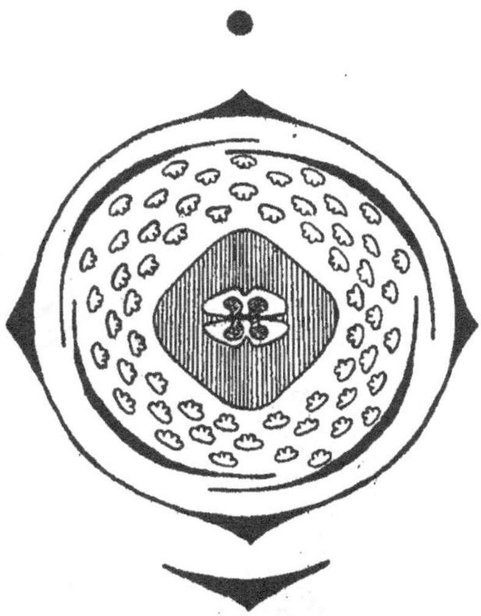

FIG. 24.—Floral diagram of *Eugenia aromatica* (Linn.) Baill.

5. Remove all the florets from a capitulum and note the numerous chaffy paleæ covering the surface of the receptacle. With a needle remove several paleæ, mount in chloral hydrate solution and examine with the 16 mm. objective. Sketch a palea as seen from the side and a second one as seen from the outside; mark on your drawing the long, undulating hairs and the numerous ovoid oil-glands.

6. Write a technical description of the chamomile flower-head, using the form given on p. 124.

7. Examine a specimen of German chamomile (the capitulum of *Matricaria Chamomilla* Linn.) and note the details in which it differs from Roman chamomile.

NOTES ON SCHEDULE XV

Cloves. These should be prepared for dissection by soaking in water for about forty-eight hours. The hypanthium is an enlargement of the torus underneath the calyx and ovary ; it is destitute of loculi. In making the floral diagram, search for a clove having the small fleshy bract attached to the stalk ; this will give the anterior position and the diagram can be immediately constructed. Indicate on the diagram the æstivation of the petals, which is not constant ; sometimes it is imbricate as shown in the

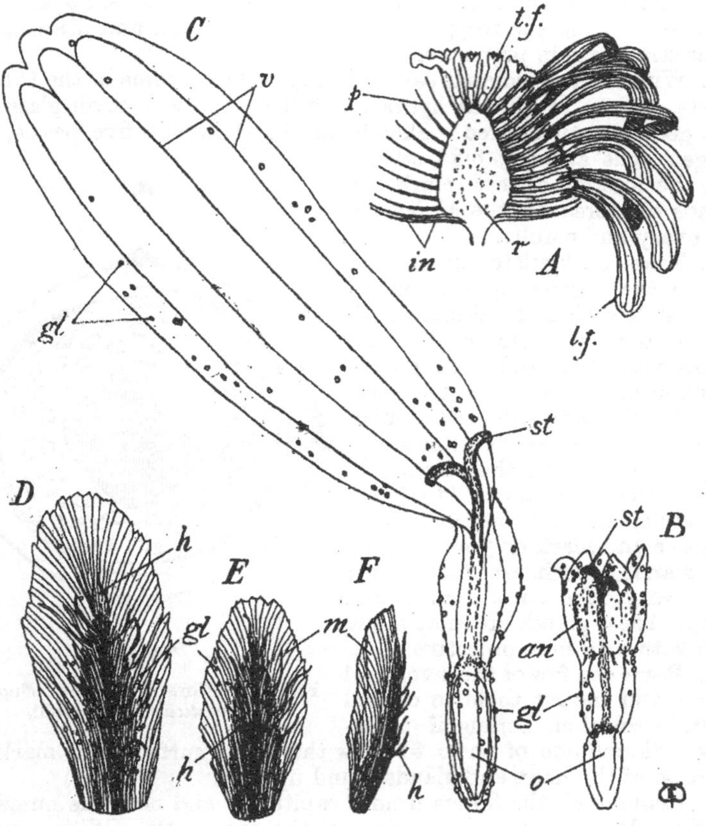

Fig. 25.—Chamomile flowers (*Anthemis nobilis*). A. An entire flower-head in longitudinal section, × 3. The florets are represented as removed from the left-hand side, so as to show the paleæ. B. A tubular floret, × 10. C. A ligulate floret, × 10. D. An involucral bract, × 10. E. and F. Outer and side views of a palea, both × 10. *an*, anther ; *gl*, glandular hair ; *h*, protective hair ; *in*, involucre ; *l.f.*, ligulate floret ; *m*, membranous margin ; *r*, receptacle of the capitulum ; *st*, stigma ; *t.f.*, tubular floret ; *v*, vein.

figure and sometimes two petals are completely outside and the other two completely inside.

The *chamomile flowers* can be rendered sufficiently supple for dissection by putting a few on to damp blotting-paper lining the bottom of a small enamelled-iron bowl and covering the bowl with a clock-glass. Stand it in a warm place for a short time or allow it to stand for a longer period at the ordinary temperature.

Vertical sections of flowers and flower-heads are, generally speaking, best cut from below upwards, because a cut made in this direction does not displace the florets or flower-parts, and also is much less apt to damage them than is the case when a section is made in any other way. In drawing the vertical section, first sketch in lightly the outline of the receptacle, then add the involucral bracts and the paleæ. All the bracts are best represented by single lines drawn somewhat heavily, as shown in the figure (Fig. 25). The florets should now be filled in and the drawing completed.

In many chamomile heads only a few tubular florets are to be found,

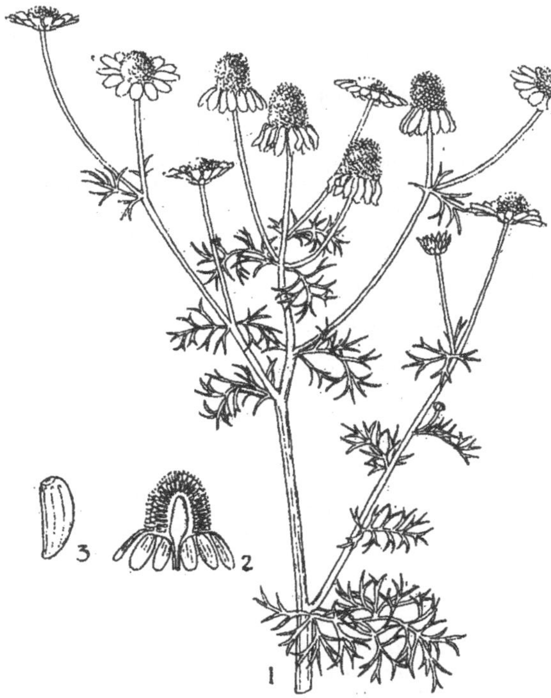

FIG. 26.—*Matricaria Chamomilla* L. 1. Upper part of a flowering plant. 2. Vertical section of a capitulum. 3. A fruit. (After Bentley and Trimen.)

and of these several are frequently distorted, showing a transition from the tubular to the ligulate type of corolla. Very frequently also, the stigmas are abnormal and possess more branches than two ; these variations are due to the effects of cultivation.

The bracts of the involucre are more strongly built than the paleæ of the receptacle, which are smaller, more delicate in texture and more boat-shaped.

The characteristics by which English or Roman chamomiles are recognised are :—

(*a*) The solid receptacle.

(*b*) The numerous paleæ, which cover the receptacle and each of which has a scarious (*i.e.*, thin and membranous) margin and a blunt apex.

(*c*) The three teeth (sometimes reduced to two, when one tooth is often larger than the other) and four veins of the ligulate corolla,

Matricaria Chamomilla L. German or wild chamomile is an annual plant with an erect and freely branched stem. Leaves glabrous, bipinnate with narrow linear segments. Inflorescence a rayed capitulum ; receptacle hollow, conical, and without paleæ. Capitula in corymbose clusters. Fruit without a pappus. The plant has a strong characteristic odour.

SCHEDULE OF INSTRUCTIONS—XVI

ARNICA FLOWERS AND SANTONICA

Arnica Flowers. The dried flower-heads of *Arnica montana* Linn., family Compositæ.

1. Dissect an Arnica flower-head and examine the receptacle and involucre. Observe the linear-lanceolate bracts and the small bristles surrounding each of the circular depressions in the receptacle. Make a sketch to show these features.

2. Soak some of the ligulate florets in water ; with a camel-hair brush spread one out carefully upon a slide and examine it with a pocket lens. Measure in millimetres the length and breadth of the strap-shaped corolla and the length of the ovary and of the corolla tube. Sketch a ligulate floret to scale and mark specially the veins and the teeth at the apex of the corolla strap.

3. Pick out a tubular floret, mount it in chloral hydrate solution and boil to remove air. Examine the preparation with the 16 mm. objective and sketch it to show all details.

4. Separate one or two of the fruits, mount them in chloral hydrate and boil gently until cleared, filling up any space by running more chloral hydrate under the cover-glass. Examine your preparation with a microscope and sketch the characteristic, appressed, two-pointed hairs of the fruit wall. Sketch also a portion of one of the barbed bristles forming the pappus.

N.B. Mark the magnification in diameters against all your drawings.

Santonica. The dried flower-heads of *Artemisia Cina* (Berg) Willkomm, family Compositæ.

1. Boil half a dozen soaked flower-heads in chloral hydrate solution about ½ in. deep in a test-tube until they sink to the bottom and air bubbles cease to escape from them. Allow to cool and pour the contents of the test-tube into a hollowed glass block.

2. Mount one of the prepared heads in chloral hydrate solution and examine it with the 16 mm. objective. Make a sketch to show the general arrangement of the parts and mark the axis, the involucral bracts and the florets. How many florets do you find ?

3. Dissect another prepared head with needles upon a glass slide and mount the preparation in chloral hydrate solution. Examine it with the ⅔ in. objective and count the number of bracts present. Make sketches to show how the bracts vary in shape and size in different part of the involucre.

4. Examine a single bract under the 4 mm. objective and observe the central midrib and its branches ; do they anastomose ? Search for stomata, hairs and glands—where do they occur and how numerous are they ? Note the scarious margin and the shape of the apex. Are there any marginal or apical hairs ? Sketch a bract to show its characteristics.

5. Examine the florets with the 4 mm. objective and note that they are all tubular; sketch one of them. What peculiarities do the stamens show? Sketch two or three pollen-grains. Are glandular hairs present; if so, where do they occur? Sketch one in detail. Determine the presence or absence of papillæ and hairs upon the apices of the corolla lobes.

6. Search for a fragment of a foliage leaf; clear it by boiling in chloral hydrate solution and sketch it to show the outline, venation, hairs and stomata.

NOTES ON SCHEDULE XVI

Arnica Flowers. Quite commonly both the rays and disc florets become separated from the receptacle, which is often found with its involucral

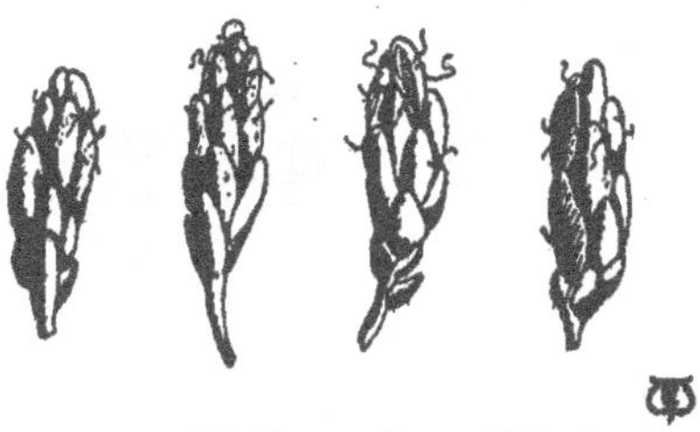

FIG. 27.—Genuine commercial Santonica. Whole flower-heads, showing the imbricated involucral bracts, × 8.

bracts in a detached condition. It will be noticed that the barbed character of the bristles of the pappus is produced by the projection of the pointed apices of the cells, of which each is composed, from the general surface of the bristle.

The receptacle should be softened by exposing it to a moist atmosphere for twenty-four hours; note that it is slightly arched and is about 8 mm. in diameter. The involucral bracts are in two rows, dark green in colour and linear-lanceolate. Make all the drawings to scale and add notes of such features as cannot be shown in the sketches.

The veins in the strap of the ligulate floret are mostly arranged in sets of three, each consisting of a vein running towards the apex of a lobe of the strap and accompanied on either side by veins which meet in an arc parallel with the curved margin of the lobe. This would give nine veins as the number typical of arnica flowers; the number may become seven by the coalescence of two neighbouring veins, or it may be larger than nine owing to abnormal development of the corolla, which occasionally shows four or five teeth, when the number of veins may reach fifteen, though the author has never seen more than fourteen in such corollas.

Arnica flowers are recognised by the following characters:—

(*a*) The deep yellow ligulate corollas of the ray florets with seven to nine veins and three teeth at the apex; occasionally the number of teeth is four or five and the number of veins may then reach fourteen.

(*b*) The appressed twin-hairs on the ovary wall.

(*c*) The well-developed pappus surmounting the fruits.

(*d*) The linear-lanceolate, hairy involucral bracts.

Santonica. Santonica may be softened by placing some in a dish and pouring hot water upon it and allowing it to soak for about half an hour.

The genus *Artemisia* is a very large one (consisting of over 260 species) and is subdivided into four divisions, that to which santonica belongs being known as *Seriphidium*. The *Seriphidium* section is distinguished by having capitula bearing only one kind of floret, all the florets being perfect; the receptacle also is quite glabrous. The *Seriphidium* division itself contains a very large number of species, so that the features by which genuine santonica may be identified are necessarily rather fine points of distinction; they are as follows:

1. The foliage leaves are linear-lanceolate with a rounded apex and an apiculus; they have a midrib with numerous, pinnately arranged branches

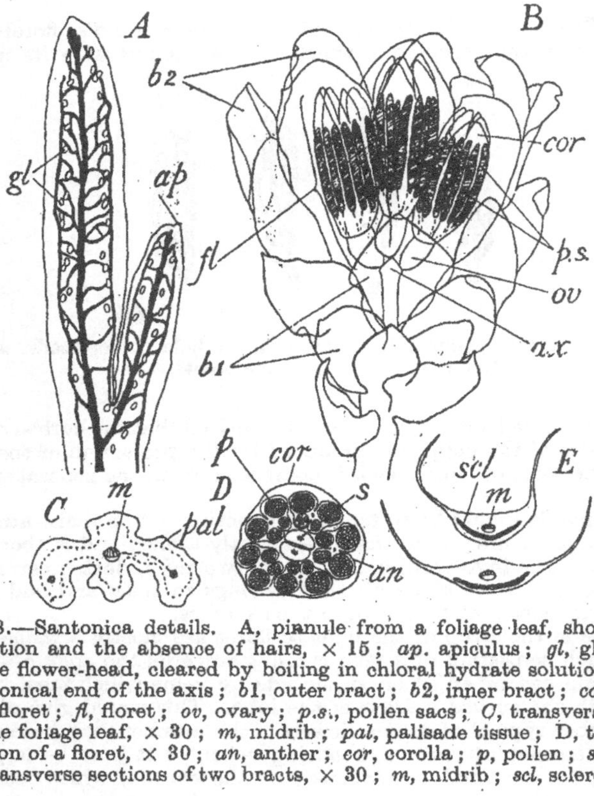

FIG. 28.—Santonica details. A, pinnule from a foliage leaf, showing the venation and the absence of hairs, × 15; *ap.* apiculus; *gl*, gland; B, entire flower-head, cleared by boiling in chloral hydrate solution, × 15; *ax*, conical end of the axis; *b*1, outer bract; *b*2, inner bract; *cor*, corolla of a floret; *fl*, floret; *ov*, ovary; *p.s.*, pollen sacs; C, transverse section of the foliage leaf, × 30; *m*, midrib; *pal*, palisade tissue; D, transverse section of a floret, × 30; *an*, anther; *cor*, corolla; *p*, pollen; *s*, stigma; *E*, transverse sections of two bracts, × 30; *m*, midrib; *scl*, sclerenchyma.

connecting it with two marginal veins, which run parallel to the margin at about one-third the distance from it to the midrib. There are no long protective hairs, but numerous sessile glands are present.

2. The involucral bracts most frequently number sixteen. The midrib branches freely and the veinlets are contorted and frequently anastomose. The number of cottony hairs is small and apical marginal hairs are always absent.

3. The flowers are all hermaphrodite and tubular and the apices of the corolla lobes are never more than slightly papillose and bear no trichomes.

SCHEDULE OF INSTRUCTIONS—XVII

FLOWERS; INSECT FLOWERS, MARIGOLD FLOWERS, SAFFRON

Insect Flowers. The unexpanded flower-heads of *Chrysanthemum cinerariæfolium* Visiana, family Compositæ.

1. Take a soaked head and cut a vertical section from below upwards. Is the receptacle solid or hollow? What is its shape? How many rows of involucral bracts do you find? Note the length of the bracts compared to the diameter of the receptacle. Are there any paleæ on the receptacle? Sketch the vertical section at a definite magnification.

2. Count the number of ligulate florets in a single head. How many rows are there? Remove a single ligulate floret and mount it in solution of chloral hydrate. Count the number of veins in the strap at about the middle point. Note the number and shape of the terminal teeth. Are there any glands present? Look for the calyx. Sketch a floret to show all these features.

3. Mount similarly some tubular florets and sketch one in detail.

4. Can you find any evidence as to whether the flowers were fully expanded or not?

5. Write out the distinguishing characters of the drug.

Marigold Flowers. The ligulate corollas of the ray florets of *Calendula officinalis* L., family Compositæ.

1. Soften some florets by soaking them in water; spread one out on a slide with a camel-hair pencil and measure the lengths of the tubular and strap-shaped portions of the corolla. What is the shape of the strap? Measure its width and note the number of terminal teeth and their shape. How many veins do you find and what is their arrangement? Sketch a floret to scale at a known magnification.

2. Using a floret mounted in solution of chloral hydrate, find the hairs on the corolla tube and sketch one or two in detail.

3. Sketch a style and stigma and a pollen grain. Is there any ovary present?

4. State how this floret differs from others you have examined.

Saffron. The dried stigmas and tops of the styles of *Crocus sativus* Linn., family Iridaceæ.

1. Examine some saffron; note the odour and record the colour and general appearance.

2. Float some saffron on water in a white dish, observe the expansion of the parts and note the coloration imparted to the water.

3. Examine the expanded stigmas and determine their arrangement. Measure the length and breadth of some of the stigmas and sketch a group to scale to show their characteristic shape and the form of the free margin at the upper extremity.

4. Search amongst the saffron for pale-coloured pieces, and examine any you can find. Are they anthers or strips of petal, or do they belong to some other plant?

Lily of the Valley Flowers. The dried inflorescence of *Convallaria majalis* Linn., family Liliaceæ.

1. Soften some of the drug by exposure for eighteen hours to a moist atmosphere. Examine and sketch an entire inflorescence. Mark, on your drawing, the scape, pedicels, bracts and flowers. Measure the length of the scape and count the flowers in the raceme.

2. Cut the scape transversely; examine and sketch the cut surface; make a note of its shape. Sketch and describe a bract.

3. Determine the dimensions of a flower. Open a corolla by cutting it

longitudinally from base to apex with the point of a needle; lay it on a slide and flatten it with a brush dipped in water so as to expose the inner surface. Sketch the corolla from the inside to show the corolla lobes and the epipetalous stamens. Sketch an ovary.

4. Write a floral formula; construct a floral diagram and make a drawing of a vertical section.

5. Note the odour and taste of the drug.

6. Write a description of the drug.

NOTES ON SCHEDULE XVII

Insect Flowers. The receptacle is nearly flat, with a slight central convexity, and is devoid of paleæ. The ligulate corollas have three teeth, the central one being small or almost flat; the number of veins is about seventeen, five or six of the main veins being more strongly marked than the remainder; oil-glands are present, scattered all over the ovary and the lower part of the corolla. The calyx is membranous and surrounds the lower third of the tubular part of the corolla. That the flower-heads are gathered unripe is evidenced by the shrunken condition of the ovaries, the unextruded stigmas of the tubular florets, and the strap of the ligulate florets folded as in the bud.

Ox-eye daisies (*Chrysanthemum Leucanthemum* Linn.), which are sometimes used to adulterate insect flowers, have ligulate corollas with seven veins and three rounded teeth, the central tooth being the largest.

Marigold Flowers. These consist of the corollas only of the ligulate florets. Typically the corolla has four veins and three acute teeth, but the number of teeth may vary from two to four and the veins from five to seven. Two kinds of hairs are present on the tube: conical, biseriate covering hairs and club-shaped glandular hairs.

SCHEDULE OF INSTRUCTIONS—XVIII

UMBELLIFEROUS FRUITS

Fennel Fruit. The fruit of *Fœniculum vulgare* Mill., family Umbelliferæ.

1. Measure the length and breadth of several fruits; record the smallest and largest measurements, and the dimensions which most frequently occur. What is the shape of the fruit? How many ribs are there and what is their colour? Are the cremocarps entire or separated into mericarps? Find the stylopods and determine their length in proportion to the total length of the fruit. Has the fruit any odour? If not immediately noticeable, rub some fruits between the hands and notice whether any odour develops. Make a sketch to scale (magnified about six times) of the fruit and mark all the features recorded.

2. Soak some fruits in water for about eighteen hours and cut transverse sections by the following method:—

(*a*) Take a small cylinder of pith, lay it on the bench, and cut it longitudinally into halves with a sharp scaplel; near the end of the flat surface of one-half of the cylinder of pith, make a small depression, using a blunt instrument, such as the handle of a scalpel, for the purpose. If the depression is cut with a knife, the pith loses its resilience, so that it is better to make the hollow by pressure with a blunt object.

Lay the fruit in this depression, apply the second half-cylinder of pith to the first and tie the two together with a piece of string.

(*b*) Smooth the top of the pith and fruit by cutting it level with a razor; then flood the razor with alcohol and cut several sections

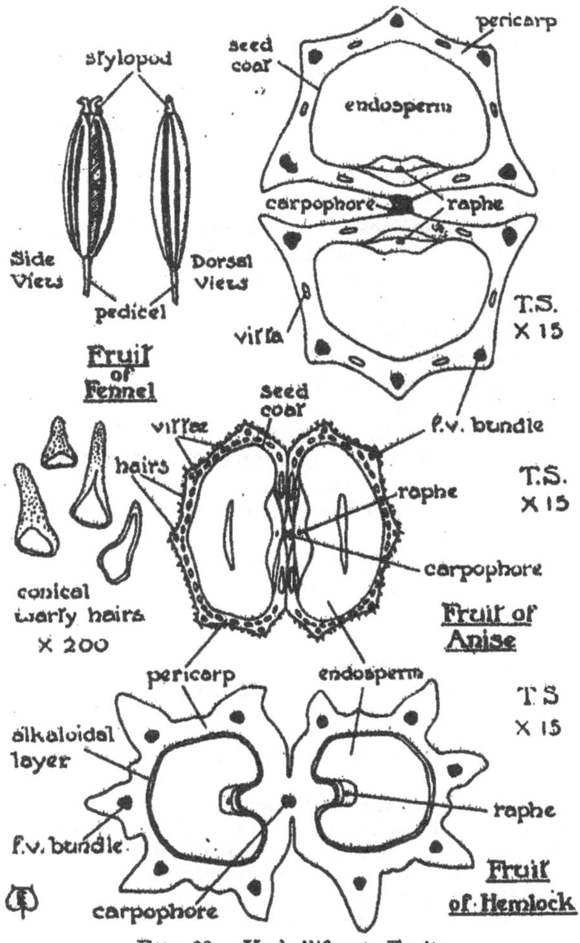

FIG. 29.—Umbelliferous Fruits.

through the fruit and pith, pushing the razor by a slow motion from toe to heel.

(*c*) Fill a hollowed glass block with alcohol, dip a camel-hair pencil into it and sweep the sections and pieces of pith into the dish. Pick out a thin section and mount it on a slide in chloral hydrate solution and boil if necessary. Mount a second section in phloroglucin and hydrochloric acid.

3. Examine the sections with the 16 mm. objective and sketch one

diagrammatically to show the number and distribution of the vittæ, the shape of the endosperm, the primary ridges and their fibro-vascular bundles, the carpophores, and the raphe.

Caraway Fruit. The fruit of *Carum Carvi* Linn., family Umbelliferæ.

Dill Fruit. The fruit of *Anethum graveolens* Linn., family Umbelliferæ.

1. Examine these two fruits as directed for fennel and note that :—

(*a*) The outline of a transverse section through a mericarp of caraway is an almost regular pentagon.

(*b*) The pericarp of dill is extended laterally to form a wing on either side of each mericarp.

Coriander Fruit. *Coriandrum sativum* Linn., family Umbelliferæ.

1. Examine the fruit externally :

(*a*) Note the shape and measure the average diameter.

(*b*) Find the somewhat inconspicuous, wavy, primary ridges.

(*c*) Find the straight, well-defined, secondary ridges.

(*d*) Look for remains of the calyx and styles at the summit.

2. Cut a transverse section and sketch it as seen under the 16 mm. objective. Note especially :

(*a*) The number and position of the vittæ.

(*b*) The form of the seed.

(*c*) The sclerenchyma of the pericarp.

3. Cut a vertical section at right angles to the commissure and sketch it as for the transverse section.

Note especially the form of the section of the seed and the position of the embryo.

4. Split open a fruit along the plane of the commissure. Sketch the commisural surface of a mericarp, noting especially the vittæ and the carpophore.

Anise Fruit. The fruit of *Pimpinella Anisum* Linn., family Umbelliferæ.

1. Examine and section fruits of anise as directed for fennel.

2. Sketch also one or two of the characteristic hairs as seen with the 4 mm. objective.

Hemlock Fruit. The fruit of *Conium maculatum* Linn., family Umbelliferæ.

1. Examine and section fruits of hemlock in the same way, noting especially the absence of aromatic odour and the presence of a well-marked alkaloidal layer as seen in the transverse section.

2. Triturate a few hemlock fruits with a solution of caustic alkali, and note the strong, disagreeable, mouse-like odour that is developed.

Cummin Fruit. *Cuminum Cyminum* Linn., family Umbelliferæ.

1. Examine the fruit as directed for fennel fruit and note the following points :

(*a*) Are the mericarps united or separate ?

(*b*) Note the colour of the primary ridges and of the spaces between them.

(*c*) Find the ridges on the intervening spaces, look for hairs and note their colour.

(*d*) Note the proportions of the different parts of the fruit (length, breadth, stylopods, etc.) and make an enlarged sketch of the fruit.

2. Cut a transverse section as for fennel fruit and sketch it as seen under the ⅔ in. objective. Mark the following features :

(*a*) The primary ridges and their fibro-vascular bundles.
(*b*) The secondary ridges and the vittæ.
(*c*) The hairs on the ridges, noting how they differ on the two kinds of ridges.
(*d*) The seed.

NOTES ON SCHEDULE XVIII

Fennel Fruit. This is a typical cremocarp, showing upon each mericarp five primary ridges and four vittæ on the dorsal or curved surface and two vittæ upon the commissural or flat surface. Note the large size of the entire, oval-oblong cremocarps and the pale straw-colour of the prominent, straight, primary ridges.

Anise Fruit. Note that the mericarps are united, the pedicel usually present, and the ridges straight. In the transverse section the most striking feature is the large number of vittæ, varying from twenty to forty-five in each mericarp. The epidermis of the pericarp bears numerous short unicellular, warty hairs, which are very characteristic, and give the fruit a rough feel when rubbed gently between the fingers.

Hemlock Fruit. Note the irregularity crenated primary ridges, and the laterally compressed forms of the cremocarp, which is usually divided into its constituent mericarps. When a transverse section is examined with a pocket lens or with a low power of the compound microscope, this fruit does not show any obvious vittæ, and this is a useful character for distinguishing hemlock from other umbelliferous fruits. The pericarp, however, does contain a large number of small and very inconspicuous vittæ, which can be seen by careful examination with the $\frac{1}{8}$ in. objective. Another useful character of the transverse section of the mericarp is the presence of a deep groove in the endosperm on the commissural surface.

The details of structure of these umbelliferous fruits are illustrated in Fig. 29, which may serve as an example of the kind of drawings which should be made, and of the way in which particulars may be recorded upon the drawing.

SCHEDULE OF INSTRUCTIONS—XIX

SENNA POD, TAMARIND, POPPY CAPSULE

Senna Pod. The dried fruit of *Cassia acutifolia* Delile and of *C. angustifolia* Vahl., family Leguminosæ.

1. Measure the length and width of several pods and determine the average size. Weight about ten pods and calculate the average weight of one pod.

2. Make a drawing of a pod and mark the dorsal and ventral sutures, the point of attachment to the pedicel, the scar left by the stigma, the veins in the carpellary wall and the raised areas over the seeds.

3. Determine the number of seeds in one pod and note how they are placed. Remove some seeds, measure them and sketch one to show its shape and the position of the radicle. Is the seed albuminous or exalbuminous ? What are its most striking peculiarities ?

Tamarind. The prepared fruits of *Tamarindus indica* Linn., family Leguminosæ.

1. From the brown, sugary mass, separate a stalk with several (about 5 to 9) tapering and branching vascular strands attached to it, and sketch it. Record the dimensions.

2. Remove also some of the seeds, each of which is surrounded by a part of the leathery endocarp, measure their length; breadth and thickness ; note the colour and shape and sketch a typical seed.

3. Note the odour and taste of the pulp and its reaction to indicators.

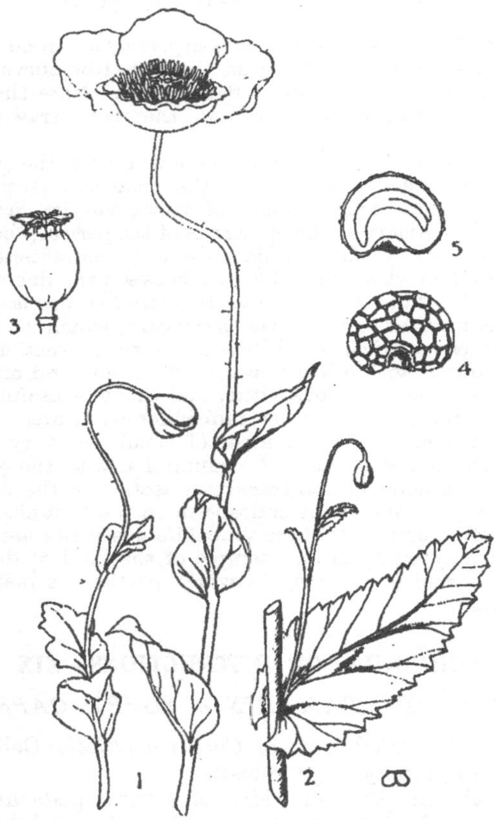

FIG. 30.—*Papaver somniferum* L. 1. Flowering stem. 2. Leaf from lower part of the stem. 3. Capsule. 4. Seed. 5. Longitudinal section of the seed.

Poppy Capsule. The fully grown, nearly ripe capsule of *Papaver somniferum* Linn., family Papaveraceæ.

1. Sketch a capsule to show the radiate stigma, the thalamus, the pores and other external features. How are the pores formed ?

2. Cut a capsule transversely and sketch it to show the loculus, placentæ, etc. How many carpels do you find and how many loculi ?

3. Cut a capsule longitudinally and sketch it to show the shape of the placentæ and the manner of attachment of the seeds.

4. Is the fruit inferior or superior, syncarpous or apocarpous, and how are the partitions placed with respect to the pores and the rays of the stigma ?

5. Measure some seeds and count the number of reticulations legnthwise and across. Note the external shape and find the hilum placed in a slight depression near one end ; the radicle points towards the hilum. Sketch to show these features and character of the reticulations.

6. Cut a section of the seed and identify the reserve food, as directed for stavesacre seed, see p 62.

Note. The reticulations are few in number, and are polygonal in shape with straight edges (*cf.* Henbane, p. 59).

Sections of poppy seeds are most easily made and examined by smearing the end of a cork with a thin layer of fish glue, as directed under Schedule XXIII., p. 59.

NOTES ON SCHEDULE XIX

Senna Pods. The seeds have very long, filiform funicles ; they are obovate-wedge shaped, compressed parallel to the cotyledons, with the hilum at the pointed end. The embryo is large and straight, with green cotyledons, and is surrounded by a scanty endosperm. Notice the wrinkling of the testa of seeds from each kind of senna pod ; Alexandrian senna seeds show a reticulate wrinkling and Indian senna seeds show wrinkles arranged in approximately parallel lines running transversely from the margins to the centre of the flat faces of the seed.

Poppy Capsule (see figure 30). The pores are formed by the excision of small tongue-shaped areas just beneath the rays of the stigma and alternating in position with its lobes ; these areas curl backwards in drying, so opening the pores. The ingrowing placentæ do not meet in the centre, so that there is only one loculus.

SCHEDULE OF INSTRUCTIONS—XX

PIMENTO, CAPSICUM, PEPPERS, CUBEBS.

Pimento. The dried, full-grown, unripe fruit of *Pimenta officinalis* Lindl., family Myrtaceæ.

1. Make a sketch from above to show the four small calyx teeth ; find the scar of the stalk below. Is the fruit superior or inferior ? Note the red-brown colour and the absence of reticulations upon the surface, which is rough from the presence of small rounded projections, due to the oil-glands, just below the surface.

2. Cut a transverse section of a soaked fruit, and sketch it to show that the fruit is bilocular and two-seeded.

Capsicum. The dried ripe fruit of *Capsicum minimum* Roxb.

1. Examine some Zanzibar chillies and sketch one to show the pedicel, calyx and elongated-ovoid berry. How many sepals has the calyx ?

2. Cut a fruit transversely ; note and sketch the thin pericarp and dissepiment. Mark also the loculi and seeds.

3. Remove some seeds and determine the diameter of several. What is the thickness ? Cut one across, parallel to the flat faces and sketch the internal structure.

4. From a few grams of a specimen of Zanzibar chillies remove the pedicels and calices and weigh them. Determine the proportion present.

5. Examine some fruits of *Capsicum annuum* and Japanese chillies ; note how they differ from fruits of *C. minimum.*

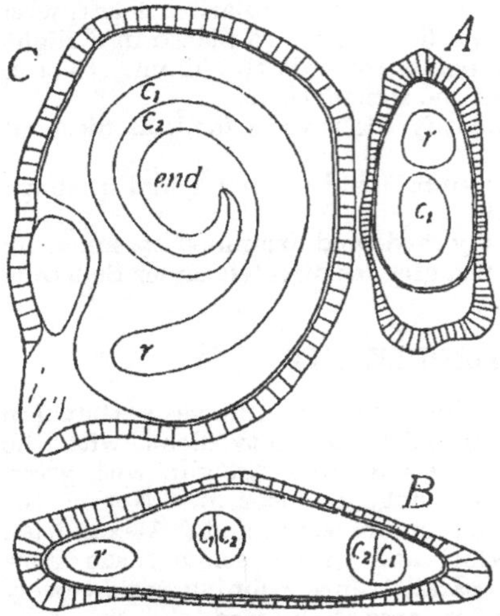

FIG. 31.—*Capsicum minimum*, sections of seeds. *A*, transverse; *B*, longitudinal, cut at right angles to the flat surfaces; *C*, longitudinal, parallel to the flat surfaces; *C*1 and *C*2, the two cotyledons; *end*, endosperm; *r*, radicle.

Black Pepper. The dried unripe fruit of *Piper nigrum* Linn., family Piperaceæ.

1. Note the wrinkled surface and find the scar marking the point of attachment of the fruit to the axis; this is the base of the peppercorn. Stick a needle into the side of the peppercorn at the equator, then roll it over and look at the pole opposite to the base and find a small papilla divided into from two to five parts; this is the remains of the stigma. Sketch a fruit as seen from the side and from above, marking the features noted.

2. Cut a vertical section of a peppercorn and note the attachment of the seed over the whole of its surface to the pericarp. Sketch to show the pericarp with the remains of the stigma and point of attachment, the seed-coat, the perisperm, the endosperm, the embryo and the central hollow.

White Pepper. The ripened fruit of *Piper nigrum* Linn., family Piperaceæ, deprived of the outer part of the pericarp and dried.

1. Note the plump appearance. Observe the conical projection below and the flattened area at the apex. Find the lines on the surface radiating from the base towards the apex; these are the fibro-vascular bundles of the inner part of the pericarp. Sketch as for black pepper.

2. Cut a vertical section and sketch the details as for black pepper. Scrape the surface and note the dark seed-coat.

Cubebs. The dried, full-grown, unripe fruits of *Piper Cubeba*, family Piperaceæ.

1. Sketch a cubeb from the side to show the wrinkled surface, the stalk, and the remains of the triradiate stigma at the apex.

2. Make a vertical section and sketch it to show the shrivelled seed attached normally at the base only.

3. *Reaction for Cubebic Acid.* Crush some fruits and sprinkle the powder upon the surface of strong sulphuric

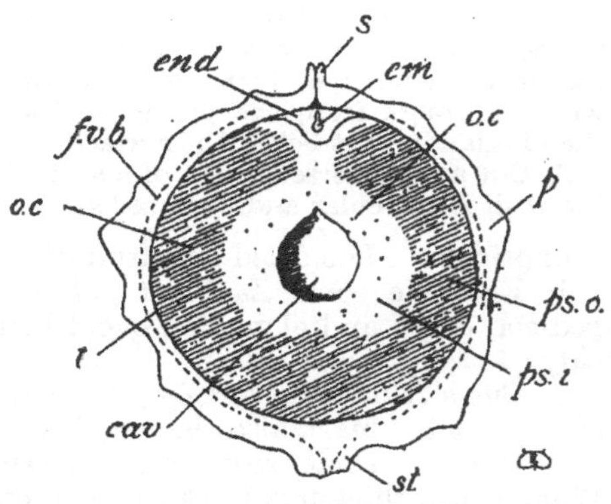

FIG. 32.—Vertical section of the fruit of *Piper nigrum* Linn. *cav.* central hollow; *em.*, embryo; *end.*, endosperm; *f.v.b.*, fibro-vascular bundle; *o.c.*, oil-cell; *p.*, pericarp; *ps.i.*, inner part of the perisperm; *s.g.*, outer part of the perisperm; *s.*, remains of the stigma; *st.*, stalk; *t*, seed-coat.

acid (sp. gr. 1·84); note the crimson colour, which is best seen when the dish is tilted.

Long Pepper. The dried fruit of *Piper officinarum* DC.

1. Measure the length and the breadth of a fruit and note the stalk. Count the number of spirals of fruits and record the phyllotaxis. Make a sketch to show these details.

2. On the outside of the fruit find two kinds of structure, viz., small areas with a dark centre and a pale-brown, wavy margin; between them rounded dark areas with a central projection. These are the bracts and fruits respectively. Draw a small piece enlarged to show the bracts and the fruits with their stigmas.

3. Cut a soaked fruit transversely and sketch the cut surface to show the small true fruits embedded in the fleshy bracts and axis. Mark the axis, bracts, fruits, perisperm, endosperm, etc. What is the reserved food in the perisperm?

NOTES ON SCHEDULE XX

Capsicum. The seed contains a strongly curved embryo, embedded in an oily endosperm (see Fig. 31).

Black and white pepper and cubebs should be soaked for twenty-four hours in cold water, so as to soften them before dissection. *Cocculus indicus* will require to be soaked for about thirty-six hours, and juniper berries should be used without soaking.

Pepper. The endosperm and embryo are only rarely definitely recognisable in either black or white pepper. In black pepper especially their presence is marked merely by a small cup-shaped hollow at the apex of the perisperm. The small conical projection at the base of white pepper is formed by the fibro-vascular bundles, which radiate in all directions from the base to enter the seed-coats, etc., thus protecting from removal the tissues in their neighbourhood, when the ripe berries are prepared for the market by the removal of the outer part of the pericarp.

Cubebs. The seed is frequently found adhering to some part of the inner surface of the pericarp other than the base. During the drying of the fruits, the seed often appears to adhere strongly to the apex, or side, of the loculus, and to be eventually dragged away from its funiculus at the base; as a consequence, it may appear to be abnormally situated in the dried fruit of commerce.

Long Pepper. The long pepper fruit is a sorosis. To determine the phyllotaxis, stick a pin into one of the fruits near the base of the sorosis; note the two crossing spirals of fruits (one right-handed and one left-handed) of which it is a member, and, beginning from this fruit, count the number of right-handed spirals of fruits in the circumference of the sorosis; count similarly the number of left-handed spirals of fruits intersecting the first set. These are the two sets of intersecting parastichies, and the phyllotaxis is expressed by writing the two numbers with a proportion sign between them, *e.g.*, 5 : 8.

SCHEDULE OF INSTRUCTIONS—XXI

COLOCYNTH, BITTER ORANGE PEEL, LEMON PEEL, COCCULUS INDICUS

Colocynth. The dried pulp of the fruit of *Citrullus Colocynthis* Schrad., family Cucurbitaceæ.

1. Examine an unpeeled fruit; note the hard, brownish outer

region of the pericarp and measure its thickness as well as the diameter of the entire fruit. Record your results.

2. Cut a peeled fruit transversely and note the three fissures united in the centre, from which they radiate, one passing through the length of each placenta. Find the six groups of seeds near the periphery of the fruit; the groups being arranged in pairs one at the end of each placental fissure. Note the pithy nature of the pulp. Make a keyed sketch to show these details.

3. Remove the seeds from a peeled fruit and determine the proportions of seed and pulp.

4. Examine a seed; note its dimensions and sketch it to show the pale brown testa and the large oily embryo, consisting of two cotyledons and a small radicle. Note also the hardness and lignification of the testa.

5. Test the cotyledons for oil by pressing them between the folds of a piece of paper and by applying staining tests for oils.

Bitter Orange Peel. The dried outer part of the pericarp of *Citrus Aurantium* Linn., family Rutaceæ.

1. Take a piece of the peel and record the colour and surface condition of the inner and outer surfaces.

2. With a razor cut a thin transverse section from a piece of soaked peel and mount it in chloral hydrate solution. Sketch it diagrammatically to show the distribution of the lysigenous oil-glands, the fibro-vascular bundles and the calcium oxalate crystals.

3. From a piece of peel softened by exposure to a moist atmosphere, cut away a portion of the white inner part, place it on a glass slide and add a few drops of 5 per cent. solution of caustic potash; record the result. To what is the observed effect due?

4. Note the odour and taste.

Lemon Peel. The outer part of the fresh pericarp of *Citrus Limonia* Osbeck, family Rutaceæ.

1. Examine lemon peel as directed for bitter orange peel and record the differences you observe.

Cocculus Indicus. The dried fruits of *Anamirta paniculata* Colebr., family Menispermaceæ.

1. Sketch a fruit, as seen from the side, to show the wrinkled pericarp, the rounded stalk scar, the pointed stigma, and the connecting ridge. (These details can be most easily seen upon a dry fruit.)

2. Make sections of soaked fruits: Cut a median vertical section passing through the ridge, a transverse section cut midway between the stigma and the stalk scar, and a longitudinal section cut at right angles to the median section. Make keyed drawings of each to show the two layers of the pericarp and its infoldings, the endosperm and the embryo.

NOTES ON SCHEDULE XXI

Bitter Orange Peel. The calcium oxalate occurs in prismatic crystals. The yellow colour produced by caustic alkali is due to the presence of the glycoside hesperidin.

Cocculus Indicus. The fruit is a variety of drupe. The seed is cup-shaped, the hollow being occupied by the two adjacent ventral infoldings of the pericarp. The cotyledons of the embryo are strap-shaped, and lie in a vertically placed slit-shaped cavity, which forms an almost complete

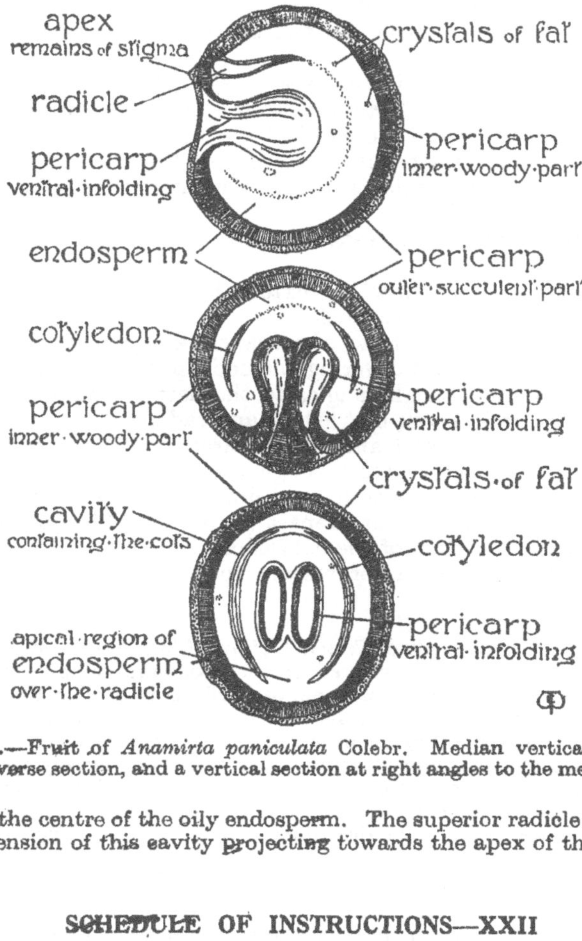

FIG. 33.—Fruit of *Anamirta paniculata* Colebr. Median vertical section, transverse section, and a vertical section at right angles to the median one.

ellipse in the centre of the oily endosperm. The superior radicle is enclosed in an extension of this cavity projecting towards the apex of the fruit.

SCHEDULE OF INSTRUCTIONS—XXII

SEEDS; NUX VOMICA, CASTOR OIL, CROTON, STROPHANTUS, LINSEED

Nux Vomica Seed. The seeds of *Strychnos Nux-vomica* Linn., family Loganiaceæ.

1. Note the rounded outline and the flattened shape; measure the diameter and the thickness in millimetres. Find the scar of the hilum in the centre of one face and a slight ridge connecting it with a projection on the edge, marking the position of the radicle. Sketch a seed to show these features and the hairs radiating from the centre.

2. Cut a soaked seed transversely and sketch the transverse surface

to show the hairy seed-coat and the horny endosperm with its central hollow.

3. Section a soaked seed by an incision along the edge parallel to the flat faces, and notice that the central hollow is disc-shaped ; find the embryo with its radicle and two small leafy cotyledons. Sketch your preparation.

4. Cut a transverse section of a soaked seed, mount it in phloroglucin and hydrochloric acid. Note and sketch the trichomes showing the lignified pitted bases and the lignified ribs in the limbs.

5. Examine Ignatius beans—the seeds of *Strychnos Ignatii* Berg.—as directed for Nux Vomica and note the similarities and differences between the two seeds.

Castor Oil Seed. The seeds of *Ricinus communis* Linn., family Euphorbiaceæ.

1. Sketch a seed to show the external features, viz., the mottled testa, the raphe, and the caruncle.

2. Carefully crack the testa of a soaked seed and remove it ; note the delicate thin tegmen covering the endosperm. Cut a longitudinal section of a kernel at right angles to the flatter surfaces, and sketch it to show the endosperm, cotyledons and radicle.

3. Take another kernel and cut it carefully round the edge by a slight incision, so as to pass through the endosperm only ; separate the two parts of the endosperm, and find the embryo lying in the flat central cavity. Sketch your preparation to show the radicle and the disposition and venation of the cotyledons.

4. Test the endosperm for reserve food by mounting sections in suitable reagents.

Croton Seed. The seeds of *Croton Tiglium*, Linn., family Euphorbiaceæ.

1. Crack the testa of a soaked croton seed and remove it. Peel off the thin, colourless inner membrane, carefully cut through the endosperm along the well-marked lateral ridges, and separate the two halves. Within the hollow find the embryo, consisting of a small radicle and two papery cotyledons, each with three clearly marked veins, and closely applied to the curved inner surface of the endosperm ; the plumule is not developed.

2. Cut a seed transversely and observe the arrangement of the parts. Test for reserve food. Make drawings to illustrate your dissections.

Strophanthus Seed. The seeds of *Strophanthus kombé*, Oliver, family Apocynaceæ.

1. Measure the length, breadth and thickness of several seeds, and record the greatest and least measurements, and also those of most frequent occurrence.

2. Note the grey-green to pale fawn colour, and the covering of silky appressed hairs, all directed towards the apex. The apex usually ends in an acuminate point, which shows evidence of having been abruptly broken off ; this is due to the removal of the large plumose awn. Find the light-coloured hilum near the apex and the raphe, extending for $\frac{1}{2}$ to $\frac{2}{3}$ down the face of the seed. Sketch the external features at a definite magnification.

3. Cut a transverse section of a seed, and sketch it to show the seed-coat, the narrow endosperm, the cotyledons, and the raphe.

4. Cut a longitudinal section of a seed at right angles to the wide faces, and sketch it to show the same details, as in (3) above. Towards which end of the seed does the radicle point ?

5. Soak a seed in hot water for about five minutes and remove the seed-coat ; boil the coat which chloral hydrate solution till clear, and examine it with the microscope for crystals of calcium oxalate. Note the presence of scattered cluster crystals and small single crystals. Only small numbers are present. Mount the testa inner side uppermost.

6. *Reaction for Strophanthin.* Take a dry strophanthus seed, cut a moderately thick section, place it on a slide, cover it with a drop of sulphuric acid (80 per cent. by volume), apply a cover-glass and observe the colour changes under a 16 mm. objective Note the deep green colour developed in the thin layer of endosperm just beneath the seed-coat, while the cotyledons may become more or less tinted green or red.

7. Remove the seed-coat from a soaked seed, embed it in pith, cut transverse sections parallel to the long axis and mount them in phloroglucin and hydrochloric acid. Note the band of lignified thickening encircling the base of the cell and the single lignified rib on the lower side of the limb of the trichome.

Linseed. The dried ripe seeds of *Linum usitatissimum* Linn.

1. Make a slit in the end of a dispensing cork and push a seed into it, so as to hold it firmly while being cut. Cut dry seeds transversely and longitudinally and examine the cut surface with a pocket lens. Note that the structure of linseed closely resembles that of strophanthus. Make sketches and write a description of linseed (see The Scheme of Description, p. 125).

2. Bruise some seeds in a mortar, place 1 g. in a test-tube and add 1 ml. of water. Cork and fix a piece of picric acid paper, moistened with solution of sodium carbonate, in the upper end of the tube ; allow to stand about 30 minutes and then warm in a water-bath. Note the brick-red colour of the paper, indicating the presence of hydrocyanic acid. (This test takes about 18 hours in the cold.)

3. Digest 1 g. of whole linseed in 20 ml. of boiling water for 15 minutes, cool, adjust the volume, strain through muslin. To 2 ml. of the liquid add 2 ml. of lead subacetate, note the abundant white precipitate. Test 4 ml. as directed under hydrolysis of starch (see p. 7). This test indicates the presence of a mucilage which is a polysaccharide derivative.

NOTES ON SCHEDULE XXII

Nux Vomica Seed. For cutting sections these seeds must be soaked for at least a week. In cutting the seed by an incision along the edge, it is well to cut a small piece from the edge of the seed on the side opposite the radicle, insert the point of a knife blade into the split in the endosperm, and work it round each way nearly as far as the radicle, and then tear the two portions apart with the fingers ; in this way one avoids damage to the embryo.

Castor Oil and Croton Seeds. Soak the seeds for eighteen to twenty-four hours before dissection. Note the general similarity in structure between the three seeds—nux vomica, castor oil and croton.

To examine the reserve foods in the endosperm of *castor oil seeds* proceed as follows :—

1. Cut thin sections of the endosperm of a castor oil seed and remove the oil by putting the sections into ether in a covered hollow glass block and allowing them to soak *for about fifteen to thirty minutes.* Mount

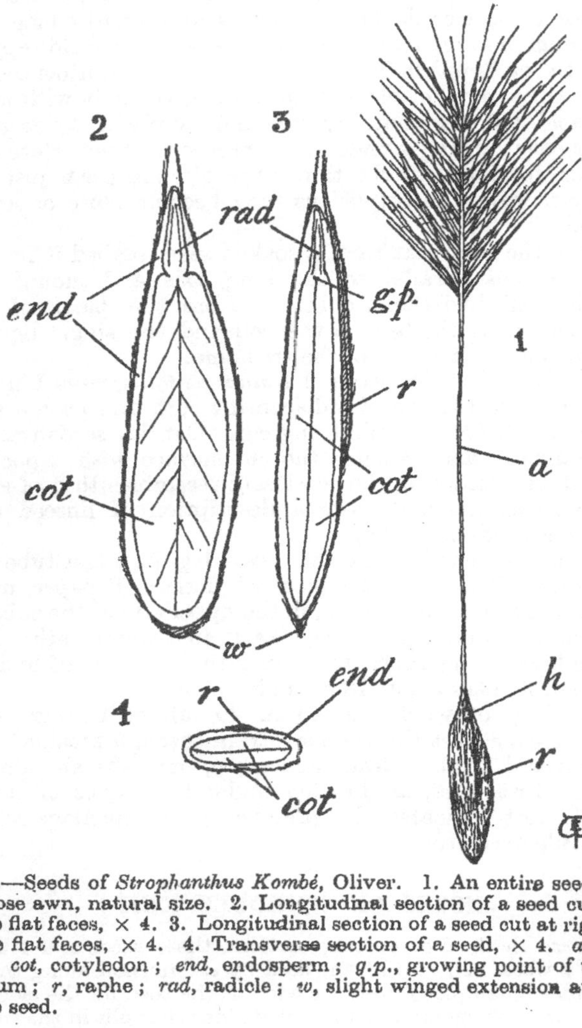

FIG. 34.—Seeds of *Strophanthus Kombé*, Oliver. 1. An entire seed with its plumose awn, natural size. 2. Longitudinal section of a seed cut parallel to the flat faces, × 4. 3. Longitudinal section of a seed cut at right angles to the flat faces, × 4. 4. Transverse section of a seed, × 4. *a*, plumose awn ; *cot*, cotyledon ; *end*, endosperm ; *g.p.*, growing point of the stem ; *h*, hilum ; *r*, raphe ; *rad*, radicle ; *w*, slight winged extension at the base of the seed.

a section in alcohol and examine with the microscope ; note the parenchymatous cells filled with ovoid aleurone grains.

2. Irrigate the preparation with iodine water and note the solution of part of the ground substance of the grains, which stain yellow, especially the well-formed crystalloids which with the colourless globoids now become evident. Sketch a few aleurone grains.

3. Irrigate the preparation with dilute caustic alkali, and note the solution of the whole substance of the grains except the globoids, which are dissolved in strong hydrochloric acid.

4. Mount another section (without treatment with ether) in tincture of alkanna. Note the staining of the fixed oil.

Strophanthus Seeds. The endosperm is a narrow layer beneath the seed-coat and completely surrounds the straight embryo, whose radicle is directed towards the awned end of the seed. The importance of establishing the paucity of crystals of calcium oxalate in the seed-coat depends upon the fact that a closely similar seed—that of *S. Courmonti* Sacleux—has numerous large single crystals in the subepidermal layer of the seed-coat. The green reaction for strophanthin distinguishes the official seed from several other varieties, which give a red coloration when submitted to the test.

SCHEDULE OF INSTRUCTIONS—XXIII

SEEDS; MUSTARD, HENBANE, ISPAGHULA, PSYLLIUM

All the seeds included in this schedule should be prepared for cutting sections by spreading some of the seeds in a single layer on a piece of paper; then smear the end of a dispensing cork with a thin layer of fish glue (such as "Seccotine"), and press the glued surface upon the seeds. Allow the cork and the adhering seeds to dry (this will take a few hours), and, when firmly fixed, the seeds may be cut in any desired direction with a razor.

White Mustard Seed. The seeds of *Brassica alba* Boiss, family Cruciferæ.

1. Determine the average diameter of the seeds, and sketch one at a magnification of about twenty diameters to show the external features.

2. Take a soaked seed, wipe it free from mucilage with a duster, and cut it all round just through the seed-coat; squeeze it gently and the coat will slip off. Make drawings of the embryo, as seen from the side and from the end, to show the radicle and the folded cotyledons.

3. Cut a seed transversely and sketch the cut surface.

Black Mustard Seeds. The seeds of *Brassica sinapioides* Roth., family Cruciferæ.

1. Fasten some seeds to each of two corks, as directed above. Cut a thin slice from the end of one of the corks and lay the slice, with its attached seeds, upon a microscope slide. Examine the seeds, illuminated from above, with a 16 mm. objective. Note the hexagonal reticulations on the surface formed by the boundary lines of the small pittings of the outer surface. Sketch the surface.

2. Take the second cork, and with a razor cut sections through several of the seeds and examine them with a lens. Look for transverse and longitudinal sections, and sketch one of each. Mark on the drawings the testa, the two-folded cotyledons, and the hypocotyl-radicle. Compare the structure with that of white mustard.

3. Weigh out 0·2 gm. of the seeds; count them and calculate the weight of 100 seeds.

Henbane Seed. The seeds of *Hyoscyamus niger* Linn., family Solanaceæ.

1. Determine the average size of the seeds, and count the number of reticulations lengthwise and across. Note the flattened shape, the

hilum on the edge, and the neighbouring slight projection over the radicle. Sketch a seed, and indicate clearly the shape and distribution of the reticulations.

2. Cut a longitudinal section parallel to the flat faces, and sketch it to show the curved embryo embedded in the endosperm. Mark the magnification against your drawings.

3. Test the endosperm for reserve food.

Ispaghula. The dried seeds of *Plantago ovata* Forskal, family Plantaginaceæ.

1. Measure the length and breadth of several seeds and determine the most usual dimensions.

2. Make a sketch of the flat face and a second sketch of the rounded surface. Key all important features.

3. Attach some seeds to a cork, as explained above, and cut them longitudinally to show the embryos embedded in the endosperm, as seen with a pocket lens or a low power of the microscope. Sketch the cut surfaces.

4. Cut some seeds transversely, and sketch the cut end. Mark on the drawing the endosperm, the cotyledons of the embryo, and the hilum.

5. Soak some seeds in water and record the effect produced. Mount two or three soaked seeds in water under a cover-glass and examine with a low-power objective. Sketch a soaked seed to the same scale as the dry seeds.

6. After removing all extraneous matter, weigh out 0·2 gm. of the seeds, and count them. Calculate the weight of 100 seeds.

Psyllium Seeds. The dried seeds of *Plantago Psyllium* Linn., family Plantaginaceæ.

1. Make the same experiments and observations with these seeds as with Ispaghula.

2. As a result of your observations, what do you consider to be the diagnostic characters of Ispaghula ?

NOTES ON SCHEDULE XXIII

White Mustard Seed. With the exception of the hilum, there are no very strongly marked external features ; but one can observe a very fine pitting upon the surface, and in the less ripe seeds the edges of the cotyledonary lobes make a set of parallel ridges and furrows, leading from the hilum, upon the opposite side of which can be dimly discerned the outline of the tip of the radicle. The embryo is folded, so as to bring the radicle against the back of one of the cotyledons, which lie face to face ; the cotyledons are also folded along their midribs, so as to partially surround the large hypocotyl radicle. The position of the radicle is described as " dorsal " and the cotyledons show " conduplicate " folding.

Black mustard seeds show the same general structure as the seeds of white mustard. They are distinguished from nearly related seeds of a somewhat similar colour, such as radish, rape, and charlock, by the well-marked, hexagonal areas seen upon the outer surface ; these areas are not present upon the epidermis of the other seeds. The weight of 100 seeds is also a good characteristic for distinguishing black mustard from other nearly related cruciferous seeds, see p. 222.

Ispaghula. The seeds are ovate in shape, and the radicle is always directed towards the broader end, where it produces a slight elevation upon the dorsal or rounded surface of the seed, extending from the extremity of the dark patch to the end of the seed. A longitudinal section shows that a perfectly straight embryo occupies almost the entire length of the seed, the remainder of the seed being filled by the endosperm. The radicle forms about one-third and the two cotyledons about two-thirds of the length of the embryo (see Fig. 35, *l.s.*). When soaked in water, the epidermis of the testa swells up enormously, so that each seed becomes surrounded by a halo-like expanse of colourless mucilage (see Fig. 35, *c.*).

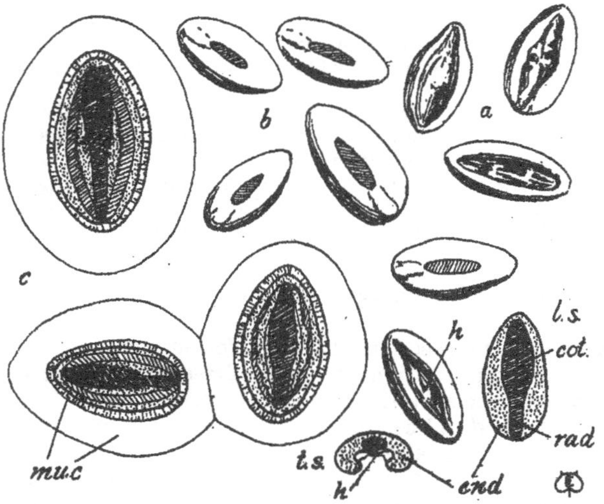

FIG. 35.—ISPAGHULA; the seeds of *Plantago ovata*; *b*, seeds showing the rounded surface with a central dark oval patch; *a*, seeds showing the flat surface with a deep groove containing the hilum, *h.*; *c*, seeds after soaking in water, showing the mucilaginous envelope, *muc.*; *l.s.*, longitudinal section of a seed; *t.s.*, transverse section; *cot.*, cotyledon; *end*, endosperm; *rad.*, radicle. All × 5.

Psyllium seeds are used on the Continent in considerable quantities in the same way as ispaghula is used in India. They are derived from a nearly related plant, and a comparison of the characters of the two seeds will enable the student to select those features of ispaghula and of psyllium which are of real diagnostic importance.

SCHEDULE OF INSTRUCTIONS—XXIV

SEEDS; STAVESACRE, FENUGREEK, STRAMONIUM, DATURA

Stavesacre Seed. The seeds of *Delphinium Staphisagria* Linn., family Ranunculaceæ.

1. Measure the length and breadth of several seeds; record the most common size and the amount of variation observed. Note that one end of the seed is more pointed; here the hilum is situated. Sketch the external appearance at a known magnification, *e.g.*, five diameters; mark the hilum and indicate the reticulations.

2. Cut a vertical section of the seed passing through the hilum, and sketch it to show the seed-coat, the embryo, and the endosperm.

3. Sketch a transverse section to show the irregularly four-sided shape of the seed.

4. Test the endosperm for reserve food. This is best done by cutting a section of the endosperm and mounting it in tincture of alkanna. One may also obtain an oily smear by rubbing the endosperm upon a piece of paper.

Fenugreek Seed. The seeds of *Trigonella Fœnum-grœum* Linn., family Leguminosæ.

1. Measure the dimensions of some seeds, and sketch a side view to show the rhomboidal outline, the hilum, and the groove separating the radicle pocket. Sketch also the edge to show the radicle pocket and the hilum.

2. Cut through the coat of a soaked seed equatorially, slip off the coat and remove the endosperm, noticing its colourless, translucent appearance; sketch the yellow embryo.

3. Cut a transverse section of a seed in a slightly slanting direction, so as to pass through the radicle and cotyledons; sketch it to show the testa, yellow cotyledons, translucent endosperm, radicle pocket and radicle. Make all drawings at a magnification of ten diameters.

Stramonium Seed. The ripe seeds of *Datura Stramonium* Linn., family Solanaceæ.

1. Measure a dry seed, as directed for stavesacre, and sketch a side view at a magnification of ten to fifteen diameters to show the reticulations, the hilum, and the general outline.

2. Cut a longitudinal section of a soaked seed parallel to the flat faces, and sketch it to show the endosperm and the curved embryo with its radicle and two cotyledons. By gentle pressure of the cut seed, the embryo may be easily removed entire, and the cotyledons and radicle are then more clearly discernible.

3. Make a longitudinal section at right angles to the flat faces, and sketch it to show the embryo cut in three places and embedded in the endosperm.

4. Determine the nature of the reserve food in the endosperm.

Datura Seeds. The dried seeds of *Datura Metel* Linn.

1. Measure the width, length and thickness of several seeds and note their average dimensions. What is their colour?

2. Sketch a seed carefully to show the general outline, the position of the hilum, the depressed lateral area, and the ridge along the curved margin. What peculiarities does the ridge show?

3. Sketch the appearance of the curved margin as seen when looking at the edge of the seed.

4. Cut a section through a soaked seed parallel to its flat faces and sketch it to show the testa, the embryo, and the endosperm. Determine the nature of the reserve food.

5. Cut a section of a soaked seed at right angles to the flat surfaces and parallel to the straight edge. Sketch it and key all its parts.

NOTES ON SCHEDULE XXIV

All the seeds in this schedule should be soaked in cold water for eighteen hours before dissection.

Stavesacre seed shows all the characters typical of ranunculaceous seeds in general—viz., the presence of a very small embryo near the hilar end, embedded in a copious oily endosperm.

Fenugreek or *Fœnugreek Seed.* To make an incision into the seed-coat "equatorially," cut it at right angles to the broad faces round the longest axis of the seed. If grasped between the finger and thumb, the two

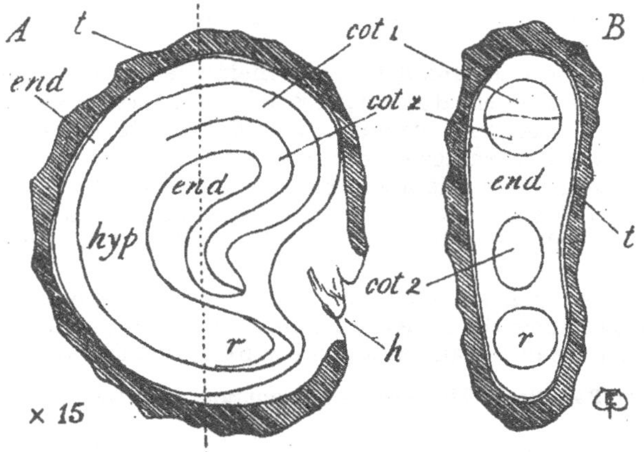

FIG. 36.—Seed of *Datura Stramonium* Linn. A. Longitudinal section parallel to the flat faces. B. Longitudinal section at right angles to the flat faces, along the dotted line marked on A. *cot* 1 and *cot* 2, the two cotyledons; *end*, endosperm; *h*, hilum; *hyp*. hypocotyl; *r*, primary root; *t*, testa. Both × 15.

halves of the seed-coat will now slip off easily without disturbing any of the interior structures.

Stramonium and *Datura seeds* show a structure similar to those of *Capsicum minimum* (See Schedule XX., p. 52).

SCHEDULE OF INSTRUCTIONS—XXV

SEEDS: COLCHICUM, CARDAMOMS, GRAINS OF PARADISE, NUTMEG

Colchicum Seeds. The dried ripe seeds of *Colchicum autumnale* L., family Liliaceæ, the autumn crocus or meadow saffron.

1. Examine some seeds externally, note and record their colour, shape, markings, etc. Find the projection on one side—what is it? Sketch a seed and key your drawing. Measure the diameter of several seeds and record the maximum, minimum and most frequently occurring dimensions.
2. Weigh out 0·5 gm. of the seeds, count the number weighed, and calculate the weight of 100 seeds.
3. Cut a median section of a soaked seed and examine the exposed surface with a pocket lens. Make a keyed sketch of your preparation to illustrate the internal structure. How is the embryo situated in relation to the hilum?
4. Test for reserve foods.
5. Write a technical description of the seeds.

Cardamom Seeds. The dried, nearly ripe seeds of *Elettaria Cardamomum* var. *minuscula*, family Zingiberaceæ.

1. Examine a fruit and note the scar at the upper end, marking the point of attachment of the flower parts ; the capsule is therefore inferior. Note also the three loculi and numerous seeds attached to an axile placenta.
2. Remove the seeds and determine their average dimensions ; find the funicle and the delicate colourless aril, best seen in soaked seeds.
3. Sketch a seed at a definite magnification to show its angular shape, the raphe, markings on the testa, the funicle, etc.
4. Cut a seed longitudinally along the line of the raphe, sketch the cut surface and mark the testa, oil layer, white perisperm, yellowish endosperm, embryo, hilum and raphe. Test the perisperm for reserve food.
5. Cut a seed transversely near the broader distal end and sketch the cut surface to show the structures named in the longitudinal section.
6. Record the odour and taste and write a technical description.

Grains of Paradise. The seeds of *Amomum Melegueta* Roscoe, family Zingiberaceæ.

1. After measuring some seeds, make a sketch at a definite magnification to show the angular shape, the papillose surface, and the fibrous remains of the funicle.
2. Dissect some soaked seeds as directed for Cardamoms.

Nutmeg. The dried kernel of the seed of *Myristica fragrans* Houtt., family Myristicaceæ.

1. Sketch a nutmeg to show the external characters, including the wrinkled, greyish perisperm, the groove along the line of the raphe, the micropyle and the chalaza.
2. Cut a seed longitudinally in the median plane and sketch the cut surface. Mark the radicle, cotyledons, ruminations of the perisperm and the whitish endosperm.
3. Put the two halves together, cut them transversely and make an annotated sketch of the cut surface.
4. Test the seeds for fat and starch.

NOTES ON SCHEDULE XXV

All these seeds should be soaked in cold water for four or five days before dissection.

Colchicum Seeds. The projection on one side of the seed is due to a local growth of tissue surrounding the funiculus and the neighbouring part of the seed. This type of growth is known as a strophiole ; a caruncle is found upon the castor oil seed. In cutting the seed, look for the strophiole or the mark left where it has broken away, and make the edge of the scalpel coincide with the long axis of the strophiole when commencing to make the section. The minute embryo has its axis lying in a radial direction, and is usually found at the periphery of the seed or sometimes directly opposite to the strophiole. The endosperm is composed of pitted, thick-walled cells composed of cellulose and containing oil and aleurone. The strophiole contains starch. These reserve foods may be identified by cutting sections and mounting one in iodine water and a second section in tincture of alkanna.

Nutmeg is the kernel of the seed, hence the testa or seed-coat is absent. The raphe and other structures in the testa are therefore not to be seen, but marks corresponding to them are impressed upon the surface of the kernel. The perisperm is infolded to form the brown ruminations and contains the volatile oil. In the cells of the endosperm there are abundant starch grains and crystals of solid fat.

SCHEDULE OF INSTRUCTIONS—XXVI

HERBS, CRYPTOGAMIC

Bladder Wrack. The entire plant, *Fucus vesiculosus* Linn., collected from the rocks and dried.

1. Make a habit sketch to show the hold-fast or attachment disc (if present), the midrib, wings, air vesicles (pneumatocysts), growing point, method of branching and the fertile tips or receptacles. Note upon the receptacles the numerous fine pores or ostioles, opening into the conceptacles.

2. Compare the fresh plant with the commercial drug, both dry and after soaking in water. Compare it also with specimens of *Fucus serratus* and of *Ascophyllum* (formerly *Fucus*) *nodosum.*

3. Write a description of the drug.

Irish Moss or **Carrageen.** The bleached alga *Chondrus crispus* Stackh., family Gigartinaceæ.

1. Soak some Irish moss in cold water for about ten minutes until it has completely softened. Spread out some of the drug, and select pieces having linear branches, others with broadly wedge-shaped branches, and a third type with a wide thallus having narrow terminal ramuli (branchlets). Sketch a typical piece of each, and note the regular dichotomous branching.

2. Search the drug for a piece showing small oval swellings, nearly as wide as the narrower ramuli and appearing dark by transmitted light. These are the fructifications (cystocarps). Sometimes small oval holes are found, being the places from which the cystocarps have fallen. Sketch a piece showing holes or cystocarps.

3. If one can be found, remove a ramulus with a cystocarp, soften it in water, embed it between two pieces of pith, and cut a transverse section : mount it in chloral hydrate solution, and observe the spores with a 16 mm. objective.

4. Cut a transverse section of a piece of softened carrageen, mount it in water and sketch the cellular tissue. Test the section with iodine water and sulphuric acid (80 per cent. by volume) ; does it react for cellulose ?

Ergot. The sclerotium of the fungus, *Claviceps purpurea* Tulasne, family Hypocreaceæ, developed in the ovary of the rye, *Secale cereale.*

1. Determine the dimensions of several ergots and note the colour, shape and fracture. Sketch one or two ergots to show the fusiform, arcuate shape and the longitudinal furrows.

2. Cut a softened ergot transversely and note the somewhat triangular or quadrilateral shape of the section. Sketch the exposed surface to show the coloured outer layer, the deep fissures, the whitish interior and the darker lines radiating irregularly from the centre.

NOTES ON SCHEDULE XXVI

Bladder Wrack. These seaweeds belong to the Phæophyceæ or Brown Algæ. *Fucus serratus* is devoid of vesicles and the thallus has a serrated margin. *Ascophyllum nodosum* bears vesicles singly.

Irish Moss. This is an alga belonging to the Rhodophyceæ or Red Algæ. This group of algæ is characterised, amongst other details by the presence of special reproductive organs. The female structure is termed a carpogonium, and, in the case of *Chondrus crispus,* this is embedded in the thallus. After fertilisation there is formed a fructification, termed a cystocarp, which contains spores called carpospores. These cystocarps are also embedded in the thallus, and are the ovoid bodies found upon certain pieces of the drug.

Ergot. Soften ergots by exposure to a moist atmosphere for about eighteen hours.

SCHEDULE OF INSTRUCTIONS—XXVII

HERBS: SAVIN, INDIAN HEMP, HOPS

Savin Tops. The young shoots of *Juniperus Sabina* L., family Pinaceæ.

1. Note the rounded quadrangular shape of the twigs. Sketch a piece of a twig at a magnification of ten to fifteen diameters, to show the closely appressed, rhomboidal leaves in opposite and decussate pairs. Find and sketch other twigs where the leaves run out into lanceolate points, and note that the leaves on these twigs sometimes occur in alternate whorls of three. In the centre of the back of each leaf find an oval depression, marking the position of the large oil-gland in the mesophyll.

2. Soak a piece of twig in water, and embed it in pith, as directed for umbelliferous fruits (see Schedule XVIII., p. 46), but without making a depression in the pith. Cut a transverse section, and mount it in phloroglucin and strong hydrochloric acid. Sketch the preparation diagrammatically to show the distribution of the tissues. Are there any stone-cells in the mesophyll ?

3. Remove a single leaf from a twig, place it outside uppermost upon a slide, and boil it in chloral hydrate solution until clear. Determine the distribution of the stomata upon the curved outer surface of the leaf. How are the stomatal openings orientated with respect to the leaf axis ?

4. Compare twigs of *Juniperus phœnicea,* French savin, with the genuine drug, noting especially the phyllotaxis and the stone cells in the mesophyll.

Indian Hemp. The dried flowering or fruiting tops of the pistillate plant of *Cannabis sativa* Linn., family Urticaceæ.

1. Take a piece of Indian hemp, which has been deprived of resin by maceration in alcohol, and soak it in cold water in a flat-bottomed porcelain dish. Dissect the drug with needles and scalpel beneath the surface of water. On the lower part of the stem search for small, palmately-compound foliage leaves ; these are rarely present, but, if found, sketch one.

2. Examine the inflorescence and notice that it is composed of bracts of various kinds and flowers in all stages of development, including the ripe fruit. Remove a bract and its two bracteoles by cutting through the floral axis above and below its point of attachment.

Sketch the bract and bracteoles and note the two red stigmas projecting from each bracteole.

3. Separate the two bracteoles from the bract and examine the bract; at its base find the narrow stipules. Sketch a bract with its stipules.

4. Take one of the bracteoles, open it, remove the enclosed flower and reserve the bracteole. Boil the flower with chloral hydrate solution until cleared. Examine the preparation under a 16 mm. objective and find the ovary enclosed in a delicate perigone (perianth); note also the stigmas and ovule and the absence of stamens. Sketch a flower to show these details.

5. Boil the separated bracteole with chloral hydrate solution; examine it with the microscope and find the numerous glandular and protective hairs. Sketch a few of the hairs. Examine also the trichomes on the bracts. Look for crystals of calcium oxalate and note that the cystoliths effervesce with acid.

6. From a mature fruit remove the seed, dissect out the embryo and sketch it. Is there any endosperm? Cut other fruits transversely and longitudinally and sketch the cut surfaces.

Hops. The dried strobiles of *Humulus Lupulus* Linn., family Urticaceæ.

1. Sketch a complete strobile, then pull one to pieces and note the zigzag axis and scales of two kinds—some with the edge folded over (bracts), and others plain (stipules); how many of each kind of leaf do you find? Observe the yellow glistening glands (lupulin) upon the folded edges of the bracts. Sketch the axis, a bract, and a stipule.

2. Remove a fruit from one of the folds, and note that it is covered by the membranous perianth (the perigone), upon which numerous yellow glands are situated.

3. Remove the perianth, cut the achenial fruit longitudinally and transversely. Note the colour of the pericarp. Make drawings of the achene with its perianth.

NOTES ON SCHEDULE XXVII

Savin Tops. The rounded quadrangular shape of the twigs distinguishes the genuine drug from those plants, like *Cupressus* (the cypress) and *Thuja* (the arbor-vitæ), which have flattened branches. The absence of stone-cells in the mesophyll distinguishes it from *Juniperus phœnicea*, where they are present (see Fig. 37, A, B and C). To mount sections in phloroglucin and strong hydrochloric acid, cover the section with a few drops of a 1 per cent. solution of phloroglucin in alcohol, and allow it to become nearly dry; then add a drop or two of strong hydrochloric acid (sp. gr. 1·16), and apply a cover-glass. All lignified structures, including stone-cells, will be coloured red. The distribution of the stomata upon the dorsal surface distinguishes it from *Juniperus virginiana*, where the stomata form a transverse band below the level of the oil-gland (see Fig. 38, E and F).

Indian Hemp. In preparing the material for dissection, macerate some pieces of the drug in alcohol for twenty-four or forty-eight hours, pour off the alcohol, and repeat the maceration twice with fresh alcohol. The dish used for the dissection may be any convenient dish, and a small enamelled-iron pie dish answers very well. By dissection under water one is able to see much more clearly what one is doing, and the parts can be separated and removed without damage. *Cannabis sativa* has an in-

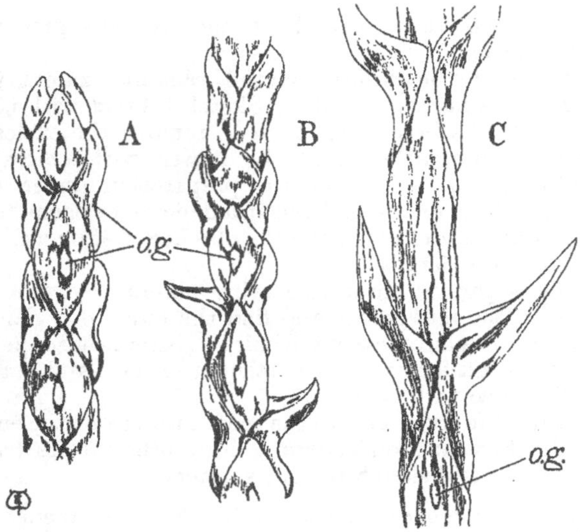

FIG. 37.—Savin Tops. A. Young twig with appressed scale leaves in opposite pairs. B. A twig similar to A, but showing some leaves with the apices standing out from the stem. C. A twig with elongated leaves, having spreading lanceolate points. *o.g.*, Oil-gland. All × 10.

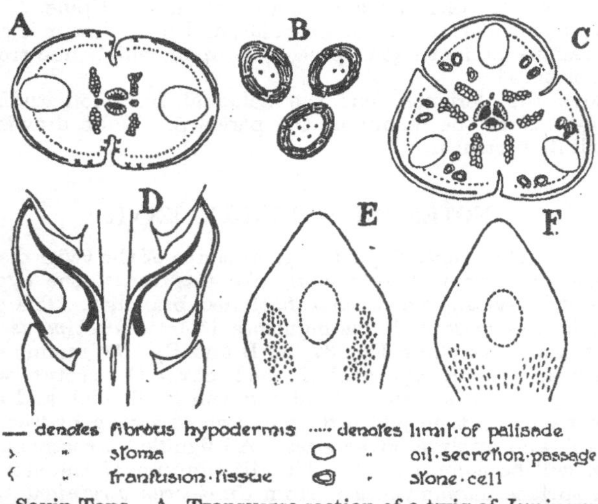

FIG. 38.—Savin Tops. A. Transverse section of a twig of *Juniperus Sabina*, showing a section of two opposite leaves; note the absence of stone-cells. B. Stone-cells, isolated from the mesophyll of *Juniperus phœnicea*. C. Transverse section of a twig of *Juniperus phœnicea*, showing sections of three leaves forming a whorl; note the large stone-cells in the mesophyll. D. Longitudinal section of a twig of *Juniperus Sabina*, showing the positions of the oil-gland and of the fibro-vascular strand. E. Outer surface of a scale leaf of *Juniperus Sabina*, showing the distribution of the stomata (rep. by short dashes). F. Outer surface of a scale leaf of *Juniperus virginiana*, showing the distribution of the stomata. All, except F, after A. J. Scholz.

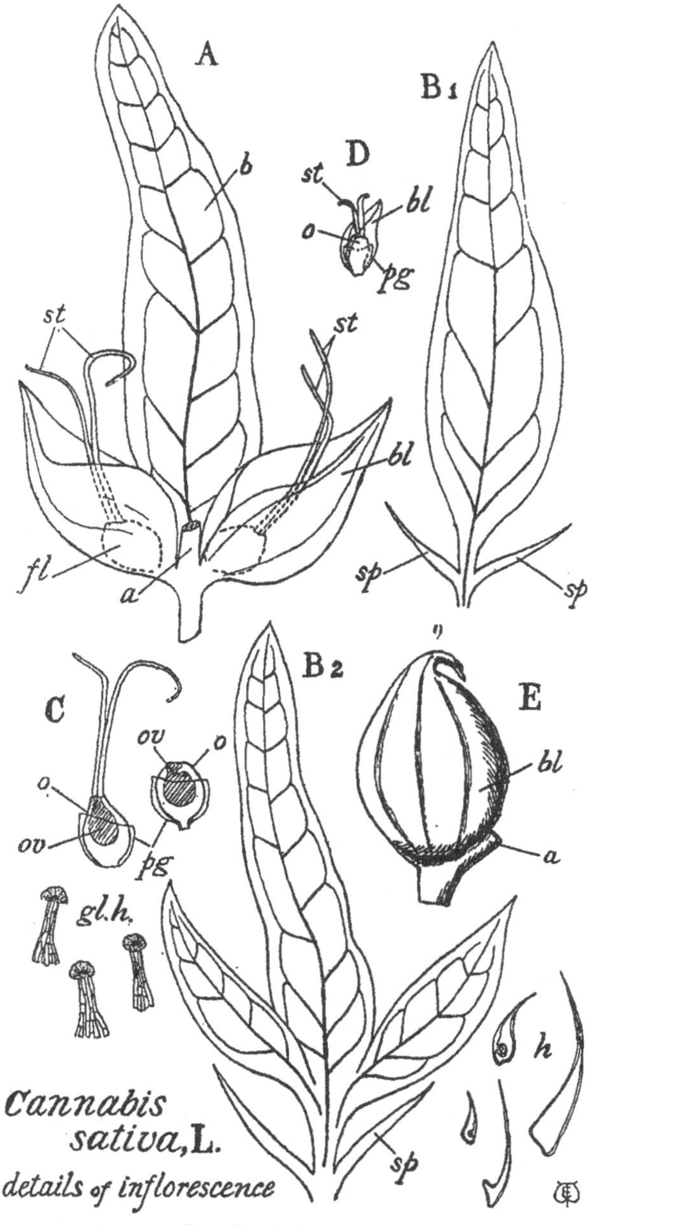

FIG. 39.—Indian Hemp. Details of the inflorescence. A. A bract with its accompanying pair of bracteoles, each having a flower in its axil. B1. A simple lanceolate bract, showing the stipules. B2. A ternate bract. C. Two pistillate flowers, one with the styles attached and the other without them. D. A much younger flower with its bracteole. *a*, axis of the inflorescence; *b*, bract; *bl*, bracteole; *fl*, flower; *o*, ovary; *ov*, ovule; *pg*, perigone; *sp*, stipule; *st*, style and stigma. All × 5. *gl.h.*, glandular hair; and *h*, protective hair; both × 50. E. Full-grown fruit surrounded by its bracteole.

florescence, the main axis of which carries bracts having a simple (Fig. 39, B1) or compound (Fig. 39, B2) leaf blade, the segments being lanceolate. Each bract has two linear stipules (see Fig. 39, B1 and B2, *sp.*). In the axil of each of these bracts is a branch which bears a pair of bracteoles (see Fig. 39, A), in the axil of each of which is a single pistillate flower, consisting of a delicate perigone (the perianth) enveloping the lower two-thirds of an ovary with two stigmas and a single ovule. The achenial fruit contains a single seed having a well-developed embryo, with thick cotyledons and a radicle, which is bent over against the back of one of the cotyledons (incumbent), and there is a small amount of endosperm surrounding the radicle.

Hops. The strobile is the pistillate inflorescence, and the zigzag axis bears a number of pairs of stipules, which are the stipules of bracts, whose blade is suppressed. The axis normally arising in the axil of the bract is also suppressed, but on either side there is a very short branch carrying two bracteoles, each of which subtends a pistillate flower, consisting of a perigone (the perianth) and an ovary. Each stipule, therefore, appears to carry in its axil two bracteoles and two flowers. After fertilisation, the bracteoles rapidly increase in size, becoming ultimately larger than the stipules. These bracteoles are referred to in the schedule of instructions as bracts. From this description it is evident that there should be twice as many bracteoles (bracts with incurved edges) as there are stipules.

SCHEDULE OF INSTRUCTIONS—XXVIII

HERBS: BROOM TOPS, EUPHORBIA PILULIFERA LOBELIA

Brroom Tops. The fresh and the dried tops of *Cytisus scoparius* Link family Leguminosæ.

1. Sketch a small piece of a green twig to show the five longitudinal ridges and the reduced leaves. What is the shape of the leaves? Do the leaves on different parts of the stem vary in form? What is the phyllotaxis?

2. Cut a twig transversely and measure its diameter. Make a sketch of the transverse section at a known magnification, as seen with a pocket lens, and mark the pith, wood, phloem, cortex, ridges with sclerenchyma, and furrows with green assimilating tissue.

Euphorbia Herb (Euphorbia pilulifera). The entire plant, dried, of *Euphorbia hirta* Linn., family Euphorbiaceæ.

1. Soften some of the drug by steaming it. Cut through the stem just above and below a node having a complete leaf attached to it; with a camel-hair pencil spread out the leaf in water and sketch it to show its characteristics, especially the unequal base and the serrated margin.

2. Hold a leaf to the light and note the pellucid areas. Examine the nature and distribution of the hairs, and observe the fine corrugations upon the surface of the leaves; make notes of your findings.

3. Boil a piece of leaf in chloral hydrate solution. Sketch a piece, as seen with the 16 mm. objective, to show the distribution and ultimate branches of the veinlets; note the sheath of special cells surrounding the veinlets and giving them additional thickness.

4. Upon the upper internodes note the long, yellowish, spreading hairs and the pubescence of short, curved hairs. Mount a piece of stem in chloral hydrate solution, and sketch one hair of each kind.

5. From a piece of the dry drug, pick out one of the tricarpellary fruits and sketch it. Remove the seeds by gently pressing the dry fruit between

the points of a pair of forceps; place them uncovered on a slide, and illuminate them from above. Note that the seeds are oblong, reddish-brown in colour, four-sided, with sharp angles and transverse wrinkles upon the flat faces.

Lobelia Herb. The dried flowering herb of *Lobelia inflata* Linn., family Campanulaceæ.

1. Observe and record the colour, shape and surface condition of the stem. Determine the phyllotaxis.
2. Examine the leaves and note especially the surface condition and the margin. Sketch a leaf.
3. Clear a small piece of leaf by boiling in solution of chloral hydrate, as directed under Senna leaf, Schedule XIII., p. 34. Sketch some of the trichomes.
4. Examine the softened fruits; are they superior or inferior? Cut one by a transverse section; how many loculi do you find? How does the fruit dehisce, and what is the placentation? Make a sketch of the whole fruit and of the transverse section.
5. Shake out a few seeds from a fruit on to a slide and examine them in the dry condition by reflected light. Sketch a seed and describe its most striking features.

NOTES ON SCHEDULE XXVIII

Broom Tops. For these dissections it is best to use fresh tops, gathered towards the end of June. Notice that the lower leaves are stalked and ternate, while the uppermost ones are simple and sessile. The leaves are always attached in the line of the grooves, and the phyllotaxis shows, therefore, five orthostichies and the two-fifths arrangement.

Euphorbia Herb. The drug may be conveniently softened by placing it in an enamelled-iron dish lined with wet blotting-paper; cover the dish with a plate, and stand it in a warm place. The curving of the smallest veinlets is very characteristic, and the accompanying sheath of parenchyma (a single enveloping layer of large rectangular cells) so greatly increases their thickness that, when the leaf dries, minute wrinkles or rugæ, corresponding in shape to the curves of the veinlets, appear upon the surface of the leaf. The pellucid dots, seen on holding the leaf to the light, are the more transparent parts of the laminæ between the veinlets. It is evident, therefore, that both the rugæ and the pellucid dots are due to the disposition of the veinlets and their accompanying sheaths. The leaves carry hairs of two types, similar to those upon the stem. The longer hairs are found chiefly near the midrib on the under surface. The wrinkles upon the seeds disappear after soaking in water, so that they should be examined dry.

Lobelia. Soften some lobelia in the same way as described for euphorbia. The capsules are bilocular and dehisce by two apical pores. The seeds are narrowly oval in outline, very small in size, and have a testa with longitudinally elongated polygonal reticulations.

To find the phyllotaxis mark any leaf by putting a pin into the stem at its base; similarly, mark a leaf vertically over this one, *i.e.*, on the same orthostichy. Count the number of leaves between the pins, calling the lower pin O and finishing with the upper pin; record the number as the denominator of a fraction. Determine the number of times the genetic spiral passes round the stem in travelling from one pin to the other through

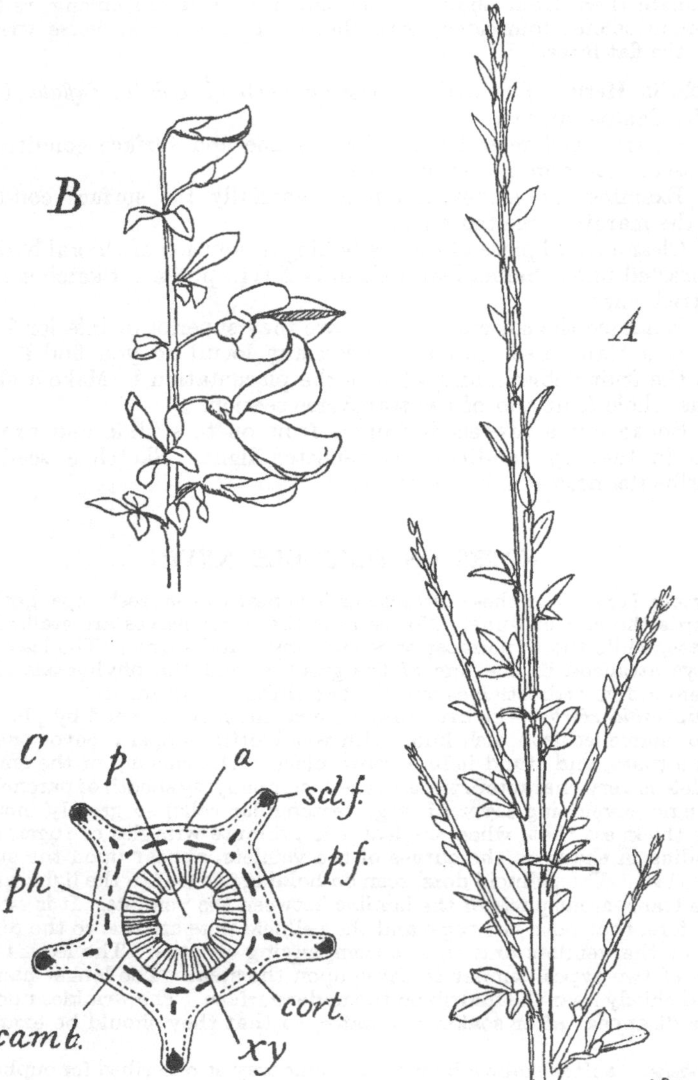

Fig. 40.—*Cytisus scoparius* Link. Broom tops. A. Young twig, showing simple sessile leaves on the upper part and compound ternate leaves on the lower part. B. Small flowering shoot. C. Diagrammatic drawing of a transverse section of a twig about one year old, × 15. *a*, assimilating tissue; *camb.*, cambium; *cort.*, cortex; *p.*, pith; *p.f.*, pericyclic fibres; *ph*, phloem; *scl.f.*, sclerenchymatous fibres; *xy*, xylem.

the leaf bases ; record this number as the numerator of the fraction. For lobelia this faction is one-third.

SCHEDULE OF INSTRUCTIONS—XXIX

HERBS, BELLADONNA, STRAMONIUM, HENBANE

Belladonna Leaves. The dried leaves and tops of *Atropa Belladonna* Linn., family Solanaceæ, collected when the plant is in flower.

1. Make a drawing of a leaf to illustrate the shape, margin, venation, petiole, etc.

2. Note the colour, texture and surface condition, and write out a brief statement of the important characters.

3. Break a leaf transversely and examine the fractured surface with a lens and find the evident white points. Cut out a piece of the

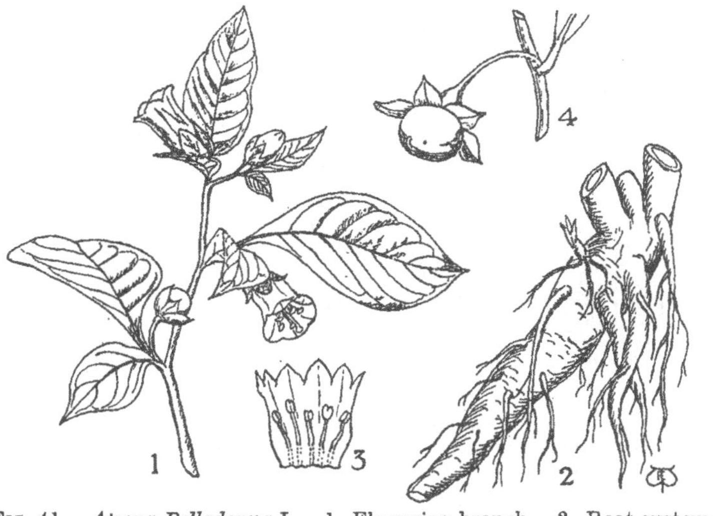

FIG. 41.—*Atropa Belladonna* L. 1. Flowering branch. 2. Root system. 3. Corolla laid open. 4. Fruit.

lamina including some of the points ; clear it by boiling with chloral hydrate solution as directed for senna leaves, and examine it microscopically to determine the nature of the whitish specks.

Make a diagrammatic sketch as seen under the 16 mm. lens to show the distribution of the veinlets and crystals. Then, using the 4 mm. lens, make a careful drawing of a few individual crystals and of the epidermis, with its characteristic glandular and protective hairs.

4. Compare with belladonna leaves the leaves of the poke-weed (*Phytolacca decandra* Linn.) and the leaflets of the Tree of Heaven (*Ailanthus glandulosa* Desf.). Sketch a specimen of each to show the differences in outline, venation, etc., making all drawings to the same scale. Make notes of the differences observed.

5. Make microscopical preparations of *Phytolacca* and of *Ailanthus* leaves similar to that for belladonna; see (3) above. Sketch any crystals present.

6. From a sample of belladonna leaf pick out some flowers and fruits; soften them by exposure to a moist atmosphere and dissect them. Make sketches to show the following details: flowers solitary, stalked, drooping, about 2 cm. long, with a livid purple, campanulate corolla and having the floral formula K (5) [C (5), A5 anthers free], G (2) obliquely placed, 2 loculi, ∞ ovules, axile placentation. Fruit

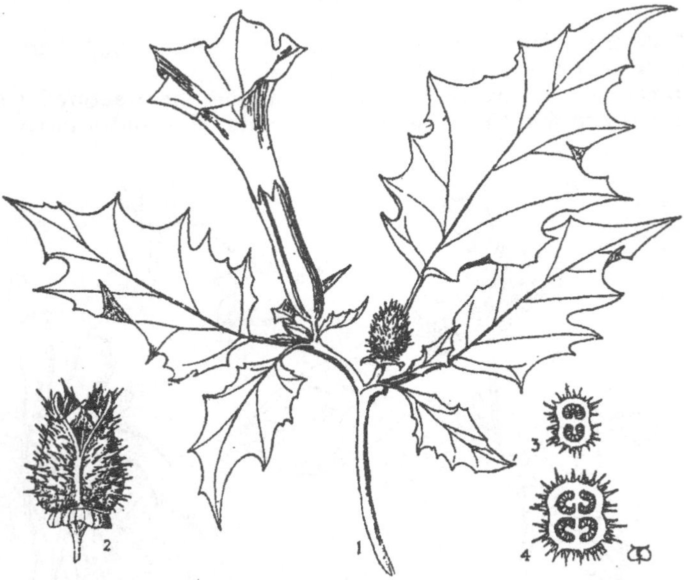

FIG. 42.—*Datura Stramonium* L. 1. A flowering branch. 2. A mature fruit. 3. Transverse section of the upper part of an unripe fruit. 4. Transverse section of the lower part of an unripe fruit.

a 2-celled berry, green when young, violet-black and about the size of a cherry when ripe.

7. Look for seeds, examine and describe them; note that they closely resemble henbane seeds (see above, p. 59).

Stramonium Leaves, the leaves and tops of *Datura Stramonium* Linn.
Henbane Leaves, the leaves and tops of *Hyoscyamus niger* Linn.

1. Make outline drawings of stramonium and henbane leaves and note the colour, texture and surface condition as directed for belladonna leaf, under (1) and (2).

2. Cut small squares from each of the leaves and prepare them as directed for senna leaves. Make for each a diagrammatic sketch showing the distribution of the veinlets and crystals, and make detailed drawings of individual crystals and of the epidermis and hairs as directed under belladonna leaf.

3. Compare stramonium leaves with those of *Xanthium strumarium*,

which are rhomboid-ovate, have small irregular teeth in the apical half and a nearly entire margin in the basal half. Note the grey-green colour, the harsh surface and the absence of calcium oxalate. Sketch a leaf.

Compare henbane leaves with those of the dandelion, *Taraxacum officinale*, see Fig. 58, p. 99. Sketch a leaf.

4. From both drugs remove flowers and fruits; soften and sketch them. Note the following details :—

Stramonium ; flowers solitary, about 7·5 cm. long, with a white plicated, funnel-shaped corolla (brownish in the dried drug); ovary

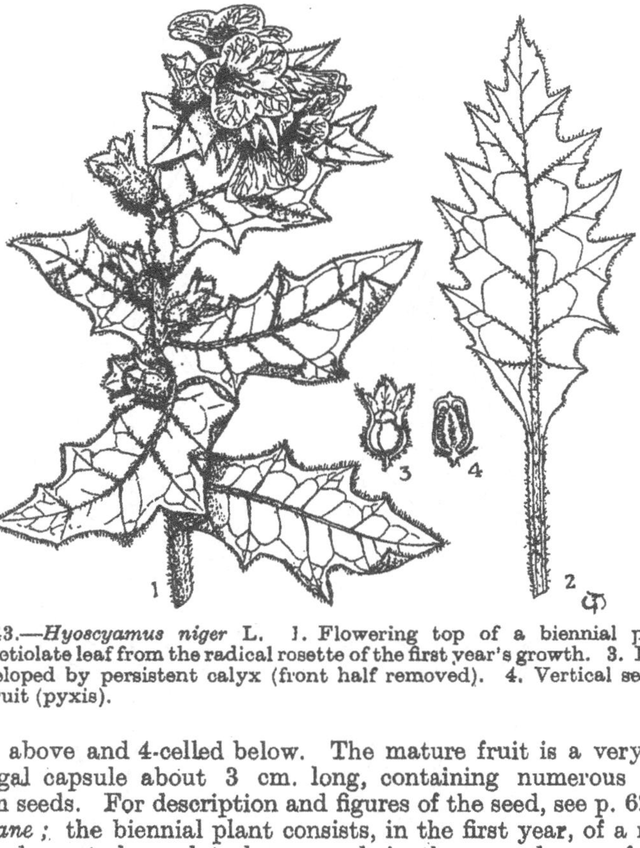

Fig. 43.—*Hyoscyamus niger* L. 1. Flowering top of a biennial plant. 2. Petiolate leaf from the radical rosette of the first year's growth. 3. Pyxis enveloped by persistent calyx (front half removed). 4. Vertical section of fruit (pyxis).

2-celled above and 4-celled below. The mature fruit is a very spiny septifragal capsule about 3 cm. long, containing numerous black, reniform seeds. For description and figures of the seed, see p. 62.

Henbane ; the biennial plant consists, in the first year, of a rosette of stalked, ovate-lanceolate leaves and, in the second year, forms a bushy plant having sessile, ovate, downy and glandular leaves with sinuate-dentate margins and a wide midrib. Flowers funnel-shaped, about 2.5 cm. in length and in diameter, corolla yellow with purple veins and five unequal lobes. Fruit a pyxis surrounded by the enlarged, persistent calyx, and containing numerous small, brown, reniform seeds. For details of the seeds, see p. 59.

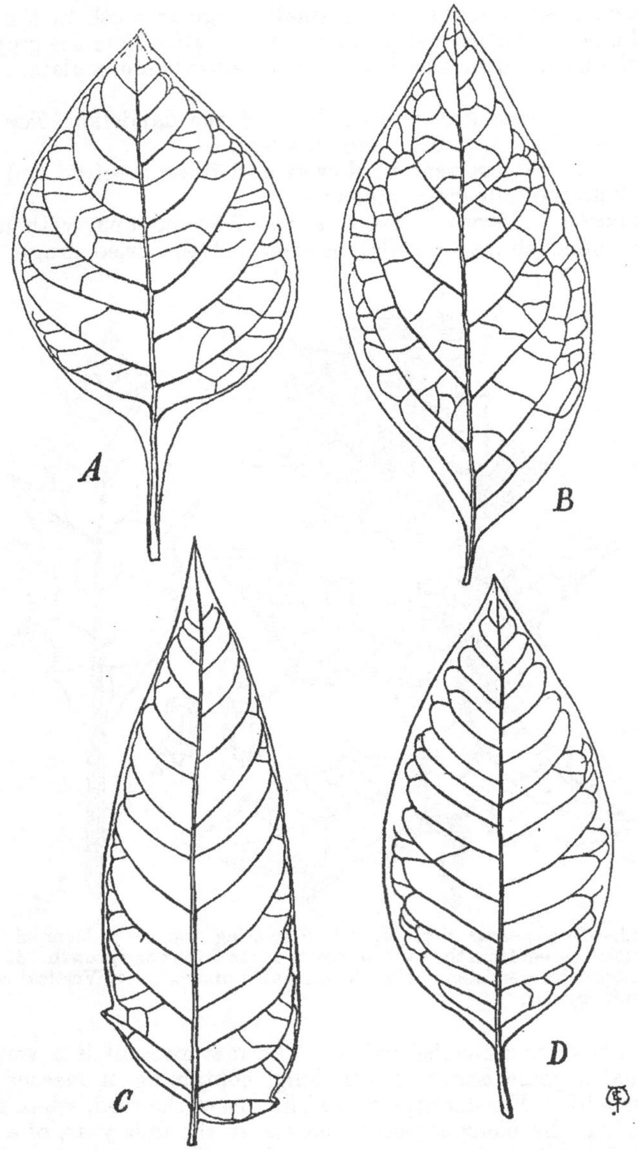

FIG. 44.—*A*. Leaf of *Atropa Belladonna* Linn. *B*. Leaf of *Scopolia carniolica* Jacq. *C*. Leaflet of *Ailanthus glandulosa* Desf. *D*. Leaf of *Phytolacca decandra* Linn. All × ½.

Capsule of Henbane. 1. Sketch a fruit and mark the persistent calyx, the membranous pericarp of the capsule, the line of dehiscence, the remains of the stigma, etc.

2. Is the fruit superior or inferior ? How many carpels are there and what is the dehiscence ?

3. Sketch a dehisced capsule as seen from above and mark the placentæ, septum and seeds.

NOTES ON SCHEDULE XXIX

Belladonna Leaves. The best characters of belladonna leaves are the thin texture, the almost glabrous surface, the entire margin, the broadly ovate shape, and the slightly decurrent lamina. The whitish points due to the cells filled with micro-crystals of calcium oxalate is a less useful

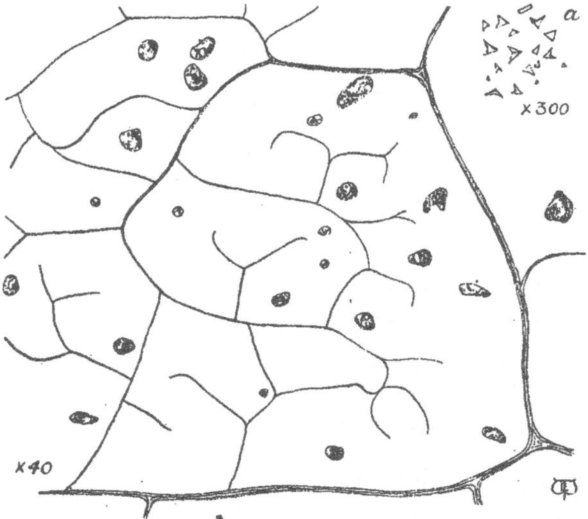

FIG. 45.—Diagram of a small piece of a leaf of *Atropa Belladonna* Linn., as seen in surface view, after clearing with chloral hydrate solution, × 40. The irregularly rounded dark areas marked by small dots are the groups of micro-crystals, often referred to as sandy crystals, of calcium oxalate. *a.* A few of the micro-crystals drawn in detail to show their form, which is most commonly sphenoidal, × 300.

character because they are not always easily found, and other minute white patches due to lichen or mould are easily mistaken for them. The curvature of the side veins, and the wide angle they make with the narrow midrib are important features, particularly for distinguishing belladonna from other solanaceous leaves. *Scopolia* leaves are ovate-lanceolate and more translucent than belladonna, and the side veins form a more acute angle with the midrib than in belladonna (see Fig. 44 (B)). *Phytolacca* leaves are more dense than belladonna ; they have a straight, strongly developed midrib (see Fig. 44 (D)), and certain cells of the mesophyll contain bundles of needle-shaped crystals (acicular raphides) of calcium oxalate. *Ailanthus* leaflets are triangular ovate (see Fig. 44 (C)) and are covered with a marked pubescence of white hairs upon both surfaces. They contain cluster crystals of calcium oxalate near the veins. The teeth near the base of the leaflets bear conspicuous glands on the under side.

The venation of belladonna leaf is more open than that of stramonium or henbane leaf and the sandy crystals appear as sparsely scattered dark or nearly black patches in the interneural mesophyll. The individual crystals separated from the sandy groups are generally triangular in shape and are frequently described as sphenoidal micro-crystals. These details are shown in Fig. 45.

Stramonium leaves show a normal reticulation of the veins, which very rarely have crystals associated with them. The crystals are found

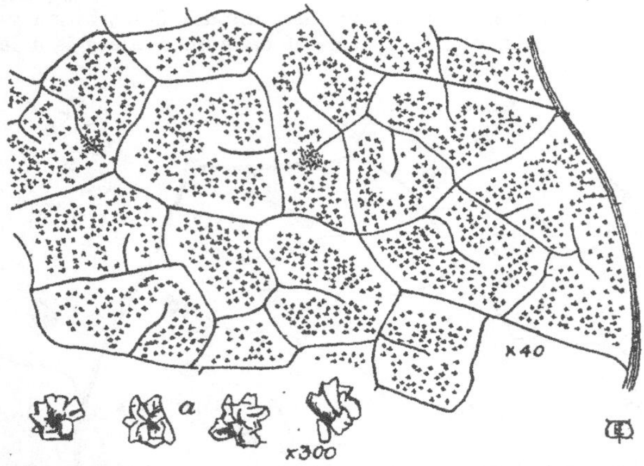

FIG. 46.—Diagram of a porton of a leaf of *Datura Stramonium* Linn., seen in surface view, after clearing with chloral hydrate solution, × 40. The crosses represent cluster crystals, and the small dots occasional groups of micro-crystals. *a*. Four cluster crystals drawn in detail, × 300.

scattered thickly throughout the interneural mesophyll, and they are almost invariably in the form of clusters. It will be noticed that these cluster crystals differ markedly from those of senna, in being composed of much larger prisms, which have comparatively blunt ends. Fig. 46 illustrates these points.

Henbane leaf has a general resemblance to stramonium leaf, but the crystals present are nearly all simple prisms. Simple cluster crystals of few components are not infrequent in some specimens.

SCHEDULE OF INSTRUCTIONS—XXX

CANTHARIDES AND MYLABRIS

Cantharides, Spanish Flies, or Blister Beetles. The dried beetle *Cantharis vesicatoria* Latreille, family Meloïdæ, order Coleoptera.

1. Take an insect which has been soaked in several changes of acetone and allow it to soak for about ten minutes in water. Remove it from the water, push a pin gently through the thorax and fix it to a piece of flat cork. Measure the length and breadth of the insect and measure the proportions of the head, thorax and abdomen. Make a sketch of the dorsal surface and mark the main divisions of the body —head, thorax (prothorax), and abdomen—the elytra and legs. Note

that the elytra almost cover the abdomen (all except the extreme hinder end), and that they exactly meet one another in a straight line along the centre.

2. Remove the pin from the cork and examine the under surface of the insect. Sketch it to show the parts named above, and note especially that all the parts of the insect are composed of joints (Arthropoda). The six legs are all attached to the thorax, one pair to each of its three segments.

3. Fasten the pin again into the cork so that the beetle stands dorsal surface uppermost, and with other pins carefully open out the elytra and wings, which are attached to the middle and hind thoracic segments respectively. Note also the segmented upper surface of the abdomen. Sketch it to show these details.

4. By means of a scalpel remove the head from a beetle and lay it face uppermost on a piece of white paper. Sketch it, as seen with a pocket lens, to show the large upper portion (the epicranium) with a central groove; the two comparatively small black eyes low down at the sides of the head, and, immediately below them, the long filiform 11-jointed antennæ or the circular scars left where they have broken off. The face terminates below in two narrow transverse plates, the upper one, called the epistome, and the lower one the upper lip or labrum, which covers over the jaws and other mouth parts; mark these upon the sketch.

5. Turn the head over and sketch the under surface, marking the following details: The foramen magnum (the large opening through which pass muscles, breathing tubes, nerves, and œsophagus); the lower lip or labium, covering the mouth parts behind; and a small portion of each eye, which is visible from behind.

6. To study the jaws in detail, insert the point of a scalpel between the labrum and the labium so that the flat of the blade is parallel with the flat surfaces of the head. Then gently force the point in and cut the head neatly into an anterior and a posterior part. Boil the pieces in a test-tube for ten minutes in a 5 per cent. solution of caustic potash or soda. If the pieces are still too dark in colour, add about 0·5 ml. of 10 vol. hydrogen peroxide and continue heating till sufficiently bleached. Cool and pour out the contents into a hollowed glass block; remove the pieces with a thin slip of wood and put them into distilled water in a second dish and soak for ten or fifteen minutes; then transfer to water acidulated with acetic acid. Mount in lacto-phenol and examine with the low power of the microscope. Sketch in detail the following parts: The labrum, the biting jaws or mandibles, the chewing jaws or maxillæ, and the labium or lower lip.

7. Examine the legs and note that each consists of a series of joints. Next to the body is a broad basal joint, the haunch or coxa, followed by a very small connecting joint, the trochanter, to which is attached the femur or thigh joint, after which come the tibia or shin, and finally the tarsus or foot, consisting of five segments in the front and intermediate feet and four segments in the hind feet. All six feet terminate in four claws each; the two external claws are large and strong, and the two internal ones are thin and less developed. Boil a leg with potash and prepare a mount as directed for the jaws. Sketch it to

show the details named, and make a separate larger drawing of the four claws of one foot.

8. Boil a piece of an elytron with 5 per cent. aqueous caustic potash, wash with water and mount in lacto-phenol. Examine in surface view. Note that the elytron is almost glabrous, and shows a delicate

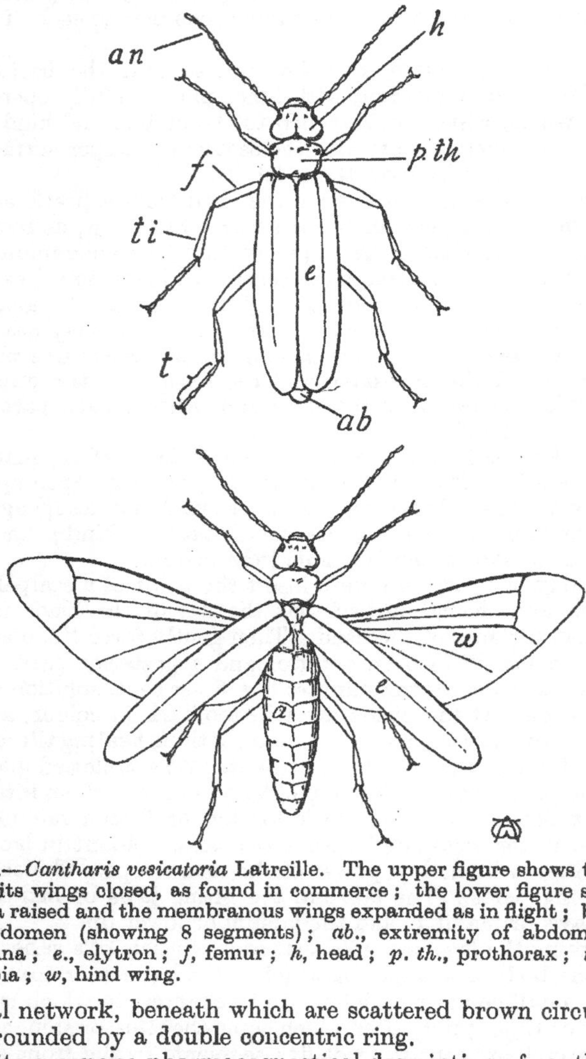

FIG. 47.—*Cantharis vesicatoria* Latreille. The upper figure shows the beetle with its wings closed, as found in commerce; the lower figure shows the elytra raised and the membranous wings expanded as in flight; both × 2. *a*, abdomen (showing 8 segments); *ab.*, extremity of abdomen; *an.*, antenna; *e.*, elytron; *f*, femur; *h*, head; *p. th.*, prothorax; *t*, tarsus; *ti*, tibia; *w*, hind wing.

polygonal network, beneath which are scattered brown circular areas, each surrounded by a double concentric ring.

9. Write a concise pharmacognostical description of cantharides

Mylabris or Chinese Blistering Flies. The dried beetles *Mylabris sidæ* Fab.; *M. cichorii* Fab.; and other species of *Mylabris.*

1. Take some Mylabris beetles and examine them as directed for cantharides. Note especially the following points :

(*a*) The elytra are black with orange-yellow transverse bands. There is a yellow pubescence upon the bands in *M. cichorii* and stiff black hairs upon the bands of *M. sidæ* (*phalerata*). Black hairs are found upon the black parts of the elytra of both species. The elytra entirely cover the abdomen, and project slightly beyond it.

(*b*) The head is more rounded in shape and has large hemispherical eyes reaching two-thirds up the sides of the head.

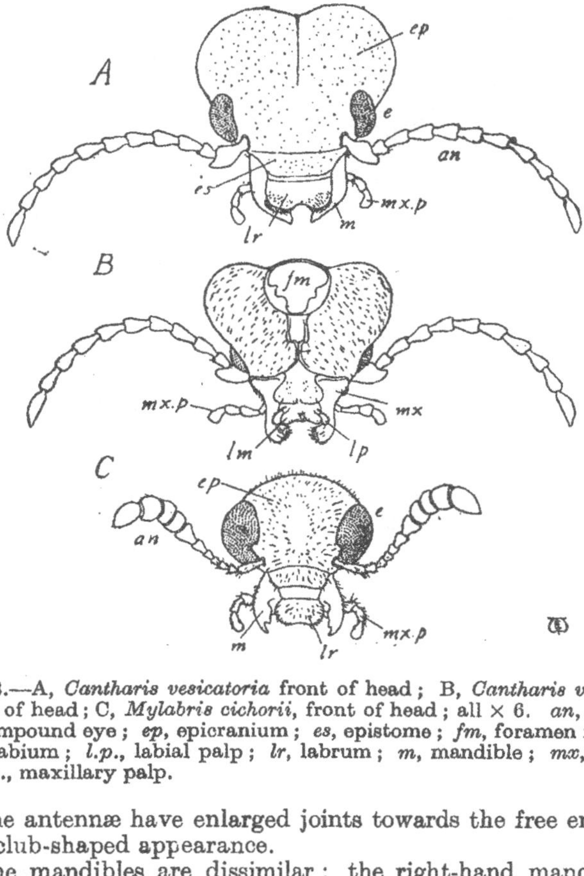

FIG. 48.—A, *Cantharis vesicatoria* front of head; B, *Cantharis vesicatoria*, back of head; C, *Mylabris cichorii*, front of head; all × 6. *an*, antenna; *e*, compound eye; *ep*, epicranium; *es*, epistome; *fm*, foramen magnum; *lm*, labium; *l.p.*, labial palp; *lr*, labrum; *m*, mandible; *mx*, maxilla; *mx.p.*, maxillary palp.

(*c*) The antennæ have enlarged joints towards the free ends, giving them a club-shaped appearance.

(*d*) The mandibles are dissimilar; the right-hand mandible has a well-developed tooth on the inner margin just behind the tip, but the left-hand mandible has no such tooth.

2. Make sketches to illustrate these details of difference. (See Figs. 48 and 50.)

NOTES ON SCHEDULE XXX

Steeping the insects in several changes of acetone removes the bulk of the cantharidin, so making the beetles safe to handle freely, and also renders them easily penetrable by water, so that they are quickly softened by immersion in water and can then be dissected with ease.

Fig. 47 shows a beetle with its wings closed as it usually occurs in commerce, and a second beetle with the wings outspread as in flight. The following points should be noted :

1. The rigid skeletal part of the body, to which the muscles are attached, is external, forming an exoskeleton, which is composed of chitin. The whole of the animal's body is made up of joints or segments ; the beetle

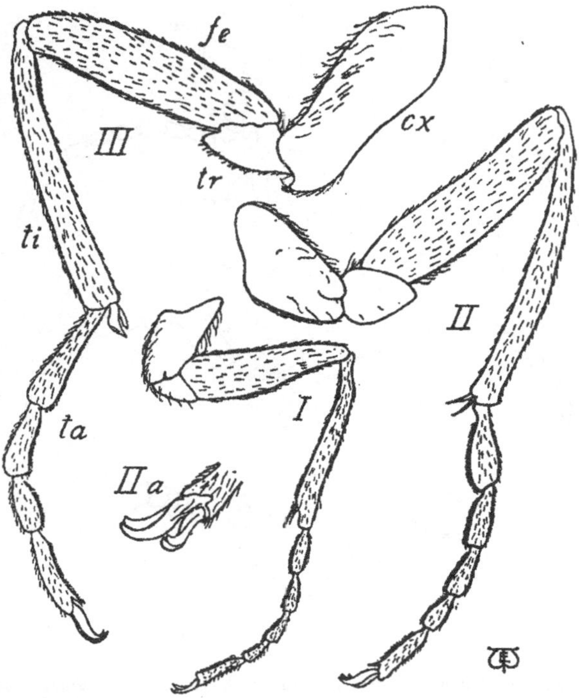

FIG. 49.—*Cantharis vesicatoria* I., II. and III., fore, middle and hind legs respectively ; all × 10. IIa, claws from the foot of the middle leg, × 20. *cx*, coxa ; *fe*, femur ; *ta*, tarsus ; *ti*, tibia ; *tr*, trochanter.

therefore belongs to the Phylum Arthropoda (Gk. *arthron*, a joint, and *pous*, a foot).

2. The division of the body into three parts—head, thorax, and abdomen —and the presence of three pairs of legs and two pairs of wings bring the beetle into the class Insecta. The structure of the two eyes is also typical of insects. The lens system of each eye consists of a very large number of lenses, termed facets, of which there are about 1,000 in each eye of this beetle ; see Fig. 48, where the lenses are indicated diagrammatically by dots. Each facet is about 28 microns in diameter.

3. The order of insects to which cantharides belong is indicated (*a*) by the modification of the forewings into hardened protecting cases, termed elytra, meeting in a straight line down the centre ; (*b*) by the presence of biting jaws (see Fig. 48, A) ; (*c*) by the fact that in the life history they

undergo a complete metamorphosis, the egg developing into a grub, which in turn becomes a motionless chrysalis, from which the fully formed insect eventually emerges. The order thus characterised is the Coleoptera. (Gk. *koleos*, a sheath, and *pteron*, a wing.)

4. If the legs are examined, it will be found that the fore and middle legs have each five joints in the foot or tarsus, while the feet of the hind legs have only four joints (see Fig. 49). This character brings the beetle into the sub-order Heteromera. (Gk. *heteros*, other, and *meros*, a part.) The genera *Cantharis* and *Mylabris* both belong to the same family Meloïdæ.

The cantharides-beetle is easily recognised by its metallic green colour, its long filiform antennæ and comparatively small eyes situated low down at the sides of the head, close to the piont of attachment of the antennæ (see Fig. 48, A and B). *Mylabris sidæ* is a very much larger

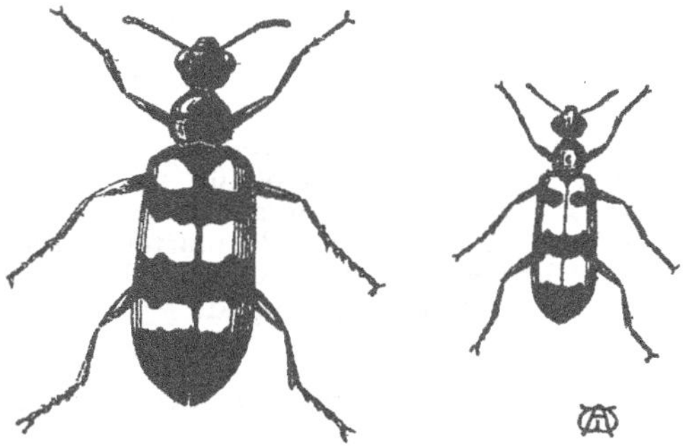

FIG. 50.—MYLABRIS BEETLES. The left-hand figure is of *Mylabris sidæ* Fab., and the right-hand figure is of *Mylabris cichorii*. Fab. Both natural size.

beetle than *Cantharis*, while *M. cichorii* is about the same size (see Fig. 50). The points for distinguishing *Mylabris* and its two common species are noted above in the Schedule of Instructions.

Characters of Powdered Cantharides

1. Abundant pieces of muscle fibres.
2. Fragments of elytra with scattered brown circular areas each surrounded by a double concentric ring.
3. Occasional fragments of mandibles, maxillæ and other mouth parts.
4. Occasional claws from the feet and other pieces of the legs.
5. Fragments of the chitinous exoskeleton and of the membranous wings.

Permanent mounts of the insect parts, prepared by treatment with potash, can be easily made by removing the parts from the dilute acetic acid and soaking them for a few hours in glacial acetic acid; then remove to clove oil and allow to soak for a short time. The parts are finally removed from the clove oil and mounted in canada balsam or in sandarac. Canada balsam makes a perfectly satisfactory mount; but sandarac is an improvement because the resin is so much less coloured. The canada balsam or sandarac medium should be used quite thin, and it is best to support the cover-glass on the top of a cork slightly smaller in diameter than the cover-glass; then arrange the insect parts on the cover-glass and add a drop or two of the medium. Put the preparation away in a place free from dust and allow the solvent to evaporate; then add more medium and put it away again, continuing the process until the objects are embedded in a mass of resin (this may take some weeks in the case of thick objects). Now take a clean slide, place a drop of medium in its centre and another drop on the cover-glass, which is then inverted upon the slide. Put the preparation away to become thoroughly hard.

Note on the Mounting of Thick Objects

For very thick objects, such as an entire head of a beetle, one should prepare the cover-glass by first attaching to its edge three or four clear glass beads, according as the cover is circular or square ; the beads should be of about the same thickness as the object to be mounted. The beads are attached by a drop of the mountant and allowed to dry before the insect parts are placed in position. The beads prevent the cover-glass from compressing the object as the mountant gradually shrinks. The cover of a mount made in this way will sometimes show a slight concave curvature after the lapse of a few months owing to the atmospheric pressure ; when this occurs, a fresh drop of medium should be added so as to run round the ledge of the cover ; this will immediately release the tension and the cover becomes again flat.

The sandarac medium is prepared as follows : Take sandarac resin, 32 gm. ; castor oil, 5 ml. ; amyl alcohol, 60 ml., dissolve, and filter through paper. The canada balsam medium is prepared by heating canada balsam on a water-bath until the volatile matter is removed and the residue sets to a hard brittle mass on cooling. Dissolve the residue in xylol or in benzol to form a thin syrupy liquid.

SCHEDULE OF INSTRUCTIONS—XXXI

COCHINEAL

Cochineal. The dried female insect *Dactylopius coccus* Costa, family Coccidæ, order Hemiptera, containing numerous larvæ.

1. Soak some cochineal insects in water for eighteen hours ; decant the water and wash once or twice by decantation Soak the swollen insects in solution of ammonia for a few hours, decant and wash by decantation with distilled water. Repeat the soaking in solution of ammonia three or four times until the insects are deprived of colouring matter. To the decolorised material add some dilute alcohol and store in a bottle.

2. Into a hollowed glass block put a little water and place in it a prepared insect. Arrange the insect so that the flat under surface is uppermost ; illuminate it by light from above the level of the dish and sketch the flat surface as seen with a pocket lens or under a low-power objective. Note the absence of divisions between the head, thorax and abdomen, and observe the marked difference between the thoracic segments and the abdominal ones as seen on the lower surface. Mark on your sketch the eyes, antennæ, suctorial mouth, legs and spiracles.

3. Take a thin slip of wood and gently press the insect so as to rupture the outer skin, when it is touched with the point of a needle at the sides, and the numerous larvæ it contains will float out into the water. Remove the collapsed insect and mount it in chloral hydrate solution on a slide. Count the larvæ lying in the water in the hollowed

glass block ; this is most easily done by standing it on a black surface having $\frac{1}{4}$ in. or 5 mm. squares ruled in white lines and counting the larvæ over each square in succession until all are counted. Then count under the 16 mm. objective the larvæ remaining in the skin mounted in

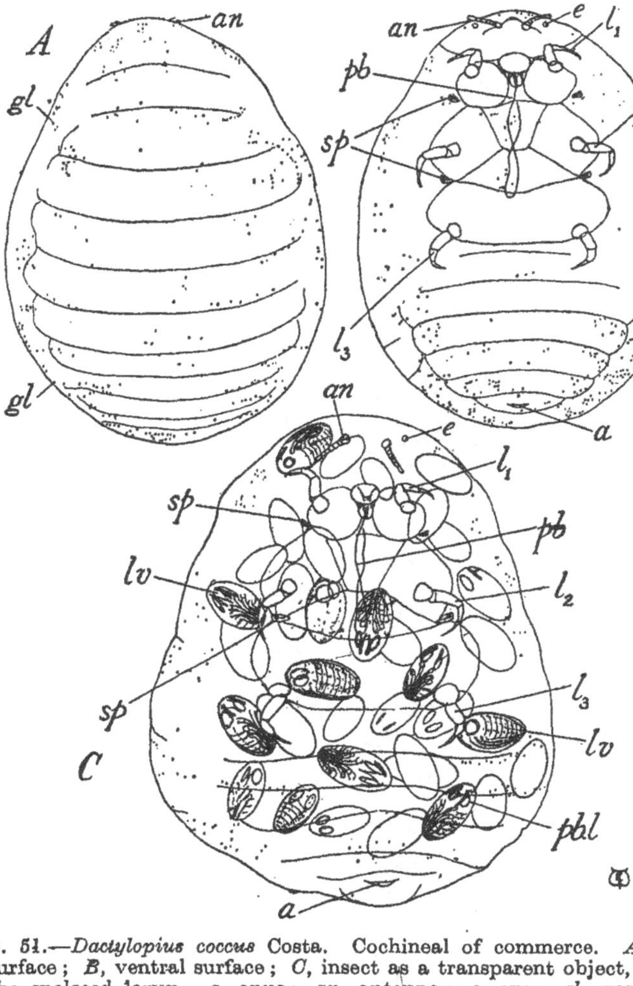

FIG. 51.—*Dactylopius coccus* Costa. Cochineal of commerce. *A*, dorsal surface ; *B*, ventral surface ; *C*, insect as a transparent object, showing the enclosed larvæ. *a*, anus ; *an*, antenna ; *e*, eye ; *gl*, wax gland ; l_1, l_2, l_3, legs of the first, second and third pairs respectively ; *lv*, larva ; *pb.*, proboscis ; *pb.l.*, proboscis of larva ; *sp*, spiracle. All × 12.

chloral, and so obtain a record of the number of larvæ in the parent insect.

4. Examine the skin of the insect under the microscope and sketch separate pieces showing respectively the wax glands, the spiracles, the legs or scars or remains of legs and the antennæ.

5. Sketch a larva and indicate the antennæ, six legs, proboscis (coiled in two spirals), wax glands in rows, etc.

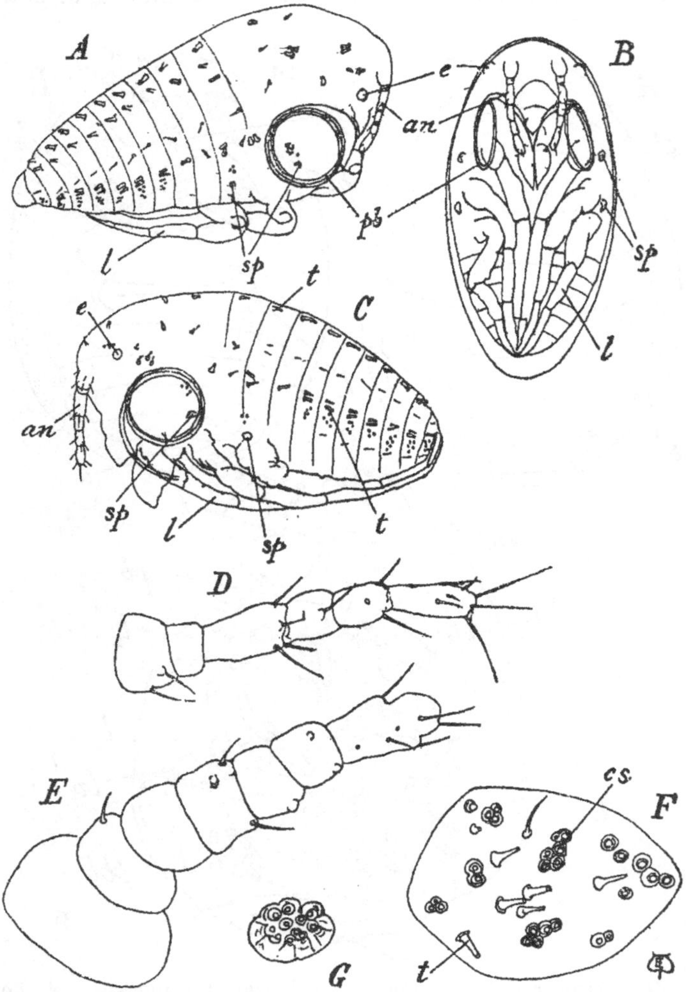

FIG. 52.—*Dactylopius coccus* Costa. *A*, *B* and *C*, larva in different positions, × 80. *D*, antenna of a larva, showing 6 joints, × 200. *E*, antenna of an adult female, showing 7 joints, × 200. *F*, piece of the dermis of an adult insect, showing hairs, truncate spines and grouped spinnerets, × 200. *G*, group of wax glands (compound spinneret), × 200. *an*, antenna. *cs*, compound spinneret. *e*, eye. *l*, leg. *pb*, probosis, *sp*. spiracle. *t*, truncate spine.

6. Examine powdered cochineal after decolorisation with solution of ammonia, and sketch pieces showing characteristic features.

7. Treat the powder with alkali and with acid, and note the change in colour.

NOTES ON SCHEDULE XXXI

Cochineal is a very highly modified type of insect. The body does not shew the usual constrictions between head, thorax and abdomen, and the antennæ and legs are so comparatively short that they do not extend beyond the margins of the flattened ventral surface to which they are attached (see Fig. 51, B). The antennæ have seven joints (Fig. 52, E), and are well developed. The eyes are very inconspicuous and quite exceptional in construction, each consisting of a single lens only (simple eyes); they are placed slightly anterior to the antennæ and nearer to the margin of the head than the points of attachment of the antennæ by a distance nearly as great as the length of the antennæ. The mouth is suctorial and more highly modified than that of the bee; externally one can see the long filiform proboscis (Fig. 51, B, *pb*), composed of four very fine chitinous styles, which are in two pairs, the anterior pair representing the mandibles and the posterior pair the first maxillæ; the origins of these two pairs can be clearly seen as club-shaped structures on focussing through the external surface. Four spiracles (Figs. 51 and 52, *sp*) are clearly visible, an anterior pair between the fore and middle legs and a posterior pair between the middle and hind legs. Within each insect of the commercial drug can be seen numerous larvæ, usually about 150, but varying in number in individual insects from about 60 to 450. A remarkable feature of the larvæ is the manner in which the two fine bristles on each side are coiled to form a conspicuous looking circle closely applied to the side of the larva (see Fig. 52, A, B and C). The wax glands, which are scattered irregularly over the dermis of the adult insect, are arranged in conspicuous longitudinal rows upon the larvæ (see Fig. 52).

Characters of Powdered Cochineal

1. Abundant pieces of muscle fibres.
2. Portions of the chitinous dermis with hairs, truncate spines and groups of wax spinnerets.
3. Fragments of larvæ showing coiled proboscides.
4. Cuticle of larvæ with rows of wax glands.
5. Occasional claws from the feet and pieces of legs.
6. Note the change in colour to purplish red with alkali and to yellow with mineral acids.

SCHEDULE OF INSTRUCTIONS—XXXII

RHIZOMES; MALE FERN, VALERIAN, RHUBARB

Male Fern Rhizome. The rhizome of *Dryopteris Filix-mas* Schott, family Polypodiaceæ.

1. Examine the rhizome, and sketch the longitudinal section to show the growing point and the young leaves with circinate vernation, the whole protected by a covering of ramenta. Note the meristeles and the leaf bases, from which the roots arise.
2. Remove a ramentum, mount it in chloral hydrate solution and sketch the margin in detail to show the two-celled projections.
3. Sketch a transverse section of a rhizome, as seen with a pocket

lens, show the distribution of the meristeles, the sclerenchyma, the ground tissue, and the leaf traces.

4. Cut across a leaf base transversely and sketch the cut surface to show the number and arrangement of the fibro-vascular strands.

5. Cut a thin transverse section of the leaf base and mount it in chloral hydrate solution. Find and sketch, under the 4 mm. objective, one of the internal secreting hairs.

Valerian. The rhizome and roots of *Valeriana officinalis* Linn., family Valerianaceæ.

1. Make a habit sketch of a rhizome of valerian and mark such of the following details as are present: main rhizome, horizontal branch with offset, adventitious roots, aerial stem.

2. Cut a rhizome transversely and sketch the cut surface to show cork, bark, cambium, xylem groups, large central pith. Test for starch. Phloroglucin and hydrochloric acid may be used to make the xylem groups more evident.

3. Cut an adventitious root transversely and sketch to show the small central xylem strand and the wide bark. Similarly cut and sketch the horizontal runner and the aerial stem and compare them with the main rhizome and the root.

4. Write a description using the scheme for rhizome and roots (p. 121).

Rhubarb. The rhizome of *Rheum palmatum* Linn., and possibly other species, family Polygonaceæ, collected in China and Thibet, deprived of most of its bark and dried.

1. Examine the outer surface of a piece of rhubarb and note the network of delicate whitish lines forming meshes, each of which is occupied by a number of alternating white and orange-yellow lines which latter are the medullary rays seen in the tangential section of the rhizome. If the rhizome has been very liberally trimmed, star spots, consisting of radiating orange-yellow lines (medullary rays) are visible externally. Make sketches to show these details.

2. Examine the smoothed surface of a transversely cut piece of rhubarb root and find the cambium line a short distance within and nearly parallel with the outer margin. All the tissue external to this cambium is secondary phloem. Within the cambium find a band of secondary xylem traversed by yellow medullary rays. In the pith, and often forming a line bordering upon the inner margin of the secondary xylem, are a number of star-spots. Make a diagrammatic sketch to illustrate these features.

3. Scrape some powder from a piece of rhubarb and mount it in solution of chloral hydrate, find and sketch the crystals of calcium oxalate.

4. *Test for Hydroxymethylanthraquinones.* Carry out the test with powdered rhubarb, as directed for cascara bark (see Schedule. IX., p. 24).

NOTES ON SCHEDULE XXXII

Male Fern Rhizome. When examining the ramentum, or scale-like hair of the rhizome and leaf bases, notice especially the margin and observe the form of the hair-like projections, which are composed in each case of two gradually tapering cells, united together, with their long axes parallel. Glandular marginal hairs are absent from the ramentum. These characteristics of the ramentum distinguish the rhizome of male fern from rhizomes of other closely allied ferns, notably from *Aspidium spinulosum*, which bears ramenta having numerous marginal, unicellular, glandular hairs. The transverse section of the leaf base is useful in a similar way, more especially for distinguishing the genuine drug from the rhizome of the lady fern, *Athyrium Filix fœmina*.

Valerian should be soaked in water for 18 hours before dissection.

Rhubarb is best examined in the dry condition.

SCHEDULE OF INSTRUCTIONS—XXXIII

RHIZOMES; PODOPHYLLUM, ARNICA, BLACK HELLEBORE, INDIAN PODOPHYLLUM

Podophyllum Rhizome. The dried rhizome and roots of *Podophyllum peltatum* Linn., family Berberidaceæ.

1. Make sketches of the upper and lower surfaces of a piece of the soaked drug to show the enlarged regions, each carrying on the upper surface a circular scar left by the aerial stem and on the under surface, numerous small circular scars left by the adventitious roots. Between the enlarged portions note the smooth, sub-cylindrical connecting portions; is there any evidence of the presence of leaves on these cylindrical parts? Key your drawing, and indicate the morphological nature of the various structures.

2. Cut a soaked piece transversely in two places, viz., through the enlarged region and through the cylindrical part; measure and record the diameter of each. Make sketches to show the distribution of the fibro-vascular bundles, and name all the parts of both sections.

3. Break a piece, and record the nature of the fracture and the horny or starchy appearance of the fractured surface.

4. Test for starch by iodine and also by scraping some dust from the cut surface and examine it microscopically. What additional information do you gain from the microscopical appearance?

5. Macerate 0·25 gm. of powdered podophyllum for ten minutes in 5 ml. of alcohol 90 per cent., filter and add to the filtrate 0·5 ml. of a 5 per cent. aqueous solution of copper acetate. Note the bright green coloration and absence of any brown precipitate; compare with Indian podophyllum.

Arnica Rhizome. The dried rhizome and roots of *Arnica montana* Linn., family Compositæ.

1. Measure the diameter of the rhizome and note the numerous curved, wiry and brittle adventitious roots and the leaf bases terminating the rhizome. Sketch to show these details.

2. Cut a transverse section of the soaked rhizome, and examine it with a pocket lens. In the centre find a large pith, which is surrounded by a narrow, yellowish ring of wood bundles, outside which is a circle of oleo-resin glands just beyond the endodermis, some of them being visible under the lens as small holes resembling pin-pricks. Sketch a transverse section at a definite magnification.

Black Hellebore Rhizome. The dried rhizome and roots of *Helleborus niger* Linn., family Ranunculaceæ, the Christmas Rose.

1. Observe and record the external colour and the odour of the drug. Measure the length of the pieces of rhizome, and record the minimum, maximum and most common sizes.

2. Sketch a piece of soaked rhizome to show its contorted shape and the numerous short, thick, ascending branches ending in cup-shaped scars left by the aerial stems. Mark also the numerous stumps or scars of the adventitious roots and the narrow scale leaves.

3. Cut a soaked rhizome transversely, and note the whitish appearance of the cut surface. Sketch the section to show the ring of elongated bundles separated by medullary rays. Test the cut surface for starch.

4. Cut a root transversely, and sketch the cut surface as seen with a pocket lens.

5. Break a dry rhizome across, and record the nature of the fracture.

Indian Podophyllum Rhizome. The dried rhizome and roots of *Podophyllum Emodi* Wall., family Berberidaceæ.

1. Note the colour of the drug and the large amount of small, loose roots. Measure the length and thickness of the pieces of rhizome, and record the maximum, minimum and most common values.

2. Sketch the upper and under surfaces of a piece of rhizome to show its contorted form and the scars of the aerial stems and of the adventitious roots.

3. Cut a soaked rhizome transversely, and sketch the cut surface, naming all the structures present.

4. Sketch also the transversely cut surface of a soaked root.

5. Carry out a test with copper acetate as directed under (5) for podophyllum, and note the brown precipitate which is formed and the absence of any green coloration.

NOTES ON SCHEDULE XXXIII

Podophyllum rhizome, also known as Mayapple root or American Mandrake, is one which produces annually, at intervals of about 5 cm., an enlarged rooting portion. This part bears on its upper surface the single large umbrella-like leaf and the flowering stem with its two smaller leaves, one such aërial stem being produced each year. Between the enlarged portions the rhizome is cylindrical, and of about half the diameter of the rooting portions. Around the margin of the large circular stem scar on the upper surface of the enlarged part note the numerous narrow scale leaves, some of which bear buds in their axils. An occasional scale leaf may be found upon the cylindrical connecting portion of the rhizome (see Fig. 53, A and B).

For cutting sections, the material should be soaked in cold water for eighteen hours. Transverse sections of the cylindrical portion (see Fig. 53, C) show a uniform white and starchy ground tissue in which a regular circle of small fibro-vascular bundles is embedded; transverse sections of the enlarged parts show a similar starchy ground-substance and a more irregular ring of bundles from which branches pass outwards into leaves and adventitious roots (see Fig. 53, D). From the appearance of the starch grains, one may discover whether or no the rhizome has been overheated in the process of drying.

Arnica rhizome should be prepared by soaking it in cold water for about eighteen hours. Arnica rhizome differs in structure from the stolons of liquorice (see Schedule XXXIV.), in that secondary development is much

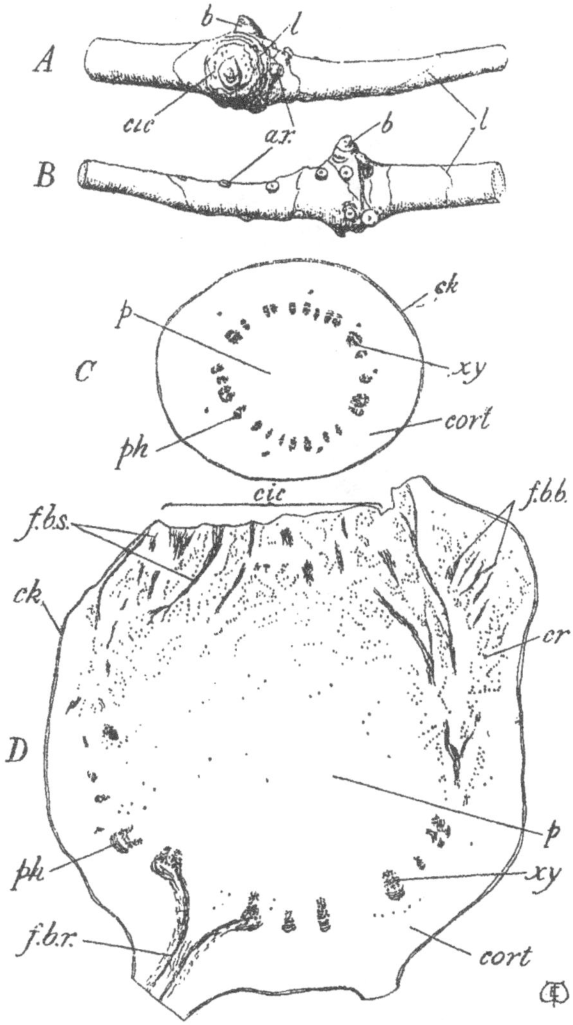

FIG. 53.—Rhizome of *Podophyllum peltatum* Linn. A and B, upper and lower surfaces respectively of a piece of podophyllum rhizome, natural size. C, transverse section through the narrow connecting portion of a rhizome, × 5. D, transverse section through one of the enlarged regions carrying the scar left by the aerial stem, × 5. *a.r.*, adventitious root; *b*, bud of a lateral branch; *cic*, scar of the aërial stem; *ck*, cork; *cort*, cortex; *cr*, calcium oxalate crystal; *f.b.b.*, fibro-vascular bundles entering a branch; *f.b.r.*, fibro-vascular bundles entering a root; *f.b.s.*, fibro-vascular bundles entering the aerial stem; *l*, scale leaf; *p*, pith; *ph*, phloem; *xy*, xylem.

less marked; the bundles always remain comparatively small and are separated by wide medullary rays.

Black Hellebore Rhizome. Hellebore rhizome is nearly black in colour,

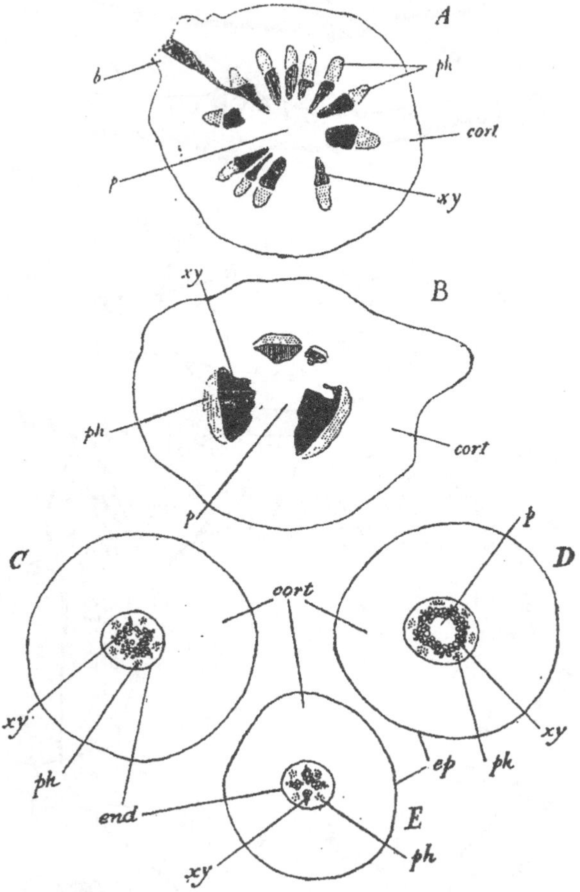

FIG. 54.—*Helleborus niger*, Linn. A and B, transverse sections of the rhizome, × 5. C, D, and E, transverse sections of adventitious roots, × 10. A is the more typical section of a rhizome, B has wider and fewer bundles. C is a pentarch root showing no pith and very little secondary structure; it is from about the middle of a root. D is a hexarch root, showing a pith and a narrow ring of xylem, mostly secondary; it is cut at a point close to the rhizome. E is a tetrarch root, and is from the lower part of a root, *i.e.*, nearer the apex. *b*, origin of a branch; *cort*, cortex; *end*, endodermis; *ep*, epiblema; *p*, pith; *ph*, phloem; *xy*, xylem.

and has a nauseous odour. The details of structure are more clearly evident in pieces of rhizome which have been soaked in water for about eighteen hours. The section (see Fig. 54, A and B) shows a ring of pale-coloured bundles usually narrow and elongated, but sometimes much wider and less numerous. There is a fair-sized pith occupying about one-third of the total diameter and a cortex whose width is about one-fourth of the diameter of the rhizome. The adventitious roots in transverse section show a wide cortex filled with starch, and a small central stele which varies from four to six-arch, sometimes having a central pith surrounded by a narrow ring of xylem, at other times without a pith, and sometimes showing a star-shaped xylem with pointed rays (see Fig. 54, C, D and E). The rhizome, collected at the proper time, in the autumn, is filled with starch; rhizomes collected when exhausted after flowering are very oily and devoid of starch.

Indian podophyllum rhizome shows a strong general structural resemblance to the rhizome of black hellebore. It is, however, externally yellowish-brown in colour, and the transversely cut surface shows a ring

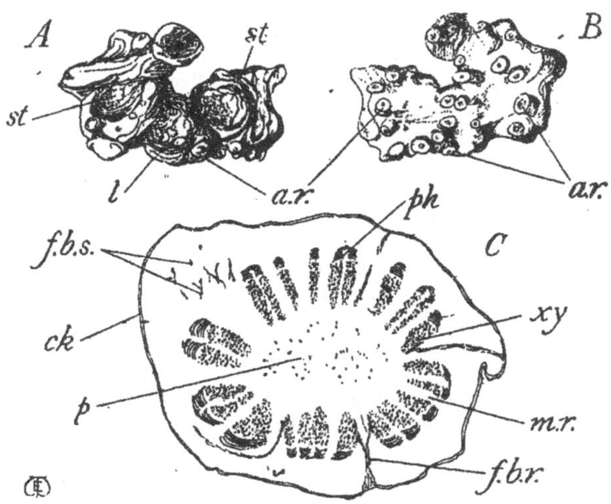

FIG. 55.—Rhizome of *Podophyllum Emodi* Wall. A, upper surface of a rhizome, natural size. B, under surface of a rhizome, natural size. C, transverse section of a rhizome, × 5. *a.r.*, adventitious root; *ck*, cork; *f.b.r.*, fibro-vascular bundles entering a root; *f.b.s.*, fibro-vascular bundles entering a stem; *l*, scale leaf; *m.r.*, medullary ray; *p*, pith with calcium oxalate crystals represented by dots; *ph*, phloem; *st*, scar left by the aërial stem.

of bundles which stand out strongly against the whitish background (see Fig. 55). The xylem of the bundles is porous, and the phloem appears as a dark-brown cap above the xylem. This rhizome should be soaked in cold water for eighteen hours before making the drawings or dissections.

SCHEDULE OF INSTRUCTIONS—XXXIV

RHIZOMES; SERPENTARY, LIQUORICE, GINGER

Serpentary Rhizome (Texan). The dried rhizome of *Aristolochia reticulata* Nutt., family Aristolochiaceæ.

1. Take a piece of soaked rhizome and find upon the upper surface the small cup-shaped scars of the aërial stems, a piece of the base of the last aërial stem, the numerous long and nearly straight roots, and the

slender horizontal rhizome. Sketch the specimen and key the drawing.

2. Cut a rhizome transversely and sketch the exposed surface, marking on your drawing the excentric pith, medullary rays, xylem, phloem, cortex, cork and origin of the adventitious roots. Stain the transverse surface with iodine water, record the result, and state your conclusion.

3. Note and record the odour and taste.

Liquorice. The root and subterranean stem of *Glycyrrhiza glabra* Linn., and other species of *Glycyrrhiza*, family Leguminosæ.

1. Compare pieces of peeled and unpeeled drug. Note the longitudinal wrinkles of the unpeeled drug and search for small buds. Sketch a piece to show these features. Note the yellow colour of the peeled piece and the fibrous nature of the exposed surface. Remove a few fibres from the outer surface, boil them on a slide in solution of chloral hydrate. Note and sketch a bundle of fibres and the accompanying crystals of calcium oxalate.

2. Cut a soaked root transversely and also a runner. Sketch each to show the cambium line, the medullary rays and the radiating rows of yellowish vascular tissue continued through the phloem as lines of dark dots (what are these ?). Determine the presence or absence of a pith.

3. Observe and record the odour and the taste. Test for starch by iodine and by examining the scrapings.

4. *Test for sugars.* Make a decoction of liquorice by putting 1 g. of liquorice in thin shavings into 20 ml. of water and bringing it to the boil. Allow to stand for 10 minutes, cool, adjust the volume and filter. To 2 ml. of the filtrate add 2 ml. of Fehling's reagent and heat on a water-bath. A red precipitate indicates the presence of reducing sugars.

5. Sprinkle some powdered liquorice on to sulphuric acid (80 per cent. by volume) and note the colour produced.

Ginger. The scraped and dried rhizome of *Zingiber officinalis* Roscoe, family Zingiberaceæ.

1. Sketch a rhizome to show the branches, called "fingers," all in one plane and forming a "hand." Note that the outer part, including the cork and the leaf and root-scars, has been removed.

2. Cut a rhizome transversely and sketch the transverse surface to show the circular endodermis, the scattered yellowish secretion cells and the greyish vascular bundles. Test for starch. Break a rhizome across and note the projecting fibres upon the fractured surface.

3. Treat the transverse surface with phloroglucin and hydrochloric acid and note that the bundles do not stain red.

NOTES ON SCHEDULE XXXIV

Serpentary. In the section the pith and medullary rays appear whitish and the wood yellow. Both pith and medullary rays contain starch. The medullary rays are usually slightly curved. The pith is usually nearer to the upper surface of the rhizome.

Liquorice. The greater part of the drug consists of the stolons, which possess a central pith and show a typical dicotyledonous structure with well-marked secondary development, resulting in the formation of a complete ring of secondary xylem. The few pieces of root which can be found show a zone of xylem reaching to the centre, pith being absent;

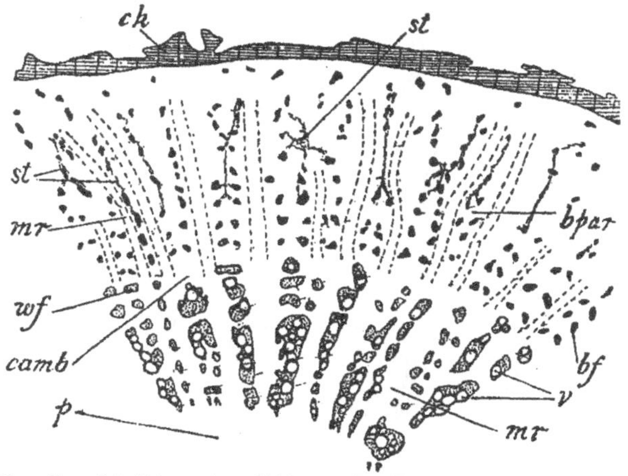

FIG. 56. Spanish Liquorice (Rhizome). Transverse section (diagrammatic). *bf*, bast fibres; *bpar*, bast parenchyma; *camb*, cambium; *ck*, cork; *mr*, medullary ray; *p*, pith; *st*, sieve tissue; *v*, vessel; *wf*, wood fibres; × 15. After Fahmy.

usually four principal medullary rays can be seen radiating from the centre at right angles to one another. The lines of dark dots visible in a transverse section of the phloem are groups of phloem fibres, see Fig. 56.

When powdered liquorice is sprinkled on to sulphuric acid, a yellow colour is formed.

SCHEDULE OF INSTRUCTIONS—XXXV

COLCHICUM CORM, SQUILL BULB

Colchicum Corm. The fresh corm of *Colchicum autumnale* L., collected in early summer.

1. Sketch a corm from the outside to show the membranous enveloping scale and the laterally placed bud for the aërial shoot.

2. Remove the brown outer scale and cut the corm by a median vertical section from below upwards. Sketch the cut surface and mark the following details upon your drawing: The corm of the present season; the point of attachment to the parent corm; the lateral flowering stem with its roots, flower-buds and leaves; the solid axis of the flowering shoot, which will become the corm of next year; and the bud for the flowering axis of next year.

3. Cut a corm transversely and sketch the cut surface to show the reniform shape of the section, the scattered fibro-vascular bundles and the deep groove in which the flowering axis lies.

4. Examine a corm gathered in June and compare its structure with that collected in the autumn.

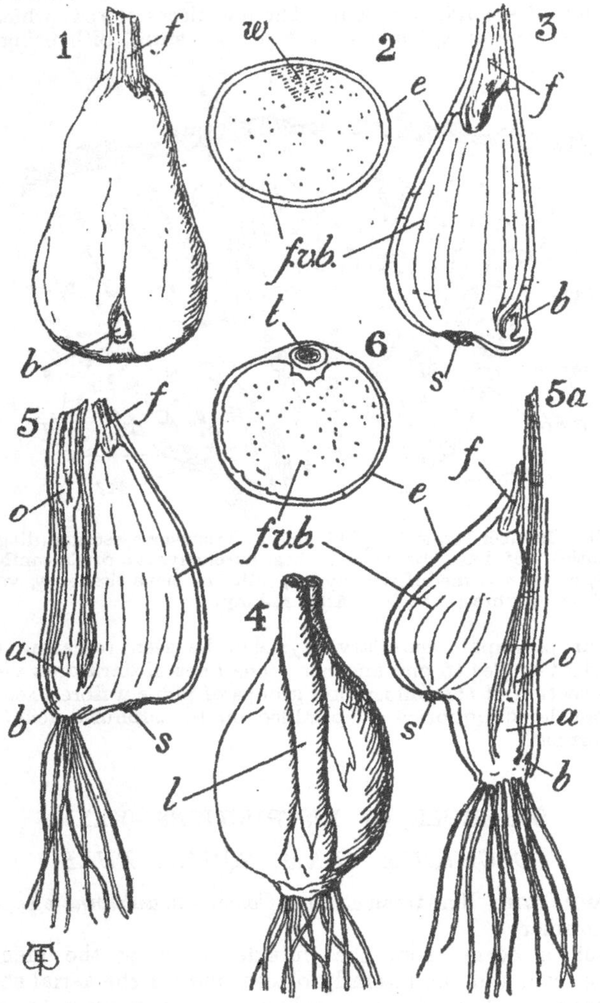

FIG. 57.—*Colchicum autumnale* L. 1. Flat surface of a corm gathered in June, after removal of the brown outer scale. 2. Transverse section of the same. 3. Longitudinal section of the same. 4. Corm gathered in October. 5. Longitudinal section of the same. 5*a*. Longitudinal section of a similar corm which had probably been planted nearer to the surface of the soil. 6. Transverse section of a corm gathered in October. *a*, axis of the flowering stem ; this axis will become the corm for next year ; *b*, bud for next season's flowering stem ; *e*, brown outer envelope ; *f*, remains of the flowering stem of last season ; *f.v.b.*, fibro-vascular bundle ; *l*, aërial shoot ; *o*, ovary ; *s*, scar where the corm has broken away from the parent corm ; *w*, the shaded area is the region that will shrink when slices of the corm are dried, giving the characteristic reniform shape to the pieces of the drug.

Dried Colchicum Corm.

5. With a sharp scalpel or a razor, smooth the surface of a dried slice and sketch it to show the epidermis, fibro-vascular bundles, ground tissue and groove. Record the shape and size of the slices. Test for reserve food.

6. Moisten the surface of a slice with 60–70 per cent. sulphuric acid and a second piece with strong hydrochloric acid. Record and explain any effects observed.

Squill Bulb. Dried transverse slices cut from the bulb of *Urginea Scilla* Steinh., family Liliaceæ, after removing the membranous outer scales.

1. Examine and sketch the preserved specimen of an entire squill bulb, note its dimensions and mark the amount of reduction against the drawing.

2. Examine slices of squill bulb. Smooth the transverse surface of a slice with a scalpel or razor and treat it with phloroglucin and hydrochloric acid. Make a sketch as seen with a pocket-lens and mark the epidermis, the fibro-vascular bundles, the inner concave upper surface and the outer convex lower surface.

3. Scrape some powder from the surface of a slice; mount it in solution of chloral hydrate and examine with the microscope. Sketch the needles of calcium oxalate.

NOTES ON SCHEDULE XXXV

Colchicum Corm. The corm of *colchicum* differs from that of the common crocus in that the bud for the aërial shoot arises laterally near the base of the parent corm, while in *Crocus* the aërial shoots are formed quite close to the apex, and are therefore found upon the summit of the parent corm. The brown membranous scale enveloping the corm is the withered remains of a leaf base of the previous season's aërial shoot. The corm for the next season will arise by an enlargement of the solid lower portion of the axis of the aërial shoot (see Fig. 57, 5 and 5*a*). The corm, gathered in early summer, will have the appearance depicted in Fig. 57, Nos. 1, 2 and 3. The bud for the flowering shoot is still quite small, and the corm shows a groove on the flat surface near the base only. Transverse slices cut from such corms show, while fresh, no notch on the flatter edge, but, as they dry, the tissue in this region (Fig. 57, 2 *w*) shrinks more than the remainder, and the dried slices show the typical reniform shape.

Acid of the strengths specified give a yellow coloration with the colchicine which the corm contains.

Squill Bulb. The needles or acicular raphides of calcium oxalate occur in bundles embedded in mucilage; they are unusually large.

SCHEDULE OF INSTRUCTIONS—XXXVI

ROOTS AND RHIZOMES: DANDELION, GENTIAN, HORSERADISH, SENEGA, ACONITE

Dandelion Root. The fresh and dried roots of *Taraxacum officinale,* Wiggers, family Compositæ.

1. Note the dark greyish-brown colour and that the drug consists of the long, nearly cylindrical tap-root with longitudinal wrinkles, crowned

by a short piece of vertical rhizome or by several branches. On the summit of the rhizome find remains of leaves. Sketch to show these details.

2. Cut a root transversely and sketch the section, as seen with a pocket lens. Mark the central, small, yellowish, porous wood surrounded by an exceptionally wide phloem, in which are numerous concentric lines marking the position of circles of laticiferous vessels. Make a similar drawing of a section of a rhizome, in which a central pith will be found, and the wood ring is frequently broken at intervals. (See Fig. 58, 5 and 6).

3. Test the drug for carbohydrate reserve foods. Cut a transverse section of the softened root, using a razor flooded with alcohol. Mount it in dilute glycerin, and observe the amorphous, irregular lumps of inulin in the parenchyma. Mount a section in water and warm gently; what happens? Mount a section in iodine water and observe the result.

4. Cut up a small piece of root about ¼ in. long, into small pieces, rejecting the central woody strand. Steep them in 5 per cent. caustic alkali, in a test-tube immersed in a water-bath, until thoroughly softened. Wash with distilled water several times by decantation; take a piece of the softened root and thoroughly tease it out with needles. Mount in dilute glycerin, and sketch a portion of the network of anastomosing laticiferous vessels with their granular contents.

Gentian Root. The dried rhizome and root of *Gentiana lutea* Linn., family Gentianaceæ.

1. Note the deep yellow-brown colour, the characteristic odour and, bitter taste (at first sweet). Pieces of root show longitudinal wrinkles while the rhizome is distinguished by leaf-scars in rings, and is often surmounted by a leaf-bud. Sketch to show these details.

2. Cut a transverse section and find the dark cambium line, the indistinctly radiate wood with a fairly large pith in the rhizome, but none in the root. Test for starch. Sketch a transverse section, as seen with a lens.

3. *Test for sugars.* Proceed as directed under Liquorice (4), see p. 94.

4. Compare gentian root with and distinguish it from pellitory root and turpeth root. Make a note of the points of distinction.

Horseradish Root. The fresh root of *Cochlearia Armoracia* Linn., family Cruciferæ, collected from cultivated plants.

1. Sketch a root to show its external features and mark the crown (a shortened stem) with scars of leaves and buds or young aërial shoots attached to it. Note the almost cylindrical shape of the tap-root and determine the number of vertical rows of fibrous lateral rootlets.

2. Examine a transverse slice cut from the root and look for the thin corky covering on the outside and the cambium, appearing as a narrow watery line which separates the outer part of the root (the secondary phloem) from the inner part (the xylem). Note also the fine lines radiating from the centre; these are the medullary rays. Make a sketch to show these details.

3. Cut across the upper portion which bears the scars of the leaves and construct a diagram to show how it differs from the root.

4. Note the colour of the root, its taste and characteristic odour when bruised. Test it for reserve food. Write a technical description.

Senega Root. The dried root and rhizome of *Polygala senega* Linn., family Polygalaceæ.

1. Sketch a root to show the large knotted crown, with the remains of the slender aërial stems, and the smaller tapering root. Note the keel and the odour of wintergreen.

2. Cut a transverse section of the root, and note the whitish wood, which frequently has a deep, wedge-shaped cleft in it. Sketch a transverse section.

3. From a soaked senega root strip off the entire outer tissues down to the cambium and examine the central woody column. Find the slit-shaped clefts in the wood; note that they are not continuous

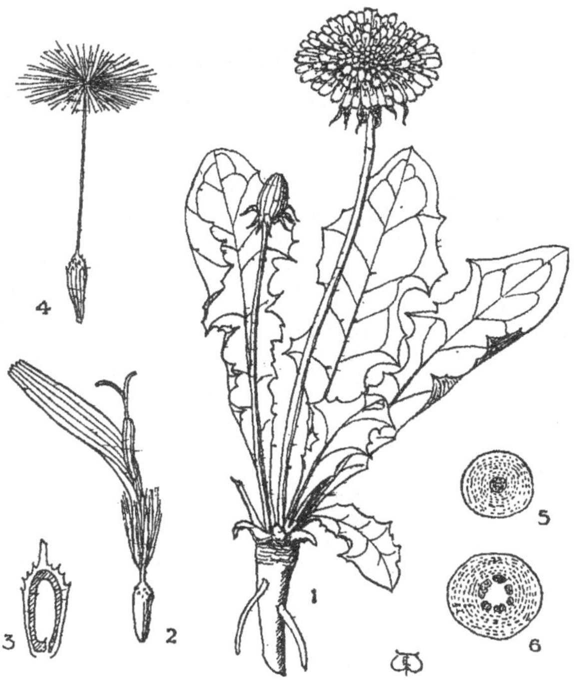

FIG. 58.—*Taraxacum officinale* Wiggers. 1. Habit sketch of flowering plant. 2. A single floret. 3. Vertical section of the ovary. 4. A fruit with its pappus. 5. Transverse section of the root. 6. Transverse section of the rhizome.

with one another, and that parts of the root are free from such clefts altogether.

4. Cut some small pieces from a root and shake them with a little dsitilled water in a test-tube. Observe the frothing; to what is it due?

Aconite Root. The dried root of *Aconitum Napellus* Linn., family Ranunculaceæ.

1. Sketch a root of English aconite; mark the terminal bud and the point of attachment to the parent plant. Record the colour of the surface and the extent of shrinkage produced by drying.

2. Sketch a root of German aconite. Mark the remains of the

aërial stem, the daughter root (if present), and the other features as for English root.

3. Cut a soaked root transversely about one quarter of its length from the crown and sketch a lens view of the exposed surface, marking the pith, cambium, xylem, phloem, cortex and suberised outer layer.

4. Test a cut surface with iodine water.

5. Gently rub the cut end of a dry root upon the tip of the tongue and note the numbing sensation which develops after a short interval.

6. Examine Japanese aconite in a similar way and record the differences you observe.

NOTES ON SCHEDULE XXXVI

The drugs described in this schedule consist of large tap-roots crowned by vertical rhizomes.

Dandelion Root. To soften the dried root for cutting sections to show the presence of inulin, the roots should be exposed to a moist atmosphere for about twenty-four hours. This is done by putting some roots on to damp blotting-paper and keeping them in a closed desiccator or other similar apparatus for the necessary time.

Gentian root gives no blue coloration when tested with iodine, owing to the absence of starch, *cf.* turpeth root. Pellitory root is distinguished by its strong radiate wood and the oil-glands scattered throughout the section. Externally pellitory root has a paler brown colour and is usually crowned by a tuft of hairs. Turpeth root frequently has a purplish tint in its brown colour, and in section the wood appears very porous, owing to the large size of the vessels. Some specimens of turpeth contain an abundance of starch.

Horseradish root is a conical tap-root reaching a length of 75 to 80 cm.; the roots sold commercially are usually about 30 cm. long and branched at the lower end. The main root (Fig. 59 *tp-r*) tapers so slowly as to be nearly cylindrical; the diameter decreases about 1 cm. in a length of about 35 cm. It attains a width at the upper end of 2·5 to 3·0 cm., and then widens out above to form a crown with from one to three or four branches (Fig. 59, *rh.*). These branches are stem structures, and are marked externally by numerous semi-amplexicaul scars left by the fall of the foliage leaves. At the summit of each branch are a number of young leaves, pale-green or nearly white in colour. The root has a pale buff colour, and carries three or occasionally four vertical rows of fibrous secondary roots. The rows of rootlets are sometimes double rows, and in rare instances one may find four rows of rootlets in the upper part of a root and three rows in the lower part of the same root, owing to the gradual convergence and ultimate coalescence of two of the rows of the upper part to form one row in the lower part. The main root sometimes becomes more or less twisted during growth, and the rows of rootlets then appear as spiral lines. The unbroken root has no odour, but when bruised or scraped it develops a strong, pungent, tear-producing odour, owing to the production of a volatile oil (allyl-isothiocyanate) by the action of the enzyme myrosin upon the glucoside sinigrin in the presence of water.

A transverse section of the root (Fig. 59, C) shows from one to three secondary roots arising at the centre and traversing the whole width of the xylem and secondary phloem. The cambium is evident as a watery-looking line, and the corky covering appears as a brown line on the outside. The crown of the root, which is a vertical rhizome, shows in transverse section a large central pith surrounded by a narrow ring of xylem bundles separated by medullary rays (see Fig. 59, B). A few adventitious roots can be seen arising in the region of the xylem and traversing the phloem and outer tissues ; they never penetrate to the centre as in the root proper.

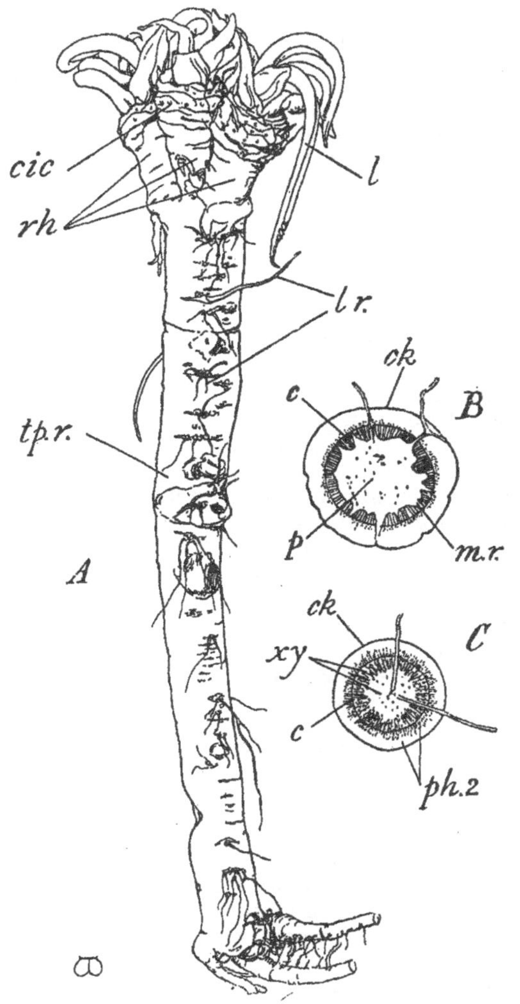

FIG. 59.—*Cochlearia Armoracia* L. A. An entire root. B. Transverse section of the crown. C. Transverse section of the root. *c.*, cambium ; *cic.*, leaf-scar ; *ck.*, cork ; *l.*, young foliage leaf ; *l.r.*, lateral root ; *m.r.*, medullary ray ; *p.*, pith ; *ph.2*, secondary phloem ; *rh.*, vertical rhizome ; *tp.r.*, tap-root ; *xy.*, xylem.

The root contains abundant starch grains, as evidenced by the blue colour produced by applying iodine water to the cut surface.

Senega Root. The odour of wintergreen is best perceived by smelling a quantity of the root in a box. The frothing with water is due to the polygalic acid which the root contains. The "keel" is evident in the dry root, but disappears on soaking.

N.B.—The diagrammatic drawings of the transverse sections of these four roots should be compared together; it will then be evident that the main differences result from the enlargement of different regions for the purpose of food storage. In dandelion the phloem is much enlarged; in gentian and horseradish the parenchyma of both xylem and phloem is generally largely developed; in senega there are abnormal local enlargements of phloem and of medullary rays; in aconite the pith and medullary rays show the greatest development, while the parenchyma of phloem and xylem is increased to a less extent.

SCHEDULE OF INSTRUCTIONS—XXXVII

ROOTS; IPECACUANHA, RHATANY, BELLADONNA, CALUMBA, ELECAMPANE, SARSAPARILLA

Ipecacuanha Root. The dried root of *Cephaëlis Ipecacuanha* Stokes, family Rubiaceæ.

1. Measure the diameter of several pieces of Brazilian ipecacuanha root, and record the maximum, minimum and average thickness.
2. Sketch a piece of the root to show the tortuous appearance and the character of the annulations.
3. Cut a soaked root transversely, sketch the cut end, and name all its parts. Test it with iodine water.
4. Scrape a little powder from the outer part, and examine it microscopically for starch grains and crystals of calcium oxalate.
5. Cut the stem of ipecacuanha transversely and compare its structure with that of the root. Make sketches to show its structure and its external features.
6. Examine and sketch Carthagena ipecacuanha root in the same way, and make a table to show the points of difference between the two roots.

Rhatany. The root of *Krameria triandra* Ruiz and Pav., family Leguminosæ.

1. Make a sketch to show the external features. Measure and record the maximum diameter.
2. Cut a root transversely and sketch the cut surface to show the cork, bark, finely radiate, yellowish wood and absence of pith. Measure the widths of the bark and the wood.
3. Separate the bark and wood from a piece of dry drug and note the difference in astringency in the two regions.
4. Test for tannin in both the bark and the wood separately, as directed for cinnamon bark.
5. Write a description using the scheme for roots (see p. 121).

Belladonna Root. The root of *Atropa Belladonna* Linn., family Solanaceæ. Collected in the autumn and dried.

1. Select, if possible, a plump root with the aërial stem or stems attached. Sketch it and note the number of rows of branch roots and the colour of the outer surface.
2. Break a piece of the dry root transversely; observe and note the short, non-fibrous fracture and the colour of the exposed surface.

Some commercial roots have a woody fracture, and are often supple, free from starch, and dark coloured within.

3. Smooth the cut end of a softened root, and sketch it to show the corky covering, the dark cambium line, the greyish, vaguely radiate secondary phloem, the scattered, yellowish groups of wood vessels and accompanying smaller tracheids and wood fibres and the small central woody group.

4. If possible make a transverse cut just below the aërial stem. Sketch it to show the central pith and the more radiate structure of the wood. What does this structure indicate ?

5. Scrape some powder from the cut surface of a root, mount it in solution of chloral hydrate, boil till clear and examine microscopically for calcium oxalate. Sketch the crystals.

Calumba Root. The dried transverse slices of the root of *Jateorhiza palmata* (Lam.) Miers, family Menispermaceæ.

1. Measure and record the diameter and thickness of some slices of the root. Sketch the transverse surface and mark the cambium line, cork, phloem, xylem, and medullary rays.

2. Describe the coloration, the manner of shrinkage and the longitudinal grooving. Note the type of fracture, the odour and taste.

3. Scrape some powder from a piece of root and mount it in iodine water ; observe the abundant, large starch granules.

Elecampane Root. The dried root and rhizome of *Inula Helenium* Linn., family Compositæ.

1. Sketch pieces of the drug to show the external form of the rhizome and root. On pieces of the rhizome look for scars left by former aërial stems, and note the longitudinal wrinkles upon the outer surface of all specimens.

2. Break a piece of dry root transversely, and record the nature of the fracture and the odour of the freshly exposed surface.

3. Smooth the cut end of a softened root, and sketch the section. Mark the cork, phloem, cambium line, xylem, medullary rays and the oil-glands.

4. Test the transverse surface with iodine water, and also examine microscopically some dust scraped from the cut end of the root and mounted in water or dilute glycerin.

Sarsaparilla Root. Jamaica sarsaparilla root is the dried root of *Smilax ornata* Hooker filius, family Liliaceæ.

1. Sketch a piece of Jamaica sarsaparilla root to show the strongly wrinkled, reddish-brown outer surface and the small branch roots.

2. Cut a soaked root transversely, and sketch the cut end to show the dark-brown cortex, the pale-yellowish, porous ring of wood, and the central pith which is sometimes largely replaced by a hollow. Test the cut surface with iodine water, and state where starch is found.

3. Cut a root transversely so as to pass through the origin of a branch root, and sketch it. What evidence do you find that sarsaparilla is morphologically a root ?

4. Make similar prepratinons and sketches of Honduras sarsaparilla. Make a note of the features by which the two varieties are distinguished from each other.

NOTES ON SCHEDULE XXXVII

Ipecacuanha Root. Brazilian or Rio ipecacuanha is the official variety, and is distinguished from all other varieties and substitutes by the characters of the annulations and the density of the central woody cylinder which contains no typical vessels. The roots should be soaked in cold water for eighteen hours before dissection.

Belladonna Root. The commercial root is often woody and dark coloured, and nearly free from starch. Some pieces become quite supple after exposure to the air. These large roots of belladonna are frequently sliced longitudinally to facilitate drying. The roots should be prepared for dissection by soaking in cold water for eighteen hours.

Elecampane root should be prepared for dissection by exposure to a moist atmosphere. Choose the uncut thinner roots and also some larger pieces which have been sliced longitudinally. The fracture is short and smooth, and the glands appear as dots scattered throughout the section. The root contains inulin, starch being entirely absent; this gives a dark, horny appearance to the section.

Sarsaparilla roots should be soaked in cold water for eighteen hours. Jamaica sarsaparilla shows in transverse section a dark-brown cortex which is much shrunken and is devoid of starch. The fact that the drug is morphologically a root is evident from the absence of any scale leaves or scars of stems on the outer surface of the specimen. The transverse section shows the endogenous origin of the branch roots, which are seen to be directly connected with the woody ring of the main root.

Honduras sarsaparilla has a yellowish-brown colour, a less wrinkled outer surface and abundant starch in the cortex. The difference in colour is best seen after carefully washing pieces of the soaked root.

SCHEDULE OF INSTRUCTIONS—XXXVIII

Jalap. The dried tubercles of *Ipomœa purga* Hayne, family Convolvulaceæ.

1. Measure the length and thickness of several tubercles and note their condition, whether whole, incised or cut into pieces. Note the odour and taste.

2. Make a habit sketch of a small tubercle to show the fusiform shape, the furrowed and wrinkled outer surface, marked with numerous transverse paler coloured lenticels. Note the colour and density.

3. Cut a softened tubercle transversely and examine the cut surface with a pocket lens. Make a sketch to show the position of the following structures: cork, a narrow layer of secondary phloem, cambium line and the central region. Find the groups of vessels scattered throughout the parenchyma of the central portion and surrounded by cambia which appear as circles, ellipses or irregularly curved lines. Throughout the section, in the secondary and tertiary phloem, find numerous small dark points, which are the resin cells.

4. Scrape some powder from a tubercle and mount it in iodine water; note the abundant starch granules and occasional cluster crystals of calcium oxalate.

Ipomœa. The dried, and usually sliced, tubercle of *Ipomœa orizabensis* (Pellet.) Ledanois, family Convolvulaceæ.

1. Measure an entire tubercle and also some slices, recording the thickness, diameter, shape, colour and density. Note the concentric circles of projecting woody strands.

2. With a scalpel smooth the transverse surface of a piece of the softened drug and examine it with a pocket lens. Sketch it to show

the external cork and the numerous concentric cambia having phloem on the outer side and xylem strands on the inner side; in the centre note a mass of wood. In all the phloem regions find numerous resin cells, appearing as dark points.

3. Examine scrapings of a slice for starch and note the odour and taste of the drug.

NOTES ON SCHEDULE XXXVIII

Jalap and Ipomœa are softened by soaking in water for several days until they can be easily cut with a knife.

SCHEDULE OF INSTRUCTIONS—XXXIX

JUICES; OPIUM, ALOES, EUPHORBIUM, KINO

Opium. The inspissated latex of the unripe capsule of *Papaver somniferum* Linn., family Papaveraceæ.

1. Sketch a piece of *Turkish* opium wrapped in poppy leaf to show the form of the mass, the midrib and veins of the leaf and the adherent fruits of *Rumex*. Record the dimensions of the mass.

2. Examine and sketch some of the fruits of *Rumex* and note their significance.

3. Sketch a cake of *Turkish Government Monopoly* opium to show the covering of broken poppy leaves and the manufacturer's mark. Note the shape and record the dimensions of a cake.

4. In a similar way examine and sketch pieces of *Persian* opium.

5. Examine some poppy capsules showing the types of incisions made in obtaining the latex from the plant.

6. Write descriptions to the samples of opium examined, using the scheme for unorganised drugs (see p. 125).

Aloes. The juice from the leaves of *Aloe vera* Linn., *Aloe Perryi* Baker, and other species of aloe, family Liliaceæ, evaporated to dryness.

1. Examine hand-specimens of Cape, Curaçao, Socotrine and Zanzibar aloes; describe each, using the scheme for unorganised drugs (see p. 125).

2. Examine Socotrine, Zanzibar, Barbadoes (Curaçao) and Cape aloes by the following method: Place a small piece, about the size of a pin's head, upon a slide, crush it to powder and add a drop of lacto-phenol. Apply a cover-glass and press it down with the finger to distribute the powdered aloes through the liquid. Examine with the microscope, and by records and sketches indicate the characteristic features of each variety. How do you account for the differences observed?

3. Prepare a clear solution of each of the four varieties of aloes by the following method: Weigh out 0·5 gm. of aloes, warm it with 50 ml. of distilled water in a beaker flask until dissolved as completely as possible, cool and add from 0·5 to 1·0 gm. of diatomaceous earth, shake and filter, repeating the filtration, if necessary, until a clear, bright filtrate is obtained.

4. *Borax Test* for barbaloin (Schouteten's reaction). Measure 5 ml.

of each of the clear filtrates from (3) into test-tubes, to each add 0·2 gm. of borax, dissolve by boiling; pour a few drops of the dark fluid formed into a test-tube three parts filled with water, and note the strong green fluorescence.

5. *Bromine Test* for aloin. Measure 2 ml. of each of the clear filtrates from (3) into test-tubes and add to each an equal volume or an excess of freshly prepared bromine water; note the copious yellow precipitate.

6. *Nitric Acid Test.* Measure 5 ml. of each of the clear filtrates from (3) into test-tubes and add to each 2 ml. of strong nitric acid (s.g. 1·42). Note the characteristic colour given to each variety.

7. *Cupraloin Reaction* for isobarbaloin. Dilute 1 ml. of each of the clear filtrates from (3) to 10 ml. with distilled water, giving a solution of 1 part of aloes in 1,000 of water. To 10 ml. of this dilute aloes solution add one drop of a 5 per cent. solution of copper sulphate, 0·5 ml. of a saturated solution of sodium chloride, and 1 ml. of alcohol; warm gently. Note the colour produced.

8. Apply the test for anthraquinone derivatives as described under cascara sagrada, see Schedule IX., p. 24.

Euphorbium. The dried latex of *Euphorbia resinifera* Berg, family Euphorbiaceæ.

1. Sketch and describe some typical pieces of the drug.

2. Remove some of the spiny stipules, some of the typical euphorbiaceous inflorescences (cyathia) and some of the tri-carpellary fruits and sketch them. Note their significance.

3. Take 1 gm. of euphorbium and 2 gm. of sand, and powder them together; transfer to a dry test-tube, add 4 ml. of petroleum spirit and shake vigorously. Filter. Into a second test-tube run from a burette 2 ml. of sulphuric acid containing 1 ml. of nitric acid in every 400 ml. (1 drop in 20 ml.); carefully pour a little of the petroleum spirit solution on to the surface of the acid and note the blood-red ring formed at the junction.

Kino. The juice obtained from incisions in the trunk of *Pterocarpus Marsupium* Roxb., evaporated to dryness.

1. Prepare a 1 in 20 aqueous solution. To the cold solution add some 20 per cent. by volume sulphuric acid. Explain the action.

2. Dilute some of the 1 in 20 solution to about one-tenth its strength and add ferric chloride solution.

3. Make similar tests with tannic acid and with red gum.

NOTES ON SCHEDULE XXXIX

Turkish Monopoly Opium is the form in which opium is now exported from Turkey. The opium is passed through a mixer which makes it fairly uniform, and is then moulded into cylindrical cakes, somewhat resembling cheeses, about 15 cm. in diameter and 10 cm. high, which are coated externally with a covering of roughly powdered poppy leaves. Each cake weighs about 2 kilos.

Aloes. Note especially the colour, the appearance of the fractured surface, and the odour of the different varieties of aloes; these characters are usually sufficient to enable one to distinguish the different kinds from one another.

Hepatic varieties of aloes show numerous fine needle-shaped crystals under the microscope, vitreous varieties are amorphous. All varieties of aloes, except Natal aloes, react to the borax test. The nitric acid test gives with Socotrine aloes a brownish-yellow, with Zanzibar aloes a yellowish-brown, with Curaçao aloes a deep brownish-red, and with Cape aloes a deep green. The cupraloin reaction gives a negative result with Socotrine aloes and only a faint evanescent colour with Cape aloes ; with Curaçao aloes a reddish-violet colour is obtained. Distilled water must be used in making the solutions of aloes ; solutions made with tap-water fail to give the cupraloin reaction.

Cape, Curaçao and Socotrine aloes all respond to the test for anthraquinone derivatives ; *Zanzibar aloes does not* give a positive reaction.

SCHEDULE OF INSTRUCTIONS—XL

EXTRACTS ; AGAR, GAMBIER, GELATIN

Agar-Agar (Japanese Isinglass). A gelatinous substance prepared from *Gelidium corneum* Lam., *G. cartilagineum* Gaill., *Sphærococcus compressus* Ag. and other algæ. Division, Rhodophyceæ.

1. Weigh out 0·5 gm. of agar, cut it into small fragments and soak it in 50 ml. of water in a conical flask, boil it until it is dissolved. Cool about 2 ml. in a test-tube and note that it sets to a firm jelly.

2. Take 4 ml. of the 1 per cent. solution ; add 0·5 ml. hydrochloric acid, sp. gr. 1·16, and heat for 30 minutes on a water-bath. Divide into two equal parts ; to one add 1·5 ml. of 20 per cent. caustic soda and 1 ml. of Fehling's reagent and warm on a water-bath. Observe the reduction. To the other half add solution of barium chloride ; the white precipitate indicates sulphates.

3. Weigh out 0·5 gm. of strip agar and boil it with 10 ml. of diluted sulphuric acid (1 volume of strong acid, s.g. 1·843, and 20 volumes of water). Stand aside for ten minutes to allow insoluble matter to settle. Remove a little of the deposit with a dipping tube (see below) and mount it for the microscope ; examine first with the 16 mm. objective and then with the 4 mm. objective. Can you find any diatoms ? What is the significance of their presence ?

4. Soak a piece of agar, about 2 mm. square, in water until quite soft, then squeeze it flat on a slide beneath a cover-glass ; examine it and search for diatoms like those separated by diluted sulphuric acid.

5. Scrape some dust from a piece of agar, mount it in ruthenium red and note the deep red stain.

6. Warm a small piece of agar with solution of caustic soda and note the canary yellow colour of the agar.

7. Write a description of the drug.

Gambier (Pale Catechu). An extract of the leaves and young shoots of *Uncaria Gambier* Roxb., family Rubiaceæ.

1. Boil 0·3 gm. of gambier in a test-tube with 2 ml. of 90 per cent. alcohol, filter, and add to the filtrate 2 ml. of 20 per cent. aqueous caustic soda, shake, and add 2 ml. of petroleum spirit, shake, allow to separate and note the brilliant green fluorescence in the upper layer.

2. Mount some powdered gambier in lactophenol for microscopical examination, and note the innumerable, rapidly soluble, small needle-shaped crystals.

3. Boil 2 gm. of gambier with 5 ml. of water until dissolved ; allow the solution to stand until insoluble matter has settled (or separate by a centrifuge) ; remove a little of the deposit with a dipping tube,

place it on a microscope slide and examine it. Sketch some characteristic particles and state the conclusion you draw from their presence.

4. Write a description of gambier using the scheme for unorganised drugs, see p. 125.

5. Compare cutch or black catechu with gambier or pale catechu.

Gelatin. The dried extract made from defatted bones and certain other animal tissues by prolonged boiling with water, concentrating and cooling the liquor.

1. Soak 1 gm. of gelatin in 50 ml. of cold water till softened, then warm on a water-bath and note that it dissolves, leaving no residue. On cooling a little in a test-tube it sets to a jelly.

2. Dilute some of the above solution with an equal volume of water and to small volumes of the solution add separately, solution of tannic

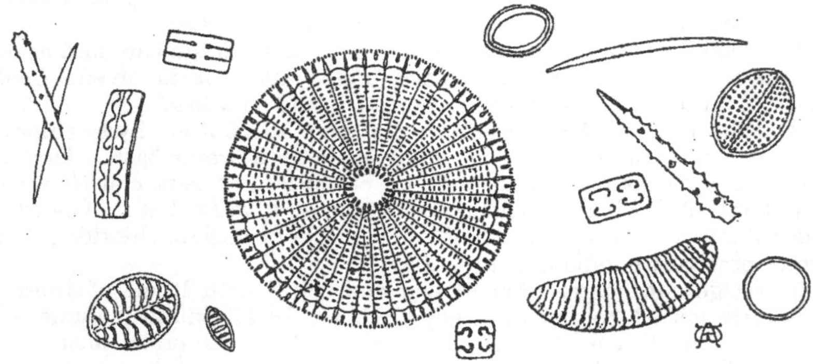

Fig. 60.—Diatoms and sponge spicules from a specimen of agar-agar, × 250. The large discoid diatom is *Arachnoidiscus Ehrenbergii*. Two sponge spicules are seen lying one over the other on the extreme left of the drawing, and two others, separate, on the right.

acid (10 per cent.) and solution of picric acid or trinitrophenol (1 per cent.). Note the precipitate formed with each reagent.

3. To further quantities of the dilute solution add solutions of alum, lead acetate and ferric chloride ; note the absence of a precipitate indicating the absence of chondrin.

4. To a little dilute solution add Millon's reagent, note the whitish precipitate ; boil and note the change in colour.

5. Heat a little gelatin in a small hard-glass tube with soda lime ; note the odour and the reaction to litmus of the vapours evolved.

6. Warm a small piece of gelatin in acetic acid (33 per cent.) and observe its solution.

7. To a dilute solution add lead acetate, then add caustic alkali and boil. Note the absence of any blackening (distinction from albumen).

8. Write a description of sheet gelatin and of strip gelatin. Note the differences from agar both in appearance and in behaviour when tested.

NOTES ON SCHEDULE XL

Agar-Agar does not consist of the algæ themselves, but is a preparation made from them.

SCHEDULE OF INSTRUCTIONS—XLII

RESINS; COLOPHONY, GUAIACUM RESIN, BENZOIN, ARAROBA

Colophony. The resin left after distilling the crude turpentine obtained by incision into the stem of various species of *Pinus*, family Pinaceæ.

1. Describe the external features of pieces of colophony, noting especially the colour, fracture and the colour of the powder.

2. Note the solubility of colophony in alcohol, chloroform, and carbon disulphide, and its insolubility in water.

3. Shake 0·05 gm. of powdered colophony with 5 ml. of light petroleum and note its solubility; filter and shake 2 ml. of the filtrate with twice its volume of 0·1 per cent. aqueous solution of copper acetate: after allowing to separate, note the coloration of the light petroleum layer.

4. Dissolve 0·05 g. of colophony by warming it with 3 ml. of acetic anhydride, cool and add one drop of sulphuric acid, s.g. 1·842. Note the production of a purplish red colour changing rapidly to violet and finally brown.

Guaiacum Resin. The resin obtained from the stem of *Guaiacum officinale* Linn., or of *Guaiacum sanctum* Linn., family Zygophyllaceæ.

1. Compare the external appearance of guaiacum resin with that of colophony, noting especially the colour of the powder and its alteration when exposed to the air.

2. *Reaction for Guaiaconic Acid.* Dissolve 0·05 gm. of freshly powdered resin in 5 ml. of 90 per cent. alcohol and add 1 ml. of a solution of ferric chloride (0·05 per cent. in water). A deep-blue colour is produced.

Benzoin. A balsamic resin obtained from *Styrax Benzoin* Dryand., family Styraceæ.

1. Write out the physical characters of benzoin, using the schedule for description of unorganised drugs (p. 125).

2. Heat a little benzoin in a dry tube; note that it melts and evolves irritating whitish fumes which condense to a white sublimate on the upper cool part of the tube; test the vapours with litmus paper.

3. Heat 0·5 gm. of Sumatra benzoin in a test-tube with 5 ml. of a 1 per cent. aqueous solution of potassium permanganate, and note the odour of benzaldehyde.

4. Treat Siam benzoin in the same way and record the result.

Araroba. The substance removed from cavities in the trunk of *Andira Araroba* Aguiar, family Leguminosæ.

Warm 1 gm. of araroba with 5 ml. of benzene in a test-tube on a water-bath, shake and filter. Evaporate the filtrate and test a little of the residue (chrysarobin) for chrysophanic acid as follows: Upon a white tile, mix about 1 mg. of chrysarobin with a drop of fuming nitric acid (sp. gr. 1·5), and note the brownish-red liquid produced. Now allow a drop or two of 10 per cent. solution of ammonia to fall upon the plate beside the nitric acid solution, and watch the two solutions as they mix. At the line of contact a brilliant, evanescent, blue-violet colour is produced, and rapidly becomes dull-reddish violet.

Note.—The nitric acid oxidises chrysarobin to chrysophanic acid, which gives the coloration with ammonia. Only traces of the free acid are present in chrysarobin.

SCHEDULE OF INSTRUCTIONS—XLIII

GUM-RESINS; MYRRH, AMMONIACUM, GALBANUM, ASAFETIDA

Myrrh. An oleo-gum-resin obtained from the stem of *Commiphora molmol* Holmes, and probably other species of *Commiphora*, family Burseraceæ.

1. Describe myrrh, using the scheme for unorganised drugs.

2. Triturate 0·03 g. of myrrh with 1·5 g. of sand; shake 1 gm. of the mixture with 3 ml. of ether, filter the solution into a porcelain dish, and allow the ether to evaporate, leaving a thin film of oleo-resin; stand for two or three minutes, and then allow the vapour of bromine to flow over the film. A violet coloration is quickly produced.

Note.—The bromine vapour may be conveniently obtained by pouring the vapour into the dish from a bottle of bromine water.

3. Rub down a small piece of myrrh in a mortar with water and note than an emulsion is formed, owing to the presence of gum with the resin and volatile oil in the drug.

Ammoniacum. A gum-resin exuded from the flowering and fruiting stem of *Dorema Ammoniacum* D. Don, and possibly other species of *Dorema*, family Umbelliferæ.

1. Make an emulsion of 1 gm. of ammoniacum with 10 ml. of water, add solution of chlorinated soda, and an orange-red coloration is produced.

2. *Test for Free Salicylic Acid.* Shake 1 gm. of powdered ammoniacum in a test-tube with ether, decant the ether into a clean test-tube, add a drop of 5 per cent. solution of ferric chloride, and a small crystal of sodium carbonate when the ether acquires a violet colour.

3. Carry out the tests for umbelliferone (free and combined), as directed under galbanum and asafetida respectively. Note the entire absence of umbelliferone.

Galbanum. A gum-resin obtained from *Ferula galbaniflua* Boissier and Buhse, and probably from other species of *Ferula*, family Umbelliferæ.

Test for Free Umbelliferone. Weigh out 0·2 gm. of galbanum, mix it with 2 gm. of sand (in No. 30 powder), and powder thoroughly; transfer the mixture to a test-tube, add 5 ml. of 90 per cent. alcohol and boil for one or two minutes, cool, filter into 5 ml. of alcohol, mixed with 0·5 ml. of 10 per cent. solution of ammonia. A blue fluorescence is produced.

Asafetida. A gum-resin obtained from the root of *Ferula fœtida* Regel, *F. rubricaulis* Boissier, and probably other species of *Ferula*, family Umbelliferæ.

1. To the newly exposed surface of a freshly broken tear of asafetida, apply a drop of sulphuric acid (sp. gr. 1·841), by means of a thin glass rod, and note the red coloration; wash off the acid and note the bright violet colour remaining.

2. Touch the surface of a freshly broken tear with a drop of dilute nitric acid (1 volume of strong acid and 1 volume of water), and note the green coloration.

3. Carry out the test for free umbelliferone, as detailed for galbanum. Note the negative result.

4. *Test for Combined Umbelliferone.* Boil 0·2 gm. of asafetida with 2 ml. of hydrochloric acid (sp. gr. 1·16) for about one minute, cool, dilute with an equal volume of water, and filter into 3 ml. of 10 per cent. solution of ammonia, and observe the fluorescence.

5. Describe asafetida, using the scheme for unorganised drugs (p. 125).

SCHEDULE OF INSTRUCTIONS—XLIV

OLEO-RESINS AND BALSAMS; COPAIBA, STORAX, TOLU, BALSAM OF PERU

Copaiba. The oleo-resin obtained from the stem of *Copaifera Lansdorfii* Desf. and other species of *Copaifera.*

1. Graduate a test-tube with water and a strip of paper gummed on the outside to read 3 ml. and 4 ml.; rinse it with 10 per cent. solution of ammonia, shake as dry as possible and fill with copaiba to the 3 ml. mark, then add 10 per cent. solution of ammonia to the 4 ml. mark stir with a glass rod and note that a clear fluid results.

2. From a burette run into a test-tube 2 ml. of a mixture of glacial acetic and nitric acids in the proportion of 1 drop of the latter to 3 ml. of the former. Allow 2 drops of copaiba balsam to fall on to the acid, shake and note the absence of a red or purple tint.

3. Repeat the experiment with copaiba containing Gurjun balsam, and observe the coloration produced.

4. Evaporate about 1 ml. of copaiba in a dish on a water-bath; note the absence of any odour of turpentine in the vapours and the brittle nature of the cooled residue of resin.

5. Describe copaiba under the headings; colour, sp. gr. (greater or less than 1·0); viscosity; odour; taste; chemical and other tests.

Storax. A viscid balsam obtained from the wounded trunk of *Liquidambar orientalis* Mill, family Hamamelidaceæ.

1. To 2 gm. of a mixture of 3 parts of sand and 1 part of storax add 2 ml. of a 10 per cent. solution of potassium chromate and 1 ml. of strong sulphuric acid. Shake, but do not boil, and note the odour of benzaldehyde.

2. To 2 gm. of the mixture of storax with sand in a test-tube add some solution of potassium permanganate (2 per cent.), warm and note the odour of benzaldehyde.

3. Gently warm 0·5 gm. storax in 1·0 mil. chloral hydrate solution and observe its complete solution.

4. Describe storax.

Tolu. The balsam obtained from the trunk of *Myroxylon toluifera* H.B. and K., family Leguminosæ.

1. Put a small piece on to the centre of a microscope slide and cover it with a second slide; warm gently over a flame and press the two slides together till the balsam forms a thin film. Examine the mount with a pocket lens or the low power of the microscope and sketch a few of the crystals of cinnamic acid visible in the mass.

2. Make a solution in alcohol and test it with litmus paper: record the reaction.

3. To some of the alcoholic solution add solution of ferric chloride note the green colour probably due to toluresinotannol.

4. Boil 0·5 gm. of tolu with 2·5 ml. of water and filter. To the filtrate add 0·3 gm. of potassium permanganate and warm. Note the odour of benzaldehyde.

Balsam of Peru. The balsam obtained from the trunk of *Myroxylon Pereiræ* (Royle) Klotzsch, family Leguminosæ.

N.B.—For the following tests use Balsam of Peru mixed with three times its weight of acid-washed sand.

1. To 2 gm. of the mixture add 2 ml. of a 3 in 2 solution of chloral hydrate, shake and allow to settle. Note that the balsam of Peru forms a clear solution.

2. To 2 gm. of the mixture add 5 ml. of light petroleum, shake and filter. Evaporate 4 ml. of the filtrate on a water-bath and examine the residue; note the absence of any odour of benzaldehyde or of turpentine.

3. To 1·0 ml. of the filtrate obtained in (2) above, add twice its volume of solution of copper acetate (0·1 per cent.), shake and after separation note the absence of any green tint in the upper layer, indicating an absence of colonhony.

4. Write a description of Balsam of Peru.

NOTES ON SCHEDULE XLIV

Copaiba. The test of miscibility with ammonia shows the absence of fatty oils. Instead of using copaiba itself, the test for gurjun balsam is often made with the volatile oil removed by distillation *in vacuo* or in steam.

Tolu. Powdered tolu shaken in the cold with 1 per cent. solution of potassium permanganate gives a strong odour of benzaldehyde.

Storax and Balsam of Peru. By mixing the balsams with sand, they become much easier to handle, and the weighing out of definite amounts is facilitated. The mixture is also more readily extracted by solvents.

SCHEDULE OF INSTRUCTIONS—XLV

TARS, OILS, FATS

Wood Tar or Stockholm Tar. A bituminous liquid obtained by the destructive distillation of the wood of *Pinus sylvestris* Linn., and of other species of *Pinus*, family Pinaceæ.

Mix wood tar with sufficient sand (in No. 30 powder) to form a stiff paste, and carry out the following tests with the mixture:

1. Shake some of the mixture in a test-tube with 5 ml. of water, which acquires a yellowish tint, but is almost colourless after filtering. Test the filtered solution with litmus paper and note the acid reaction. To a cubic centimetre of the filtrate add one or two drops of a 0·05 per cent. solution of ferric chloride and observe the red coloration produced.

2. Put a little of the mixture into a test-tube and shake it vigorously with 15 ml. of light petroleum and filter. To 3 ml. to 5 ml. of the filtrate add an equal volume of a 5 per cent. solution of copper acetate and shake. Allow to separate, and pour off a little of the upper layer into a clean

in a dish; to the residue add 1 drop of a 1 per cent. *w/v* solution of resorcinol in hydrochloric acid (s.g. 1·16).

Make the test with pure honey and note the absence of any persistent herry-red colour. Repeat with honey containing artificial invert ugar and note the cherry-red colour produced.

3. Remove any scum present on the surface of the honey; mount me in lactophenol and examine it microscopically for pollen grains.

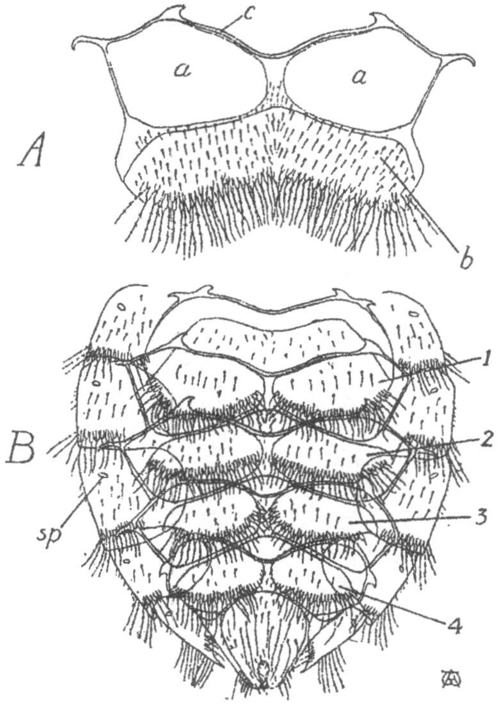

.—*Apis mellifica*, the worker bee. *A*, ventral plate of a worker bee. wer surface of the abdomen of a worker bee. *a*, transparent area which wax is secreted; *b*, portion of the plate carrying hairs and pping the plate immediately posterior to it; *c*, chitinous frame; iracle; 1, 2, 3 and 4, the four overlapping ventral plates upon wax is secreted. All × 8.

x. The wax from the honeycomb of the hive bee, *Apis* inn., family Apidæ.

for fatty substances and resin. Into a 100 ml. conical flask n. of wax and add 20 ml. of 10 per cent. aqueous caustic k the level of the liquid by a strip of paper on the outside k. Boil for ten minutes, being careful to avoid spurting, up the volume with water. Cool, filter through a small estos in the throat of a funnel and acidify the clear filtrate chloric acid. Make the experiment with genuine beeswax, when no turbidity appears, and make a second experiment using wax containing 10 per cent. of Japan wax, stearic acid, fat or resin, when a turbidity will form.

2. *Test for paraffin and similar waxes.* Weigh out 1 gm. of wax and put it into a flask with 10 ml. of seminormal alcoholic caustic potash and 10 ml. of alcohol (95 per cent.). Attach a water-cooled reflux condenser and boil for one hour. Detach the flask, insert a thermometer and allow the liquid to cool with constant stirring. Note the temperatures at which the liquid becomes cloudy and at which large flocks

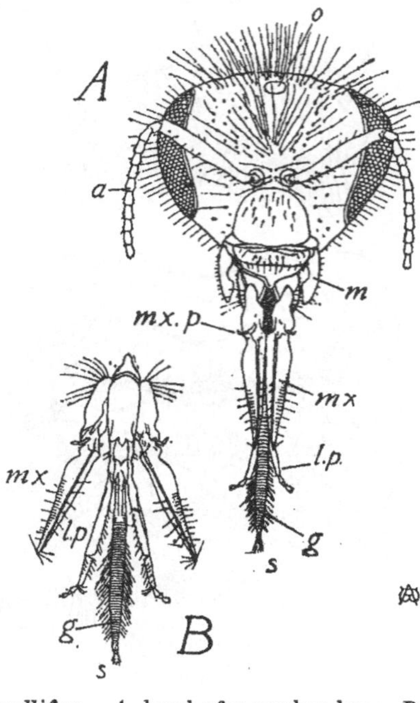

Fig. 62.—*Apis mellifica.* *A*, head of a worker bee; *B*, proboscis, showing the constituent parts separated. *a*, antenna; *e*, compound eye; *g*, glossa or tongue; *l.p.* labial palp; *m*, mandible; *mx*, maxilla; *mx.p*, maxillary palp; *o*, ocellus or single eye. *s*, spoon-shaped tip. All × 8.

are precipitated. There should not be more than 2 degrees between these two temperatures and the cloudiness should not occur above 61°.

Make this experiment with genuine wax and with wax containing 10 per cent. of paraffin.

3. Write a description of beeswax.

Spermaceti (Cetaceum). A solid wax obtained from the sperm whale *Physeter macrocephalus* Linn.

1. Weigh out 0·2 gm. of spermaceti and boil it in a small conical flask with 15 ml. of alcohol. Note that complete solution takes place.

Note.—Stearin, paraffin wax, tallow and similar fats are all insoluble in alcohol.

NOTES ON SCHEDULE XLVI

Hive bees should be preserved in alcohol until required for dissection. The wax-secreting areas occur in pairs, one pair on each of four of the sterna, or ventral portions of the chitinous segments, of the abdomen. The areas upon which the wax is secreted are perfectly plain, slightly sunk,

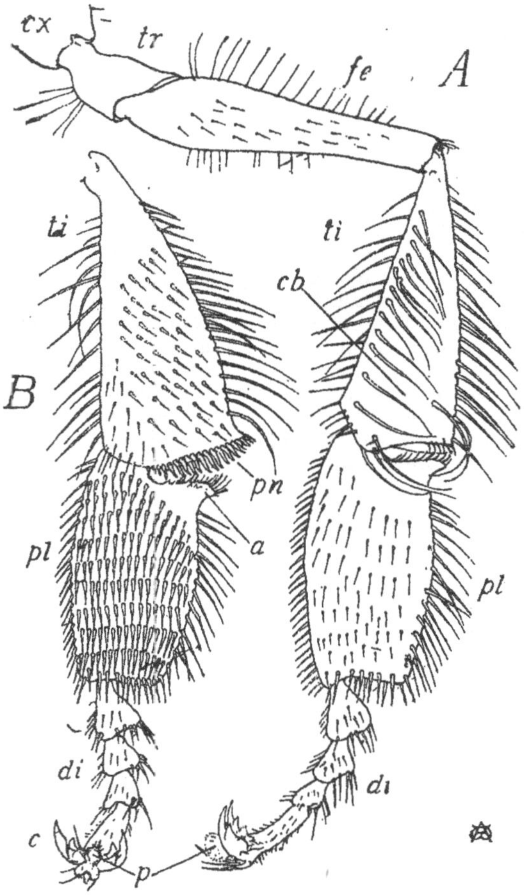

FIG. 63.—*Apis mellifica.* Hind legs of a worker bee. *A*, outer surface of a leg. *B*, inner surface of the tibia and tarsus of a leg. *a*, auricle; *c*, claw; *cb*, corbiculum or pollen-basket; *cx*, coxa; *di*, digiti or small joints of the tarsus or foot; *fe*, femur; *p*, pulvillus or cushion between the claws; *pl*, planta or first joint of the foot; *pn*, pecten or comb; *ti*, tibia; *tr*, trochanter. All × 15.

and are surrounded by firm chitinous margins, the posterior of which are fringed with feathered hairs and overlap the anterior portions of the plates of the sternum posterior to them. Fig. 61, A, shows an isolated sternum with its pair of wax-secreting areas, and Fig. 61, B, shows the whole series of overlapping sterna from the abdomen of a bee. The mouth parts of the bee are modified to form a proboscis, up which nectar may be drawn into the honey stomach. This suctorial mouth is derived from a mouth of the biting type, such as is found in *Cantharis*, and the corresponding parts are indicated in the drawings in Fig. 62. The mandibles are strongly constructed, and are used for manipulating the plates of wax secreted beneath the abdomen; the maxillæ and labium are modified in such a way that, when closed together, they form a long hollow tube, up which the nectar travels (Fig. 62). The hind leg is remarkable in the construction of the tibia and the basal joint of the tarsus or foot. The tibia (Fig. 63) widens rapidly downwards towards the distal extremity, which is provided with a row of stiff bristles, named the pecten or comb. The outer surface of the tibia is strongly concave, the edges being fringed with long curved hairs, so forming a receptacle in which the bee places the pollen removed from its body by the pollen-brush upon the foot of the opposite leg. The first joint of the tarsus or foot is hinged to one margin of the wide end of the tibia, and is itself very broad and flat, being only about twice as long as wide; this basal joint is named the planta (see Fig. 63). The inner surface of the planta carries ten rows of stiff hairs, forming a brush with which the bee cleans the pollen from the hairs which thickly clothe its body. The articulation of the planta to the tibia being at the interior margin only, the remainder of the opposing surfaces between the two joints forms a pair of pincers (see Fig. 63), with which the bee seizes hold of the edges of the plates of wax protruding between the abdominal sterna; at the same time, the teeth of the tibial comb pierce the plate, which is thus firmly held while it is being drawn out to be passed on to the anterior legs and so to the mouth, where it is masticated and rendered plastic before incorporation in the comb of the hive.

PART II

DRUG DESCRIPTION AND HABITATS

DESCRIPTION OF DRUGS

An important function of the pharmacognosist is to write adequate descriptions of the drugs which he studies, and for this purpose a scheme for the description of parts of plants is necessary. Such a scheme in very brief outline is given below, and by following it the worker will acquire a uniform method of expression, and will tend to avoid the accidental omission of characters, which may be of diagnostic importance.

The particulars suggested sometimes differ from those required for purely biological descriptions, because one is frequently concerned with dried structures, which may have been subjected to manipulation during preparation for the market, and also because certain points of pharmacognostical importance may possess too small a value for inclusion in the descriptions of systematic biology.

Skeleton Plan for the Description of Plant Members

ROOTS AND RHIZOMES

1. **Size and Colour.** As seen in bulk.
2. **Shape.** (*a*) Cylindrical, conical, fusiform, napiform, etc.
(*b*) Straight, tortuous, knotted, etc.
3. **Branching.** Fibrous, tuberous, fascicled, etc.
4. **Condition.** Fresh, dry, peeled, unpeeled. Whole : cut vertically, longitudinally, into transverse slices, etc.
5. **Rootlets.** (*a*) Present or absent.
(*b*) Kind—true, adventitious, etc.
(*c*) Attached, loose, thin, thick, wiry, brittle, etc.
6. **Direction of Growth.** Horizontal, ascending, inclined, vertical, etc.
7. **Surface Characters.** Scale leaves, scars of stems or roots, lenticels, etc.
8. **Transverse Section.** Arrangement of vascular tissues, pith, cortex, woody cylinder, medullary rays, secretory structures, etc.
9. **Food Storage.** Starch, inulin, sugar, etc.
10. **Fracture and Texture.** Starchy, horny, fibrous, etc.
11. **Odour and Taste.**
12. **Peculiarities.** Abnormalities of xylem, or of leaf traces, etc.
13. **Chemical Tests.**

STEMS

1. **Kind.** Herbaceous, shrubby, woody, rhizome, annual, biennial, etc.
2. **Direction.** Upright, spreading, creeping, climbing, etc.

3. **Shape.** Terete (cylindrical), angular, square, ribbed, winged, etc.
4. **Surface.** Colour, smooth, hairy, rough, etc.
5. **Phyllotaxis.** Opposite, decussate, whorled, alternate ($\frac{1}{2}$, $\frac{1}{3}$, $\frac{2}{5}$, $\frac{3}{8}$, etc.), sets of crossing spirals (3 : 8, etc.).
6. **Transverse Section.** General arrangement of the tissues.

BARKS

1. **Shape of Pieces.** Quills, channelled, flat, recurved, etc.
2. **Dimensions.** Length, breadth, thickness, etc.
3. **Colour.** As seen in bulk.
4. **Outer Surface.** Cork, rhytidoma, colour, surface condition (*i.e.*, cracks, furrows, etc.), etc.
5. **Inner Surface.** Colour and surface condition.
6. **Fracture.** Short, fibrous, granular, etc.
7. **Transverse Section.** General arrangement of the tissues, *e.g.*, cork, cortex, phloem, medullary rays, etc.
8. **Odour and Taste.**
9. **Peculiarities and Chemical Tests.**

WOODS

1. **Colour and Density.**
2. **Grain.** Straight, behaviour when split, etc.
3. **Annual Rings.** Present or absent, width, etc.
4. **Vessels.** Diffuse porous, ring porous, etc.
5. **Medullary Rays.** Appearance, width, number per millimetre, etc.
6. **Wood Parenchyma.** Tangential bands, etc.
7. **Odour and Taste.**
8. **Peculiarities and Chemical Tests.**

LEAVES

1. **Dimensions.** Length, relative length and breadth.
2. **Colour.** As seen in bulk.
3. **Condition.** Fresh, dry, whole, broken, shrivelled, flat, etc.
4. **Lamina.** (*a*) *Composition.* Simple, compound, palmate, etc.

(*b*) *Incision.* -fid, -partite, -sect, etc.

(*c*) *Venation.* Parallel, reticulate, etc. Number of principal veins (uninerved, two-nerved, etc.).

(*d*) *Margin.* Entire, dentate, serrate, etc.

(*e*) *Apex.* Acute, obtuse, acuminate, etc.

(*f*) *Base.* Entire, cordate, etc.

(*g*) *General Outline.* Ovate, lanceolate, linear, etc. If compound, describe also the leaflets.

(*h*) *Surface.* Smooth, hairy, etc.

(*i*) *Texture.* Coriaceous, papery, etc.

5. **Petiole.** Long, short, grooved, cylindrical, flattened, etc. If absent, the leaf is sessile.

6. **Leaf Base.** *Stipules,* absent or present. If present, describe as lamina of leaf.

Sheath, if present, describe it.

Pulvinus, etc.

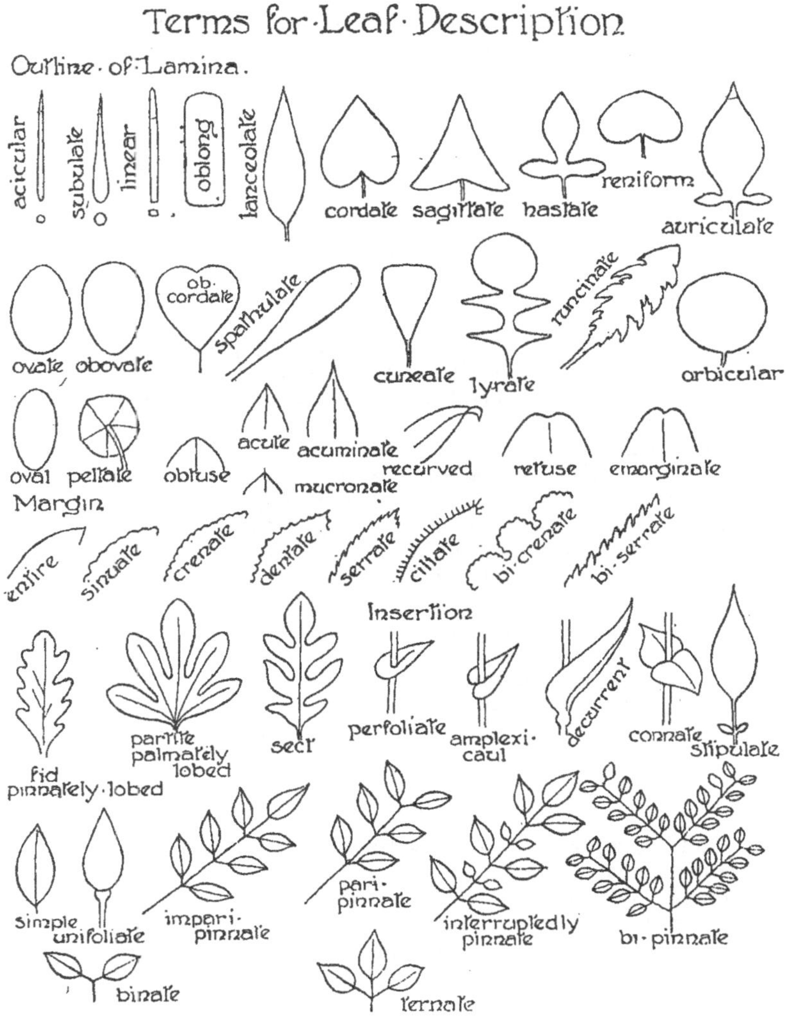

FIG. 64—Terms for leaf description.

7. **Insertion.** Radical, cauline, etc.

8. **Phyllotaxis.** Opposite, whorled, alternate, one-half, one-third, 5 : 8, etc.

9. **Peculiarities.** (*a*) Presence of glands, special adaptations, etc.

(*b*) Taste and Odour.

INFLORESCENCE

1. **Kind.** Racemose, cymose, simple, compound, etc.
2. **Axis, or Receptacle.** Elongated, flattened, conical, solid, hollow, etc.
3. **Bracts.** Shape, size, colour, etc. Involucre, involucel, etc.
4. **Distribution of Flowers.** Ray and disc florets, etc.

FLOWERS

1. **General Features.** Regular, zygomorphic, complete, perfect, unisexual, etc.

2. **Calyx.** (*a*) *Number* of sepals or of divisions, if gamosepalous.
(*b*) *Cohesion.* Gamosepalous or polysepalous.
(*c*) *Insertion.* Superior or inferior.
(*d*) *Peculiarities.* Colour, shape, etc.

3. **Corolla.** (*a*), (*b*), and (*d*) as calyx.
(*c*) *Insertion.* Hypogynous, perigynous or epigynous.
N.B.—If a perianth, describe as the calyx.

4. **Corona,** or other appendages between the corolla and stamens, *e.g.*, disc, glands, etc.

5. **Androecium.** (*a*) *Number* of stamens.
(*b*) *Cohesion.* Free, monadelphous, etc.
(*c*) *Insertion.* Hypogynous, perigynous, epipetalous, etc
(*d*) *Peculiarities.* Tetradynamous, didynamous, etc.
(*e*) *Filament, Anther,* and mode of dehiscence.

6. **Gynæcium.** (*a*) *Number* of carpels.
(*b*) *Cohesion.* Apocarpous, syncarpous, etc.
(*c*) *Insertion.* Superior or inferior.
(*d*) *Peculiarities* of :—
Style. Long, short, simple, branched, etc.
Stigma. Sessile, capitate, radiate, etc.
Ovary. Number of loculi, placentation, number of ovules, etc.

FRUITS

1. **Kind.** Simple, aggregate, compound, succulent, dry, etc.
2. **Dimensions.** Length, breadth, etc.
3. **Shape.** Globular, ovoid, flattened, etc.
4. **Insertion.** Superior, inferior, etc.
5. **Dehiscence.** Dehiscent or indehiscent. If dehiscent, mode of dehiscence.

6. **Pericarp.** (*a*) *Colour.*
(*b*) *Texture.* Woody, papery, etc.
(*c*) *Markings.* Ridges, stigma, scars, etc.
(*d*) *Sutures.* Ventral and dorsal.
(*e*) *Differentiation.* Epicarp. Thin, tough, etc.
Mesocarp. Fleshy, fibrous, vittæ, etc.
Endocarp. Woody, parchment-like, etc.
(*f*) *Loculi.* Number.

(*g*) *Placentation.* Axile, parietal, etc., seeds adherent to pericarp or loose.

7. **Seeds.** Number.

8. **Peculiarities.** Odour, taste, special adaptations to dispersal, etc.

SEEDS

1. **Physical Characters.** Shape, dimensions, hardness, etc.
2. **Seed coats.** Number, markings, hilum, raphe, aril, arillode, etc.
3. **Perisperm.** Present or absent, nature of reserves.
4. **Endosperm.** Present or absent, nature of reserves.
5. **Embryo.** (*a*) Position, shape, dimensions.

(*b*) *Cotyledons.* Colour, outline, venation, straight, curved, folded, etc.

(*c*) *Radicle.* Accumbent, incumbent, etc.

6. **Odour and Taste.**
7. **Weight** of 100 seeds.
8. **Peculiarities.** Adaptions to dispersal, etc.
9. **Chemical Tests.**

Skeleton Plan for the Description of Insects

INSECT

1. **Dimensions** and **Colour.**
2. **Shape** and **Division** of the body.
3. **Head.** Shape and position.

Appendages to the head.

(*a*) *Antennæ.* Filiform, club-shaped, number of joints, colour, etc.

(*b*) *Eyes.* Simple or compound.

(*c*) *Mouth parts.* Biting, suctorial, etc.

4. **Thorax.** Shape and dimensions.

Appendages to the thorax.

(*a*) *Wings.* Number, texture, arrangement, markings, etc.

(*b*) *Legs.* Number, special features, *e.g.*, modification of tibia or other joints, number of joints in the tarsus, number of claws, etc.

5. **Abdomen.** Shape and proportion to the whole body, number of segments ; special adaptations.
6. **Peculiarities.** Blistering property ; colouring matter, etc.
7. **Odour.**

Skeleton Plan for the Description of Unorganised Drugs, *e.g.*, *Resins*, *Gum-resins*, *Juices*, *etc.*

1. **Size and Form.** In tears, lumps, agglutinated masses, etc., approximate dimensions.
2. **Colour.**
3. **Packing.** In skins, paper, leaves, etc.
4. **Surface Condition.** Shining, clean, dusty, etc.
5. **Fracture and Hardness.** Conchoidal, brittle, granular, etc.

6. **Odour and Taste.**
7. **Solubility.** In water, alcohol, etc.
8. **Chemical Tests and Peculiarities.**

Skeleton Plan for the Description of Starch and Calcium Oxalate

STARCH

1. **Colour.** Usually white with a slight tint, such as yellowish.
2. **Feel.** Behaviour when pressed firmly between finger and thumb.
3. **Fineness.** Appearance under pocket-lens ; mobility.
4. **Shape** of the granules.
5. **Hilum.** Position in granule, shape, etc.
6. **Striations.** Concentric, transverse, etc.
7. **Dimensions.** Length, breadth and thickness of the granules measured in microns.
8. **Aggregation.** Simple or compound granules ; number of components in compound granules.
9. **Polarised Light.** Behaviour of the granules with crossed nicols.
10. **Neutrality.** *p*H value as determined by a universal indicator.

CALCIUM OXALATE

1. **Shape.** Prisms, needles (acicular raphides), clusters, microsphenoidal, etc.
2. **Size.** Measured in microns.
3. **Distribution.** In scattered idioblasts, accompanying the veins, in a special crystal layer, forming a crystal sheath, associated with bundles of fibres.
4. **Envelope.** Presence of a lignified envelope.

HABITATS

The usual method of indicating habitats is to mark the area or areas of production upon a map. The area is generally shaded and the districts producing the larger amounts are more heavily shaded. For this purpose, blank outline maps of the world on Mercator's projection are most commonly used, but where the commodity is limited to a very circumscribed area, blank maps of single continents or of lesser extent are also employed, so as to show greater detail.

For the purpose of studying the habitats of drugs, small blank maps of the world are most generally convenient and, if each map is printed in the form of a gummed label, about 6·5 by 9·0 cm., they can be used freely and attached to the note-boook in convenient places. It would be ideal to adopt graduated shading of areas for marking the habitats and to use a separate map for each drug, but such a method is perhaps rather more elaborate than is necessary for elementary instruction. A simpler method, and one which answers well in practice, is to use one map for several drugs and for each drug to draw a line from the place of production to the outer margin of the map and to write the name of the drug and also the name of the habitat on the paper against the map, see Fig. 65.

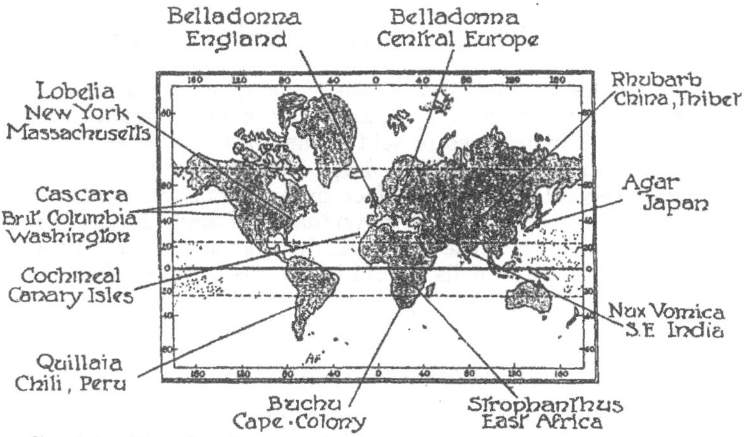

FIG. 65.—Map showing a method of indicating the habitats of drugs.

PART III

HISTOLOGICAL SCHEDULES

THE schedules in this part of the book give instructions for the histological examination of a number of the more important drugs, chiefly those which are used or sold in the form of powder. There are three stages in the study of each drug: first, to examine it by means of sections; second, to make surface preparations and to disintegrate the tissues so as to separate the individual cells, and, third, to examine a specimen of powder of the authentic drug, so as to learn the appearance of the tissues and cells, found in the dissections, after the drug has been reduced to a No. 60 or 90 powder.

HISTOLOGICAL SCHEDULE—I

Starches, Micrometers, Camera Lucida

1. By means of a stage micrometer, calibrate the scale of the eye-piece micrometer, following the directions given in the notes to this schedule.

2. Construct a scale of microns at a magnification of 600.

3. Soak in water, grains of wheat, barley, rice, maize and oats. Take a soaked grain of wheat, cut it in two portions and remove some of the endosperm on the point of a needle; mount some in water and a further quantity in lactophenol. Measure the size of a typical granule and sketch that granule at a magnification of 600, using the scale already constructed; measure other granules from the wheat starch and sketch them also to scale.

4. Measure the diameters of several of the largest grains of commercial wheat starch you can find and record their sizes.

5. Make other measurements, using a Camera Lucida, as explained in the appended notes. Use potato starch for this exercise.

6. Examine, by polarised light, wheat starch mounted in lacto-phenol. Rotate the analyser and note the changes produced. Record also the intensity of the polarisation effects for potato, maize and rice starches.

7. Examine starch from grains of maize, rice and oats and from a tuber of potato and confirm the identity of the commercial samples.

8. Write out descriptions of the starches of potato, maize and rice, recording your observations in the following order: shape, hilum, striations, size, compound grains, polarised light.

9. Examine some materials, such as the following, and report upon the presence or absence of starch and, if present, state the kind found, giving your reasons in full: custard powders, bloom of Ninon, papier poudré, infants' foods, acetanilide tablets.

10. Mount potato, maize and rice starches in 0·9 per cent. solution of potassium hydroxide; observe and record the behaviour of the

granules. Treat Maranta starch (West Indian Arrowroot) in a similar way, comparing it carefully with potato starch.

NOTES ON HISTOLOGICAL SCHEDULE I

Micrometers. Two scales are needed for making microscopical measurements. One of them, termed a stage micrometer, takes the form of an ordinary mounted microscopic object, and consists of a scale 1·1 mm. long, 1 mm. being divided into tenths and the odd tenth divided into hundredths. This scale is engraved or photographed upon an ordinary microscope slide, and mounted under a cover-glass like any other object. It is intended to

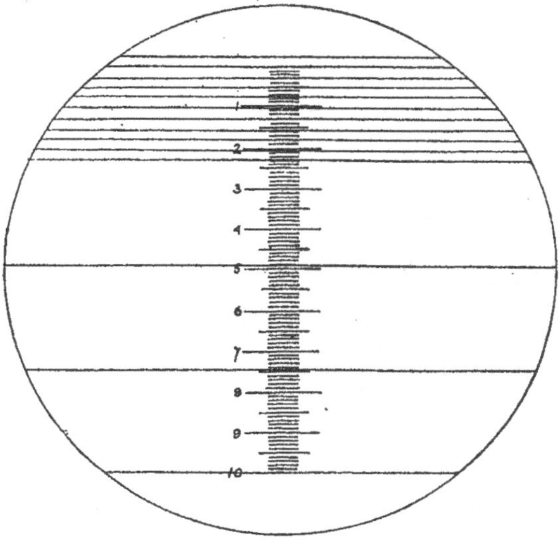

FIG. 66.—Appearance of eyepiece and stage micrometer scales as seen through the microscope with a 4 mm. objective and a × 6 eyepiece. One hundred eyepiece scale divisions (marked 1 to 10) are seen to be exactly equal to 3·9 of the stage micrometer divisions, *i.e.*, to 0·39 mm.

be placed upon the stage of the microscope, and is viewed through the instrument.

Other types of ruling are also common, sometimes a millimetre or 2 mm. are divided into tenths and hundredths throughout the entire length and either numbered at every tenth or engraved with lines of different lengths for tenths and hundredths.

The second scale, named an eyepiece micrometer, consists of a small disc of glass to be dropped on to the diaphragm of an Huyghenian eyepiece. Across the centre of the disc is engraved or photographed a scale divided into units and tenths of units. The exact size of the unit chosen is immaterial, but it is customary to make the scale 10 mm. long, each millimetre being divided into tenths.

It is most convenient to set aside a special eyepiece for the micrometer scale, which is allowed to remain permanently in position upon the diaphragm in the middle of the eyepiece tube. If the scale is not properly in focus, this should be rectified by readjusting the eye lens. When one wishes to make a measurement, this eyepiece is exchanged for that ordinarily in use.

Before a *measurement can be made*, the value of the divisions of the eyepiece micrometer must be determined. This is accomplished by placing the stage micrometer upon the stage of the microscope and focussing the lines engraved upon it, using for the purpose the objective with which the measurements are to be made and the ocular containing the eyepiece micrometer. The appearance of the field of view will resemble that shown in Fig. 66.

In this figure, the lines reaching quite across the field represent the image of the rulings upon the stage micrometer, while the shorter lines of the numbered scale represent the rulings of the eyepiece micrometer. If there should be no exact coincidence between the extremities of the eyepiece scale and two of the rulings of the stage micrometer, the draw-tube of the microscope must be extended until coincidence occurs. One now determines the number of stage micrometer divisions which are exactly equivalent to the hundred divisions of the eyepiece scale; in the figure this number is 3·9 divisions. Since the rulings of the stage micrometer

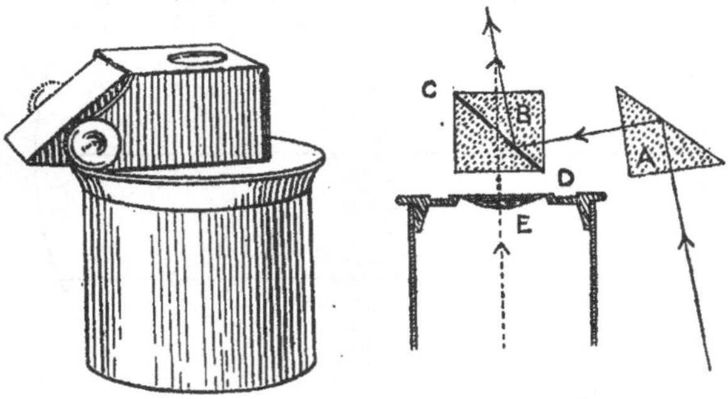

FIG. 67.—The Swift-Ives camera lucida and a diagram to explain the path of the light rays through the instrument. (See text.)

are 0·1 mm. and 0·01 mm. apart respectively, we have the result that 100 eyepiece divisions are equivalent to 0·39 mm., or each division of the eyepiece scale represents, with this particular optical combination, 0·0039 mm. or 3·9 μ (1 micron—μ—is 0·001 mm.).

If now the stage micrometer is removed and any ordinary object is viewed through the same lenses, without altering the tube-length, one can read off its dimensions in terms of the divisions of the eyepiece scale, and these numbers multiplied by 3·9 give the actual dimensions in microns.

Camera Lucida. Another way of making measurements is by means of a camera lucida, such as is used for drawing. There are many types of this instrument, and the better ones are those which permit of the microscope being used in a vertical position. The Abbe model is a very good pattern, but is rather heavy, and hence liable to strain the microscope. The most convenient type of camera lucida is the Swift-Ives pattern, which is quite a small instrument, and may be attached to the cap of a capped eyepiece, as shown in the figure (Fig. 67), or can be adapted to fit over the upper or eye lens of an ordinary eyepiece, and is then clamped in position by a small screw. With this instrument, the paper, lying upon the table or upon a drawing-board beside the microscope, is reflected by the small movable right-angled prism A into a second prism, B, above the eye lens E of the ocular. The face CD of this prism is silvered, and reflects the light vertically upwards into the observer's eye, while the microscope image is viewed directly through a small central opening in the silvered surface (see dotted line in the figure). As a result of this optical arrangement, the image in the microscope and the paper are seen superposed one upon the other, while a pencil used on the paper also comes into the field of view, so that one can easily trace over the image seen in the microscope.

The whole instrument is quite small, and measures about 35 × 17 × 18 mm.; the total weight, including the eyepiece cap, is less than 50 gm. (1·75 oz.).

One should, if possible, keep an eyepiece specially for use with the camera lucida; such an eyepiece should have a low magnifying power of about six diameters.

When *using a camera lucida*, place the stage micrometer on the microscope stage and trace its divisions as seen on the drawing-paper and measure the distance between them. Now tilt the drawing-board by raising the edge farthest from the microscope until the divisions drawn on all parts of the board are equally spaced. In this position drawings and measuremnets can be accurately made.

To make measurements first trace off the stage micrometer scale as seen in the microscope and the drawing obtained will represent tenths and hundredths of a millimetre at the magnification of the drawing. Next trace the outlines of the objects to be measured and determine their dimensions against the scale already traced. To find the magnification measure in millimetres the distance between two adjacent tenth graduations of the drawing and divide by 0·1.

Wheat Starch. This starch so closely resembles barley starch that the two starches cannot be distinguished by simple inspection. Barley starch never contains granules exceeding 40 microns in diameter, whereas there are always a few such granules in wheat starch, hence, for the exact identification of a starch as being derived from wheat one must measure the diameter of the larger granules and find some greater than 40 μ. To prove that the wheat starch is pure, it is further necessary to determine the number of granules per milligram which exceed 40 μ in diameter; this number is greater than 400.

Gelatinisation by 0·9 *per cent. Caustic Potash.* Potato starch is very rapidly gelatinised by this reagent, whereas Maranta starch is practically unaffected. In a similar way rye starch gelatinises rapidly, while wheat starch, which is closely similar, is attacked only slowly.

HISTOLOGICAL SCHEDULE—II.

Oil, Lycopodium, Kamala

Oil, microscopical identification of. 1. Take up a very small drop of oil by dipping the point of a needle into some olive oil and place it upon a glass slide; mix it on the slide with a similar droplet of mucilage of acacia to form an emulsion. Add a drop or two of water, mix and transfer a droplet of the diluted emulsion to a clean slide and apply a cover-glass and compare together the droplets of oil and bubbles of air as seen under the microscope. Air bubbles show a central bright area surrounded by a dark circle, and, on focussing down, the dark line becomes wider and the bright area is reduced to a point. Oil droplets somewhat resemble air bubbles, but, on focussing down, the dark circle diminishes in thickness and finally disappears.

2. Place a drop of diluted emulsion upon a slide, and near it put a drop of tincture of alkanet root, and beside this a drop of water. Mix the water and tincture of alkanna, and then either mix with the emulsion or apply a cover-glass to the emulsion, and draw the tincture of alkanna beneath it by irrigation. Note the red colour acquired by the oil globules.

3. Make three fresh mounts of the diluted emulsion ; to one, add a drop of solution of Scharlach R, to the second add a drop of solution of Soudan III., and to the third add a drop of a freshly prepared

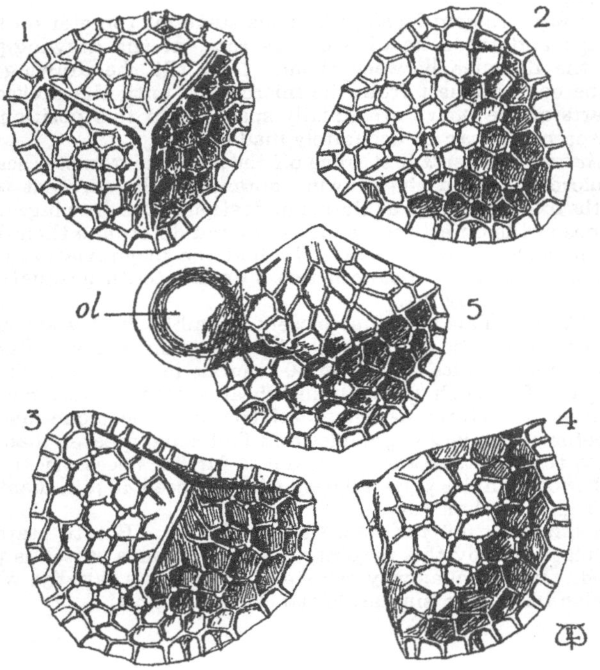

FIG. 68.—Spores of *Lycopodium clavatum* L. 1. Spore seen from above to show the apex. 2. Base of a spore. 3. Spore partly turned over. 4. Side view of a spore. 5. A spore burst by pressure upon the cover-glass and a globule of oil, *ol*, emerging from the split. All × 1200.

solution of chlorophyll in alcohol. Note the colorations given to the droplets of oil. (For the reagents, see Appendix.)

Lycopodium, the spores of *Lycopodium clavatum* Linn., family Lycopodiaceæ.

1. Dip the point of a glover's needle into some lycopodium, and remove the spores which adhere to it by tapping it upon a slide. Moisten the spores with alcohol, and mount them in dilute glycerin. Examine with the microscope, using the 4 mm. ($\frac{1}{6}$ in.) objective ; observe the shape of the spores, and the raised network upon the surface. Sketch a few spores to show different aspects of their shape,

and the number and form of the reticulations. Make the drawings 2·5 to 3 cm. (1 to 1·25 in.) in diameter, corresponding with a magnification of about 1,000 diameters.

2. Moisten some lycopodium with alcohol, and mount it in a small drop of water; crush the spores by pressing them firmly between the cover-glass and the slide. Identify as oil the globules that escape by

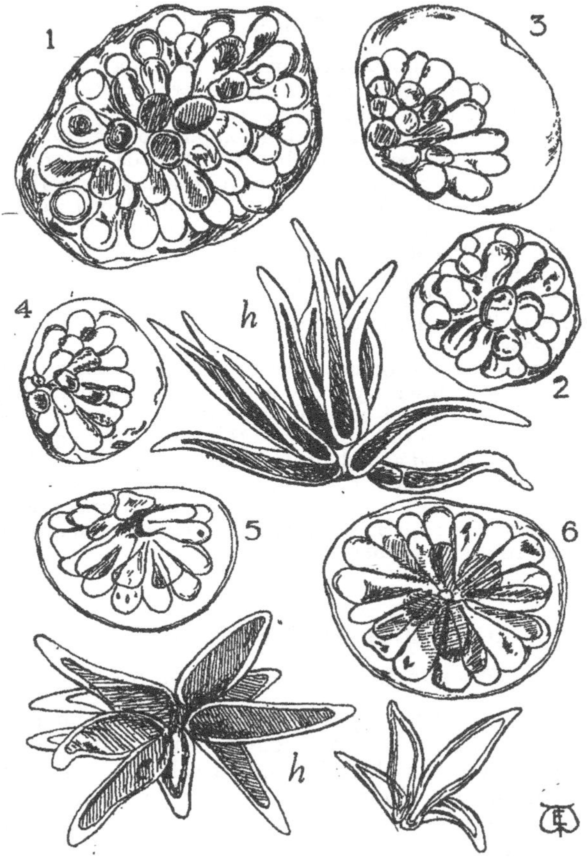

FIG. 69.—Hairs and glands from kamala. 1 and 2. Glands seen from above. 3, 4, 5. Glands seen from the side. 6. Gland seen from below. *h*, Radiating groups of protective hairs. All × 400.

staining them with alkanna in the following way: Place a drop of tincture of alkanna against the edge of the cover-glass and run it underneath by irrigation, or by raising the edge of the cover-glass with a needle and then replacing it.

Kamala, the hairs and glands from the fruits of *Mallotus philippinensis* Mull.-Arg., family Euphorbiaceæ.

1. Take some kamala as directed for lycopodium, moisten it with alcohol, and mount it in solution of potash, which forms a soluble soap with the resin. Irrigate with water and examine first with the 16 mm. and then with the 4 mm. objective. Observe and sketch the thick-walled unicellular hairs arranged in radiating groups and the rounded glands each composed of a group of radiating club-shaped cells enveloped by the delicate raised cuticle.

NOTES ON HISTOLOGICAL SCHEDULE II

Oil. The difference in appearance between oil drops and air bubbles is due to the different refractive indices of the two substances relative to water, oil having a higher and air a lower refractive index than water.

Lycopodium is derived from a plant belonging to the Pteridophyta or fern-like plants. The spores are produced in tetrads or groups of four, each group being formed by the sub-division of a single spherical mother-cell. The sub-division is brought about by the formation of walls radiating from the centre of the spherical cell, so that each spore has three flat triangular faces, which were in contact with neighbouring spores during their development, and a fourth rounded surface, which was moulded by the spherical surface of the mother-cell. The form of the reticulations and their number afford characters which distinguish spores from different species of *Lycopodium*.

Kamala. The red colouring matter of the glands consists of red resins, which are acidic in nature; they are secreted by the club-shaped cells and accumulate between the cuticle and the inner layers of the outer cell-wall, and between the radial walls of the cells. The common cuticle of all the cells is thus raised as a delicate bladdery structure filled with the red resinous secretion. Caustic alkali unites with the resin to form soaps, which are soluble in water, and, for this reason, treatment with caustic potash or soda followed by irrigation with water clears the glands so as to make the structure easily visible.

HISTOLOGICAL SCHEDULE—III

Ergot of Rye (*Claviceps purpurea*)

1. Soften some ergots by exposure to a moist atmosphere for about eighteen hours. Cut transverse and longitudinal sections of a softened ergot and mount them in chloral hydrate solution. Sketch a small piece of each so as to include the outer layers and also some of the central region. Describe the pseudo-parenchyma of each region.

2. Mount a section in sulphuric acid and a second one in 5 per cent. caustic alkali; note the behaviour of the colouring matter.

3. Mount a section in chloral hydrate solution and warm it; wash out the chloral hydrate with water and stain with tincture of alkanna. Note the colour taken by the globules of fixed oil.

4. Soak a section for some time in ether in a covered hollowed glass block. Remove the section and mount it in iodine water. Note the reaction for protein and the absence of starch.

5. Cut a surface section from an ergot, mount it in chloral hydrate solution and sketch a portion to show the character of the tissue in surface view.

6. Test sections for cellulose and for lignified walls and record your observations.

7. Heat ergots at 120° to 150° with concentrated aqueous caustic alkali for thirty minutes. Remove them from the alkali and wash them thoroughly with alcohol and then with water; the residue is chitosan. Place a piece on a slide, tease it out and soak it in decinormal iodine solution, remove excess of iodine and add 5 per cent. sulphuric acid, note the deep reddish-violet coloration produced (reaction for chitin).

8. To a piece of the chitosan in a test-tube add 50 per cent. nitric acid and boil. Note the solution of the mass.

9. Prepare some insects by digestion in potash as was done for the ergots and note that the exoskeleton reacts in the same way as ergot. Test cellulose similarly treated and note the absence of any colour reaction or solubility.

10. Examine some powdered ergot and some defatted powder, using the same reagents as for the sections. Write out the diagnostic characters of the powder.

NOTES ON HISTOLOGICAL SCHEDULE III

Ergots may be softened by exposure to a moist atmosphere for eighteen hours, as explained under Foxglove Leaves (see Schedule XIV., p. 38).

A convenient form of cellulose to use for digestion with caustic alkali, as directed under (10) above, is the endosperm of date stones, which can be soaked for a week or more in water and then cut up into small pieces for the digestion experiment.

Characters of Powdered Ergot. 1. Ergot consists chiefly of small, unequal, rounded cells with thick, highly-refractive walls, which give no reactions for cellulose or for lignin.

2. Occasional patches of purplish-brown, narrow, rectangular cells in rows from the outer layers. These give a blood-red with sulphuric acid, and a violet with caustic alkali.

3. Abundance of oily drops released by heating with chloral hydrate solution.

4. Protein matter, which stains with iodine.

5. Starch, calcium oxalate crystals, spores and vascular tissues are absent.

6. Moistened with caustic alkali the powder develops an odour of trimethylamine.

HISTOLOGICAL SCHEDULE—IV

Galls (*Quercus infectoria*)

1. Soak galls in several changes of water until soft and preserve them in a mixture of alcohol containing 20 per cent. of glycerin. Cut a gall across and sketch the naked-eye appearance to show the limiting outer layer, the parenchyma, the sclerenchymatous layer and the central hollow containing the grub or insect.

2. Cut transverse sections of a prepared gall to include all the tissues from the outside to the centre. Mount separate sections in chloral hydrate solution, phloroglucin and hydrochloric acid and in iodine water. Note the two or three outer layers of small cells with suberised walls, followed

by numerous layers of parenchyma with pitted walls and containing both prisms and cluster crystals of calcium oxalate which in the inner part often occur in cells arranged in radial rows. Next is found a wide band of stone-cells, within which is more parenchyma, which contains starch, cluster crystals of calcium oxalate and, in the inner cells, so-called lignin bodies, which stain red with phloroglucin and hydrochloric acid.

3. From a gall, which has been softened by exposure to a moist atmosphere for about forty-eight hours, cut some transverse sections. Mount one section in clove oil and search for the characteristic angular plates of tannic acid with which the parenchymatous cells are filled. Irrigate a second section with ferric chloride solution (B.P. tincture diluted 1 to 10) and note the reaction.

4. Cut a thin surface section and test the nature of the walls by the following tests for suberised walls: Mount in sulphuric acid (80 per cent. by volume) and warm gently; mount in 20 per cent. caustic potash and warm. For these experiments use the 16 mm. objective.

5. Examine the insects and grubs removed from the central hollows of some of the galls.

6. Prepare some authentic powder of galls by grating a gall on a rasp file and mount preparations in the same reagents as were used for the sections. Identify the structures present and sketch typical pieces. Write out a list of the characters of powdered galls.

NOTES ON HISTOLOGICAL SCHEDULE IV

Characters of Powdered Galls. 1. Fairly numerous sclerenchymatous cells.

2. Lignin bodies.
3. The presence of only a few small vessels.
4. A few starch grains.
5. Abundance of tannin flakes, visible in clove oil mounts.
6. Abundance of fairly thick-walled, pitted parenchyma with both cluster and prismatic crystals of calcium oxalate.
7. Occasional insect fragments.
8. Coloured bluish-black by ferric chloride solution.

HISTOLOGICAL SCHEDULE V

Wood of Pine (*Pinus sylvestris*)

1. From a piece of red deal (*Pinus sylvestris*) cut some small cubes of about 1 cm. edge, so that two surfaces are transverse to the grain of the wood, two surfaces at right angles to the medullary rays, and two surfaces parallel with the medullary rays. Soak the cubes in water for an hour or two and then boil them for about thirty minutes to expel air and allow to soak until sufficiently softened to cut easily.

2. With a razor flooded with alcohol cut several transverse sections; mount sections separately in chloral hydrate, in iodine and sulphuric acid, in aniline hydrochloride, and in phloroglucin and hydrochloric acid. Make a note of the action of the reagents used and sketch in detail a small portion including an annual ring as seen with a 4 mm. objective. Mark the following details on your drawing: Spring wood, autumn wood, medullary rays, bordered pits and a resin duct with its accompanying parenchyma. Where do the bordered pits occur?

3. Cut tangential longitudinal sections and mount them in chloral hydrate solution and in phloroglucin and hydrochloric acid. Examine the preparations under the 4 mm. objective and sketch a small piece to show the wood tracheids with bordered pits, which are here seen in section, and the medullary rays which appear as narrow lenticular areas, usually one cell wide. Include in the sketch a multiseriate ray with its resin duct.

4. Cut some radial longitudinal sections. Mount and examine them as above. Sketch to show the following details : Tracheids with bordered pits, which are now seen in surface view, medullary rays with starch cells and the tracheidal edge cells and resin ducts cut longitudinally, which will be seen traversing the wood longitudinally, and also running through the centre of the occasional large medullary rays and at right angles to the tracheids.

5. Cut some thin shavings of the wood along the grain and soak them in solution of chromic and nitric acids (10 per cent. of each) for about three quarters of an hour, using a hollowed glass block and cover for the purpose. Wash by decantation with water and tease out a piece with needles. Sketch the various elements present, viz., tracheids with bordered pits, tracheids with pits of different types, cells of the medullary rays with simple pits and others with small bordered pits. Remove the water from a small amount of the disintegrated wood and apply phloroglucin and hydrochloric acid and record the result.

6. Examine the powder of pinewood and search for the characters observed in the sections and other preparations.

7. Scrape a little dust from the inside of a cardboard pill-box, mount it in chloral hydrate and determine its nature.

8. Examine some "cellulose wadding" and determine the nature of the fibres present (see Schedule IV, p. 15).

NOTES ON HISTOLOGICAL SCHEDULE V

Characters of Powdered Pine Wood. 1. Absence of fibres and of vessels.

2. Consists almost entirely of four-sided tracheids, with large, circular. bordered pits, mostly in a single row on each of the radial walls.

3. Medullary rays heterogeneous, showing starch cells and tracheidal cells. They are mostly uniserate, a few being multiseriate, and then each contains a resin duct.

4. Cross-field (in *Pinus sylvestris*) usually with one large, rectangular, simple pit only. (The "cross-field" is the area enclosed by the intersection of a tracheid and a medullary ray starch cell.)

5. All elements are lignified, except after treatment with oxidising reagents when they react for cellulose only.

HISTOLOGICAL SCHEDULE VI

Quassia Wood (*Picraena excelsa*)

1. Split some quassia wood into small pieces, about the size of a matchstick, and cut them into lengths of about ½ in. Digest the pieces of wood in 50 per cent. nitric acid to which small quantities of powdered

potassium chlorate are added from time to time, to maintain a gentle effervescence. When thoroughly softened and washed, tease out a small piece of the wood upon a slide with needles. Find and sketch the following elements : Wood fibres, wood parenchyma, vessels, cells of the medullary rays.

2. From the radial surface of a piece of soaked wood, cut several sections and mount one in chloral hydrate solution and a second one in iodine water. Identify the above elements and observe their arrangement. Note the crystals of calcium oxalate, their form and manner of occurrence. Sometimes small starch grains and (in the

NUT-SHELLS and FRUIT-STONES

Name and Source.	Shape of Cells.	Colour and Character of Walls, when mounted in Chloral Hydrate.	Lumen and Contents.	Action of warm 5% Caustic Potash.
Olive Stones. *Olea europea.*	Mostly elongated. A few small spiral vessels and thin-walled parenchyma from the pulp are present.	Colourless and mostly very thick, numerous pits.	Linear lumen. Contents colourless.	Walls coloured bright yellow.
Coco-nut shells. *Cocos nucifera.*	Both isodiametric and elongated. A few spiral and reticulate vessels ; very few fibres and silica nodules.	Deep yellow, thick with branching pits. A few thin-walled with circular pits.	Narrow lumen. Dark brown contents.	Contents coloured dark red-brown.
Almond Shells. *Prunus communis.*	Some isodiametric and rather thin-walled. Others elongated and thick-walled.	Nearly colourless.	Fairly large lumen in many cells. Linear lumen in thick-walled cells.	No marked colour change.
Walnut Shells. *Juglans regia.*	Mostly isodiametric. Some cells with rather thin walls which are slightly concave.	Nearly colourless, mostly very strongly thickened.	Small lumen in thick-walled cells.	No marked colour change.
Hazel-Nut Shells. *Corylus avellana.*	Both isodiametric and elongated. Some unicellular trichomes with thick walls and linear lumen.	Nearly colourless.	Brown contents.	Walls coloured pale yellow. Contents coloured deep brown.

vessels) yellow amorphous masses may be observed. Sketch a small typical piece of the section.

3. Cut sections from a tangential surface; mount them as directed in (2). Sketch one to show the structures previously found. Note especially the height and width of the medullary rays. Sketch a typical piece.

4. Cut sections from a transverse surface and sketch as for the two other sections. Stain a section with phloroglucin and hydrochloric acid, another with chlorzinciodine, and a third with aniline sulphate. Sketch a small portion to show the arrangement of the fibres, wood parenchyma, vessels and medullary rays.

5. Examine genuine quassia powder and identify the elements found in the above preparations. Make a note of the characteristic features.

6. Examine some powdered olive stones and powdered coconut shells sketch them and compare them with the woods you have examined.

NOTES ON HISTOLOGICAL SCHEDULE VI

Characters of Powdered Quassia Wood. 1. Fragments of vessels showing minute bordered pits with an oval outline and slit-shaped opening.

2. Portions of rather thin-walled fibres with linear, oblique, slit-shaped pits.

3. Occasional prisms of calcium oxalate, either free or sometimes enclosed in rectangular parenchymatous cells, arranged in files accompanying the fibres.

4. Small pieces of medullary rays, usually crossing fibres; sometimes as in tangential section.

5. Entirely lignified.

6. A very few round starch grains are present.

7. Bitter taste; pale buff colour.

HISTOLOGICAL SCHEDULE VII

Cascara Bark (*Rhamnus Purshianus*)

1. Cut transverse sections of the soaked bark, mount one in solution of chloral hydrate, warming if necessary, and a second section in iodine water. Make a diagrammatic sketch to show the distribution of the tissues, viz., cork, phellogen, primary cortex, medullary rays, primary and secondary phloem, calcium oxalate crystals, sclerenchymatous cells and fibres.

2. Sketch small portions of the transverse section as seen under the 4 mm. objective to show the following details: Cork cells and phellogen; cortex with collenchyma, thin-walled parenchyma, sclerenchyma, crystals, etc.; phloem with medullary rays, sclerenchymatous cells, fibres, crystals of calcium oxalate and sieve tubes. Note the absence of companion cells to the sieve-tubes.

3. Mount a further section in corallin soda and note the staining and distribution of the callus of the sieve areas.

4. Stain a section with phloroglucin and hydrochloric acid; record the results.

5. Cut several radial sections and mount one in chloral hydrate solution and another in corallin soda. Identify the elements named above and sketch small portions to show details of the sclerenchymatous cells, fibres, crystal sheaths, etc.

6. Digest a small piece of bark upon a water-bath for ten to fifteen minutes in a 5 per cent. solution of caustic alkali. Wash thoroughly by decantation with distilled water and tease out some of the material upon a slide. Sketch isolated cells from the various tissues.

7. Cut transverse sections from a piece of bark which has been softened by exposure to a moist atmosphere, mount them in caustic potash and record the colour changes.

8. Examine powdered cascara bark by mounting in suitable reagents. Decolorise some of the powder by soaking it in chlorinated soda solution and then examine it microscopically. Identify the structures seen in the dissections and make a list of the diagnostic features. To find the sieve-plates in the powder, select a fragment consisting of parenchyma and focus carefully any wider elements present.

9. Prepare pieces of the epiphytic bryophytes by boiling them in solution of chloral hydrate and examine them with the 16-mm. objective.

10. Compare powdered bark of *Rhamnus Frangula* with powdered cascara.

NOTES ON HISTOLOGICAL SCHEDULE VII

Characters of Powdered Cascara Bark. 1. Bundles of slender phloem fibres, accompanied by files of crystal cells with prisms of calcium oxalate.

2. Groups of stone-cells accompanied by prisms of calcium oxalate in the adjacent cells; these groups appear as large dark masses.

3. Yellowish colouring matter, which is soluble in chloral hydrate solution and becomes purple with caustic alkali.

4. Calcium oxalate crystals, both clusters and prisms.

5. Cork cells with thin colourless walls, containing dark brown masses.

6. Minute starch grains in the chloroplastids of the cortical parenchyma.

7. Sieve-tubes with sieve-areas embedded in colourless masses of parenchyma, often showing also crossing cells due to medullary rays.

Alder Buckthorn bark (*Rhamnus Frangula*) will be found to resemble cascara bark, excepting that it contains no stone-cells.

Epiphytes of Cascara. Liverworts are dorsiventral and usually foliose; the leaves are in 2 rows, the laminæ being one cell thick and without a midrib. Mosses are radially constructed, the leaves being one cell thick except at the midrib, which is always present except in the Sphagnaceæ.

HISTOLOGICAL SCHEDULE VIII

Cinchona Bark (*Cinchona succirubra*)

1. Soak fairly thin pieces of red cinchona bark in several changes of water for about three days. From a piece of the soaked bark cut several transverse sections; mount one in chloral hydrate solution, one in phloroglucin and hydrochloric acid, and a third in iodine water.

2. Make a diagrammatic drawing of a transverse section, indicating the following particulars: Cork, phellogen, cortex with secretion cells,

secondary phloem with large bast fibres, mostly isolated or in short radial rows, and medullary rays. Indicate the distribution of the idioblasts containing sandy calcium oxalate and also the occurrence of starch grains. Sketch characteristic portions of each tissue in detail under the 4 mm. objective. Note that the sieve tubes are accompanied by companion cells.

3. Make some radial longitudinal sections and mount them as for the transverse sections. Sketch important details such as fibres and the calcium oxalate idioblasts.

4. Digest small pieces of the bark in 5 per cent. caustic alkali for about thirty minutes upon a water-bath. When sufficiently softened, pour off the alkaline fluid and wash by decantation with distilled water. Tease out a piece of the treated bark and examine and sketch the isolated fibres and other cell forms. Stain a piece with corallin soda and find the callus plugs of the sieve tubes.

5. Measure the lengths and maximum diameters of some of the isolated phloem fibres, including the largest present. Record the range of size and the maximum width. To measure these dimensions, use drawings made with a camera-lucida.

6. Examine powdered cinchona bark mounted in chloral hydrate solution and also in lacto-phenol. Bleach some powder with sodium hypochlorite solution, wash and stain for callus.

7. Write out a list of the characters you consider most useful for the identification of the powder.

NOTES ON HISTOLOGICAL SCHEDULE VIII

Characters of Powdered Red Cinchona Bark. 1. Fibres, spindle-shaped and isolated and of a large size, attaining a diameter of 80 to 90 microns.

2. Microcrystals of calcium oxalate, usually in idioblasts.
3. Thin-walled cork cells.
4. Starch in small grains not very abundant.
5. Red-brown colour ; bitter taste.
6. Absence of stone-cells and of oil-cells.

HISTOLOGICAL SCHEDULE IX

Cassia, Cinnamon, Witch-hazel and Quillaia Barks

Cassia (*Cinnamomum Cassia*) and **Cinnamon** (*Cinnamomum zeylanicum*) **Barks.** 1. Make transverse and radial longitudinal sections of the soaked barks ; bleach some sections with chlorinated soda solution, wash and mount in lacto-phenol. Mount other sections directly in chloral hydrate solution and in phloroglucin and hydrochloric acid.

Observe, sketch and note the characters of the starch grains, sclerenchymatous cells, phloem fibres, secretion cells, cork, medullary rays and calcium oxalate crystals. Make a diagrammatic sketch of the transverse section of each bark.

2. Digest pieces of each bark in 5 per cent. solution of caustic alkali and tease them out and sketch characteristic elements. Measure the maximum diameters of the isolated fibres.

3. Examine powdered cassia bark, mounting preparations in the same reagents as were used for the sections. Measure the diameter of the starch grains.

4. Examine powdered cinnamon bark and determine any differences from cassia, noting especially the starch grains, the fibres and the absence of cork.

5. Test for oil and mucilage in sections cut with a dry razor from material exposed to a damp atmosphere.

6. Place a little powder on a slide, slightly tilted lengthwise; add ether in drops from a glass rod and allow the ethereal solution to flow to the centre of the slide and evaporate. Remove most of the exhausted powder and to the ethereal extract add a drop or two of Scharlach R. reagent. Apply a cover-glass and examine for stained oil droplets—the staining may require about 5 minutes.

Note. Tincture of alkanet is *not* a suitable reagent for volatile oils.

7. Write out the characters of the two powders.

Witch-hazel Bark (*Hamamelis virginiana*). 1. Cut sections of the soaked bark, mount them in suitable reagents. Make a diagrammatic sketch of a transverse section and detailed sketches of characteristic elements.

2. Digest pieces of bark with 5 per cent. solution of caustic alkali and tease them out.

3. Digest pieces in the cold with a mixture of 10 per cent. of chromic anhydride and of nitric acid dissolved in water, and tease them out.

4. With a dry razor cut sections of the bark softened by exposure to a moist atmosphere and mount them in ferric chloride solution and in Braemer's reagent.

5. Examine powdered witch-hazel bark and write out its characters.

Quillaia Bark (*Quillaia sp.*). 1. Cut transverse sections and mount them in suitable reagents. Make a diagrammatic drawing of a transverse section and mark the cork, medullary rays, bast fibres, sieve tissue, bast parenchyma. Look for stone-cells, starch grains and crystals. Find well-formed sieve tubes with companion cells.

2. Cut longitudinal radial sections and identify the structures found in the transverse sections. Sketch characteristic elements.

3. Tease out a piece of bark after treatment with caustic alkali. Sketch fibres, stone-cells, crystals, etc. Stain some of the teased material with corallin soda and identify the sieve tubes. Measure the length and breadth of a few of the crystals, including the largest you can find.

4. Examine the powdered quillaia in various reagents.

5. Write out the characters of powdered quillaia bark.

NOTES ON HISTOLOGICAL SCHEDULE IX

Cassia and cinnamon barks should be soaked in water for about eighteen hours before use. Further quantities of each should be softened by exposure to a moist atmosphere.

Most of the secretion cells are empty, the contents having become dispersed amongst the tissues; an occasional cell stains with alkanna. A satisfactory reaction for mucilage is rarely obtained.

Witch-hazel bark should be soaked for about eighteen hours in *distilled* water in a glass or porcelain dish. Some pieces should also be prepared by exposure to a moist atmosphere.

A mixture of chromic and nitric acids is used for the disintegration of witch-hazel bark, because this bark contains a large amount of sclerenchyma in the pericycle. Such woody tissues can only be separated into their constituent cells by means of oxidising agents ; caustic alkalis will not effect any disintegration.

Quillaia bark should be soaked in cold water for three or four days.

Characters of Powdered Cassia Bark. 1. Isolated phloem fibres, often 30 to 40 microns in diameter.

2. Sclerenchymatous cells, having one wall thinner than the remainder.
3. Patches of cork cells.
4. Starch grains abundant and often over 10 microns in diameter.
5. Calcium oxalate in minute needles in the cells of the parenchyma.
6. Characteristic odour and taste.

Characters of Powdered Cinnamon Bark. Similar to cassia bark, except that :

1. Cork is absent (except in very small amounts).
2. The phloem fibres are usually under 30 microns in diameter.
3. The starch grains are mostly under 10 microns in diameter.

Characters of Powdered Witch-hazel Bark. 1. Fibres in groups accompanied by crystal cells in files.

2. Prismatic crystals of calcium oxalate in the parenchyma.
3. Abundant stone-cells, evenly thickened.
4. Ferric chloride solution gives a bluish-black with the parenchyma.
5. Cluster crystals are absent, and only a very little starch, in rounded grains, is present.

Characters of Powdered Quillaia Bark. 1. Phloem fibres in bundles, tortuous and irregularly enlarged at intervals.

2. Calcium oxalate in very large prisms up to 170 microns long and 31 microns wide.
3. A few stone-cells, sub-rectangular with fairly large lumina and circular simple pits. They occur in small groups or singly.
4. Fairly abundant starch, small grained.
5. Froths when shaken with water. Sternutatory.

HISTOLOGICAL SCHEDULE X

Bearberry Leaves (*Arctostaphylos Uva-ursi*)

1. Soften some bearberry leaves by soaking them in cold water for about thirty hours. Mount one in pith, cutting the leaf to a suitable size if necessary, and make several thin transverse sections. Mount one section in chloral hydrate solution and a second one in phloroglucin and hydrochloric acid. Make a diagrammatic sketch including the region of the midrib and mark the limits of the various tissues, viz., upper and lower epidermis and position of the stomata, palisade and spongy parenchyma, xylem and phloem of the meristele of the midrib, collenchymatous parenchyma containing crystals above and below the meristele. Sketch a few cells from each tissue in detail.

2. Mount a transverse section in chlorzinciodine and another section in tincture of alkanna diluted with an equal volume of water and warm it gently. Record the staining effects you observe and draw conclusions as to the nature of the materials present.

3. Hold a soaked leaf over the finger and carefully cut surface sections from both faces of the leaf. Mount them in chloral hydrate solution and sketch a few cells from each.

4. Cut up some leaves and put them into a test-tube with a little 5 per cent. solution of caustic alkali and heat on a water-bath until the epidermis is easily separable (about half an hour). Wash several times by decantation with distilled water. Mount a piece of each epidermis and compare with the appearance of the sections. What difference do you observe ? Make sketches to illustrate the distribution and grouping of the stomata and their relationship to the surrounding cells.

5. Examine the teased out tissues of the midrib itself and sketch fibres, vessels and crystal cells.

6. Find a group of young leaves attached to the tip of a twig. Remove one of the leaves carefully and note with a pocket lens the fine hairs at the base of the upper surface of the lamina and on the short petiole. Cut off this basal part of the leaf and boil it with chloral hydrate solution in a small test-tube till clear. Mount it on a microscope slide and sketch a few of the covering and glandular hairs.

7. Examine the powdered leaf mounted in reagents as used for the sections. Identify the elements seen in the dissections and write out the diagnostic features of the powder.

NOTES ON HISTOLOGICAL SCHEDULE X

Characters of Powdered Bearberry Leaves. 1. Epidermis of straight-walled polygonal cells. Stomata in the lower epidermis only, and without any special subsidiary cells.

2. Irregular prismatic crystals of calcium oxalate in the cells of the collenchyma ; no crystals in the interneural mesophyll.

3. Palisade layer of three to five rows ; mostly three rows.

4. Small oil droplets in most of the cells.

5. Very occasional hairs, which are mostly unicellular, conical and smooth, with thick walls. A few glandular hairs, consisting of a short two-celled stalk carrying an ovoid multicellular secreting head.

6. A few fibres from the veins and a few small spiral vessels.

HISTOLOGICAL SCHEDULE XI

Senna Leaves (*Cassia acutifolia* and *Cassia angustifolia*)

1. Soften some senna leaves by exposing them to a moist atmosphere for about eighteen hours. Take two or three leaves and place them together between two pieces of pith and cut transverse sections, using a razor flooded with alcohol. Mount one in chloral hydrate solution and another in phloroglucin and hydrochloric acid. Make a diagrammatic sketch to show the limits of the tissues, viz., upper and lower epidermises, and the position of stomata, upper and lower palisade, spongy mesophyll, bundle of the meristele, pericyclic fibres, cluster and prismatic crystals, hairs and collenchyma. Sketch a small portion of the interneural lamina in detail.

2. Mount a section in ruthenium red and note the staining of the mucilage in the epidermis.

3. Cut two small squares of leaf, about 2 mm. side, and place them upon a slide, one with the upper and the other with the lower surface

uppermost, moisten with alcohol and mount in chloral hydrate solution, apply a cover glass and boil till clear. Sketch a portion of each epidermis, taking special note of the stomata with their subsidiary cells and the hairs. On part of the sketch fill in the underlying palisade cells.

4. Cut out midribs from two or three leaves, digest them on a water-bath in some 5 per cent. aqueous caustic alkali and tease out when sufficiently softened. Sketch the isolated elements.

5. Examine the powdered senna leaves and identify the elements observed in the dissections. Write out the diagnostic characters of the powder.

6. Boil a little confection of senna with water in a test-tube; allow the insoluble matter to settle; remove a little of the sediment with a dipping tube, mount it in chloral hydrate solution and find the particles of powdered senna leaves.

NOTES ON HISTOLOGICAL SCHEDULE XI

Characters of Powdered Senna Leaves. 1. Warty, unicellular, thick-walled hairs, often slightly contracted and bent near the base; apex acute. Length 70 to 260μ; breadth 12 to **18** to 25μ.

2. Pieces of epidermis with stomata, each having usually two subsidiary cells with their long axes parallel to the porus, *i.e.*, rubiaceous type.

3. Strands of fibres, accompanied by rows of cells each containing a single prism of calcium oxalate, 4 to **15** to 25μ in diameter.

4. Hyaline angular masses, which stain with ruthenium red (mucilage).

5. Pieces of leaf showing a transverse section with isobilateral structure.

6. Cluster crystals, 8 to **15** to **20** to 30μ in diameter, in the mesophyll.

HISTOLOGICAL SCHEDULE XII

Foxglove Leaves (*Digitalis purpurea*)

1. Soften some foxglove leaves by exposing them to a damp atmosphere for twenty-four hours. Cut transverse sections from a piece of leaf so as to include the midrib; mount one in iodine water, another in chloral hydrate solution and a third in phloroglucin and hydrochloric acid.

2. Make a diagrammatic sketch to show the distribution of the tissues in the midrib and lamina. Make sketches to show details of the two types of trichomes.

3. Cut a piece about 2 mm. square so as to include one of the marginal teeth. Boil with chloral hydrate till clear and sketch to show the shape of the tooth and the water pore or pores.

4. Cut a small square from the middle of the lamina and clear it by boiling in chloral hydrate solution. Sketch in detail a piece of both upper and lower epidermis. Look for calcium oxalate crystals.

5. Examine powdered foxglove leaves and write a list of the diagnostic characters.

6. Make surface preparations of primrose, comfrey and mullein leaves ; sketch epidermal cells, hairs and crystals in each case.

Red Rose Petals (*Rosa gallica*)

1. Soften some red rose petals by exposure to a moist atmsophere.
2. Mount a piece of petal in acid and another in caustic alkali. Note the colour changes.
3. Boil a piece of petal with chloral hydrate solution and sketch a few cells of both the upper and lower surfaces ; look for stomata near the base of the petals and for hairs on the margin and near the veins on the under surface. Search also for pollen grains.
4. Examine the confection of roses as directed for confection of senna, p. 145.

NOTES ON HISTOLOGICAL SCHEDULE XII

Characters of Powdered Foxglove Leaves (*Digitalis purpurea*). 1. Epidermal cells with wavy walls.

2. Stomata not very numerous on the upper surface, but abundant on the lower surface ; no special subsidiary cells, *i.e.*, ranunculaceous type.
3. Covering hairs 3 to 5 cells long, apex acute, finely warty surface ; cells often collapsed alternately in planes at right angles to one another.
4. Glandular hairs, mostly with a short unicellular stalk and a two-celled head.
5. One large water pore on the tip of each tooth.
6. Calcium oxalate and fibres absent.

Comfrey (*Symphytum officinale*) has typical covering trichomes, which are narrowly conical, with thick walls and very sharp apices ; many of them are strongly curved like a crook near the tip.

Mullein (*Verbascum Thapsus*) is densely covered with large candelabra hairs.

Primrose (*Primula vulgaris*) has hairs 4 to 12 cells long abundant on the lower surface ; also numerous small glandular hairs with a short one-celled cylindrical stalk and a one-celled spherical head. Calcium oxalate absent.

Characters of Powdered Red Rose Petals (*Rosa gallica*). 1. Upper epidermis with papillose outer walls.

2. Lower epidermal cells have wavy walls with small internal projections.
3. Stomata few and on the lower surface only.
4. Long, narrow, waved and twisted hairs on the margin and near the veins. A few glandular hairs near the base.
5. Only small spiral vessels present.
6. Colour red with acid and green to blue with alkali.

HISTOLOGICAL SCHEDULE XIII

Solanaceous Leaves

1. Make sections, surface preparations and an examination of the powder for each of the three leaves—Belladonna, Stramonium and Henbane. Proceed as directed for Foxglove leaves (see Histological Schedule XII.).

2. Make diagrammatic sketches of the transverse sections through the midribs of the three leaves.

3. Using surface preparations, made by boiling pieces of the leaves in chloral hydrate, sketch in detail cells from the upper and lower epidermises, trichomes—both covering and glandular—and calcium oxalate crystals. Find and sketch stomata.

4. Write out the diagnostic characters for the powder of each of the leaves.

5. Examine surface preparations of leaves of *Phytolacca* and of *Ailanthus* and state how each may be recognised in the form of powder. Cut transverse sections of the midribs and make diagrams.

6. Examine the following materials and report upon them :—

(*a*) Extractum belladonnæ siccum.
(*b*) Laminated stramonium.
(*c*) Asthma cigarettes.

NOTES ON HISTOLOGICAL SCHEDULE XIII

All three of these *solanaceous leaves* show :—

1. Stomata on both surfaces, but more numerous on the lower surface. They have 3 or 4 subsidiary cells, one of which is smaller than the others, *i.e.*, cruciferous type.

2. Perimedullary phloem in the meristeles of the midribs.

3. Palisade consisting of one row of cells.

4. Absence of lignified fibres.

Characters of Powdered Belladonna Leaves. 1. Epidermal cells with wavy walls and striated cuticle.

2. Idioblasts in the mesophyll containing numerous microsphenoidal crystals of calcium oxalate.

3. A few trichomes of two kinds—covering, uniseriate trichomes 3 to 4 cells long, and glandular trichomes of various forms.

Characters of Powdered Stramonium Leaves. 1. Upper epidermal cells have nearly straight walls. Lower epidermal cells have wavy walls.

2. Crystal layer under the palisade ; calcium oxalate clusters in all the cells except those adjacent to the veins. Occasional idioblasts with microsphenoidal crystals near the veins.

3. Trichomes—(*a*) covering, uniseriate, 3 to 4 cells long, cuticle warty, not numerous ; (*b*) glandular having a pear-shaped head of about 7 or 8 cells and a unicellular stalk.

Characters of Powdered Henbane Leaves. 1. Epidermal cells of both surfaces have wavy walls.

2. Crystal layer under the palisade ; mostly prisms, sometimes clusters of a few components and occasionally microsphenoidal crystals.

3. Few covering trichomes. Numerous glandular trichomes with a long uniseriate stalk and usually a large ovoid pluricellular head.

Phytolacca leaves are glabrous ; they contain idioblasts filled with acicular raphides of calcium oxalate. The epidermal cells are straight-walled or slightly wavy (on the lower surface), and the stomata have no special subsidiary cells, *i.e.*, ranunculaceous type.

Ailanthus leaves have straight-walled epidermal cells with a strongly striated cuticle ; large, unicellular, sharply conical covering trichomes ; clusters of calcium oxalate near the veins ; stomata which have no special subsidiary cells, *i.e.*, ranunculaceous type.

HISTOLOGICAL SCHEDULE XIV

Determination of Palisade Ratio

1. Clear a piece of a leaf by boiling in cloral hydrate solution (use Hamamelis, Belladonna, Hyoscyamus or Stramonium).

2. Arrange a drawing board and sheet of paper for use with a camera lucida as explained in the notes on Histological Schedule I., p. 131, and, using the 4 mm. objective, trace off the outlines of four cells of the upper epidermis and then focus down to the palisade layer and trace off sufficient cells to cover the tracings of the epidermal cells, completing the outlines of those palisade cells which are intersected by the epidermal walls ; ink the outlines of the epidermal cells.

3. Count the palisade cells under the four epidermal cells, and where a cell is intersected, include it in the count when more than half is within the area and exclude it when less than half is within the area of the epidermal cells.

4. Calculate the average number of palisade cells beneath a single upper epidermal cell ; this figure is the " palisade ratio."

Determination of the Vein-Islet Number

1. From an Indian senna leaflet cut a transverse strip about 6 mm. wide to include the central region. Cut a similar piece from an Alexandrian senna leaflet. Put each piece into a test-tube, add about 2 ml. of solution of chloral hydrate and heat them for thirty minutes on a water-bath, to clear the tissues. Mount each on a slide in chloral hydrate solution and add a small drop of glycerin.

2. Arrange a camera lucida and drawing board for making drawings to scale ; place a stage micrometer on the microscope and, using the 16 mm. objective, draw a line equivalent to 1 mm. as seen through the microscope. Construct a square on this line.

3. Move the paper so that the square is seen in the eyepiece, in the centre of the field. Place the slide with the cleared leaf on the stage and trace off the veins which are included within the square, completing the outlines of those islets which overlap two adjacent sides of the square.

4. Count the number of vein-islets in the square millimetre. Where the islets are intersected by the sides of the square, include those on two adjacent sides and exclude those on the other two sides.

5. To obtain a critical result for a leaf, 4 sq. mm. should be used, preferably in one large area of 4 sq. mm.

Determination of the Stomatal Number

1. By means of a stage micrometer, measure the diameter of the field of view of the microscope, using a 4 mm. objective. Calculate the area in sq. mm.

2. Clear a piece of leaf, square in shape and not less than 5 mm. edge, by heating it on a water-bath in a test-tube with solution of chloral hydrate—this requires about 10 to 15 minutes. Mount it on a slide and count the stomata present in ten fields selected by means of a counting field finder. Use an eyepiece with a net-ruled disc.

3. Record the result for each of the ten fields and calculate the average number of stomata per sq. mm.

4. If the stomatal index is to be determined, count also the number of epidermal cells in each field.

NOTES ON HISTOLOGICAL SCHEDULE XIV

Palisade Ratio. After an exhaustive study of 53 species of plants belonging to the Compositæ, it was shown by Zörnig and Weiss (1925) that the palisade ratio is one of the most reliable anatomical characters for the identification of leaves, and this conclusion has been confirmed by more recent workers in England and in America, dealing with quite different material. The value is very simply determined and can be used for drugs in powder as fine as No. 90, in which portions containing four adjacent epidermal cells are easily found.

Vein-Islet Number. The term "vein-islet" was introduced in 1915 by Benedict, who directed attention to this character as being of specific significance. A vein-islet is the area of photosynthetic tissue surrounded by the ultimate ramifications of the conducting strands of a leaf; the term "vein-islet number" is the average number of vein-islets per sq. mm. calculated from 4 contiguous sq. mm. in the central part of the lamina, midway between the midrib and the margin.

Permanent mounts may be made in Berlese Mountant, see p. 226.

Stomatal Number is the number of stomata per sq. mm. of epidermis. The "stomatal index" is the percentage that the stomata form of the total number of epidermal cells and stomata together, *i.e.*, $S \div (E + S) \times 100$, where S = No. of stomata per unit area and E = No. of epidermal cells in the same unit area.

Use senna leaves and stramonium leaves for the counts.

HISTOLOGICAL SCHEDULE XV

Cloves (*Eugenia aromatica*)

1. From a clove which has been soaked in water for forty-eight hours, remove the petals and stamens, and place them in a separate hollowed glass block containing water.

2. Cut transverse sections through the middle region of the hypanthium or stalk-like solid portion (the so-called gynophore) and mount them separately in chloral hydrate solution, phloroglucin and hydrochloric acid, dilute glycerin, tincture of alkanna and alcoholic ferric chloride. Record the effects produced and make a diagrammatic sketch to show the epidermis, cortical region with oil-glands, region with intercellular spaces and the central solid strand; mark also the fibro-vascular bundles and the position of the calcium oxalate crystals. Sketch details from each region as seen with the 4-mm. objective.

3. Mount a fairly thick transverse section (cut with a dry razor from a clove softened in a moist atmosphere) in 50 per cent. caustic potash. Note and sketch the crystals of potassium eugenate.

4. Steep a clove in hot dilute caustic potash on a water-bath till quite soft and tease out the tissues with needles. Sketch isolated fibres and vessels and measure their dimensions.

5. Cut a surface section from the hypanthium and from one of the calyx teeth, mount them in chloral hydrate solution and sketch the epidermis in surface view.

6. Mount a petal in chloral hydrate solution and sketch a portion of each epidermis. Note the oil-glands in the mesophyll.

7. Mount a stamen in chloral hydrate solution. Examine the filament; note and sketch the glands and the numerous small cluster crystals of calcium oxalate. Sketch some pollen grains and a portion of the fibrous layer of the anther wall in surface view. Measure the diameter of the pollen grains.

8. Cut transverse and longitudinal sections of a clove stalk, which has been soaked in water for forty-eight hours, and mount as for the hypanthium. Make a keyed diagram of a transverse section and sketch characteristic elements in detail. Sketch a piece of a longitudinal section to show the prisms of calcium oxalate, which are often found in rows of cells adjacent to the fibres.

9. Digest clove stalks in caustic potash on a water-bath and tease out the tissues. Sketch some isolated stone-cells.

10. Examine powdered cloves in the same reagents as were used for the sections, and identify the structures seen in the dissections. Write out a list of the diagnostic characters of the powder.

NOTES ON HISTOLOGICAL SCHEDULE XV

Characters of Powdered Cloves. 1. Epidermis of the hypanthium and calyx teeth composed of straight-walled cells, with a very thick cuticle; large stomata.

2. Pollen grains, which are biconvex with a rounded edge, the edge being triangular in outline. Diameter 15 to 20 microns.

3. Fibrous layer from the anther walls.

4. Petals with straight-walled epidermal cells without papillæ or stomata and containing numerous cluster crystals of calcium oxalate and oil-glands.

5. Pericyclic fibres up to 40 microns in diameter and 650 microns long; small spiral and annular vessels up to 20 microns wide.

6. Spongy tissue from the hypanthium.

7. Absence of stone-cells, starch, prisms of calcium oxalate and reticulately-thickened vessels.

Clove stalks show numerous stone-cells, up to 120 microns in size, reticulately-thickened vessels and prisms of calcium oxalate. The prisms are well-formed diamond-shaped octahedra, chiefly in the secondary phloem. There are a few small starch grains in the pith.

The stalks also contain an abundance of cluster crystals of calcium oxalate.

HISTOLOGICAL SCHEDULE XVI

Flowers of Belladonna, Henbane and Stramonium

1. Dissect a flower of belladonna; determine the number and arrangement of the floral members, construct a floral diagram and white the floral formula.

2. Remove a corolla and clear a piece of the upper part by boiling

it in solution of chloral hydrate. Sketch surface views of the upper (inner) and lower (outer) epidermises. Note any colour changes and draw conclusions as to the nature of the colouring matter.

3. Clear and mount a piece of the basal part of the corolla. Note that the epidermis here forms a band of sclerenchyma and that the epidermal cells just above the sclerenchyma contain small clusters of calcium oxalate.

4. Examine the trichomes at the bases of the filaments and at the same level on the inside of the corolla tube.

5. Remove some pollen from an anther and mount in lactophenol. Sketch some grains to show the pores and cuticular markings. Measure the diameters of several grains and find the average diameter.

6. Examine flowers of henbane and stramonium in a similar way.

NOTES ON HISTOLOGICAL SCHEDULE XVI

The flowers are prepared for dissection by exposure to a moist atmosphere. The upper epidermis of the corolla is papillose for about half its length and the cells are polygonal with straight anticlinal walls. The under (*i.e.*, outer) epidermis has cells with very wavy walls and no papillæ.

The outer epidermis of the corolla has numerous uniseriate glandular trichomes having stalks of about 2 cells and one or up to three spherical glandular cells.

The pollen grains of the three flowers should be carefully compared as to size and markings.

HISTOLOGICAL SCHEDULE XVII

Lobelia Herb (*Lobelia inflata*)

Prepare some lobelia herb by exposing it to a moist atmosphere for about eighteen hours.

1. Cut transverse sections of a softened leaf, mount sections in chloral hydrate solution, phloroglucin and hydrochloric acid and in tincture of alkanna. Make a diagrammatic sketch to show the meristele with its laticiferous vessels, the distribution of the tissues of the mesophyll, the hairs and stomata. Look for pollen grains in the groove above the midrib; measure their diameter and sketch one or two.

2. Sketch a small piece of the interneural mesophyll in detail. Mark the papillose upper epidermis, the large curved hairs and the oily drops in the cells of the mesophyll.

3. Boil a small piece of leaf (about $\frac{1}{8}$ in. square) with chloral hydrate solution and sketch part of both the upper and lower epidermises in surface view.

4. Cut a piece from the margin of a leaf so as to include three or four teeth. Place it on a slide and boil with chloral hydrate solution till transparent. Sketch to show the specialised epidermal cells and the distribution of the water pores in the upper epidermis of a tooth.

5. Cut transverse sections of the stem internode, softened by soaking in water for twenty-four hours; mount sections separately in chloral hydrate solution, chlorzinciodine and in phloroglucin and hydrochloric

acid. Sketch diagrammatically to show the distribution of the tissues (epidermis, cortex, endodermis, phloem, xylem and pith).

6. Digest a piece of stem in 5 per cent. caustic alkali on a water-bath for about twenty minutes or until quite softened. Tease out some of the phloem from the stem, wash with distilled water, mount in iodine water and examine. Sketch some of the laticiferous vessels. Take the woody core, disintegrate it with nitric acid and potassium chlorate, and sketch the elements.

7. Cut surface sections of the stem and sketch a piece of the epidermis in surface view.

8. Remove a flower bud and boil it on a slide in solution of chloral hydrate until clear. Sketch the calyx, ovary and style. Find and sketch some pollen grains and measure their diameter.

9. Shake some seeds from a fruit; boil some in chloral hydrate solution and sketch one or two and measure their length and breadth. Mount some seeds also in phloroglucin and hydrochloric acid; note the thickening of the epidermal cells and their lignification, which is easily seen on crushing the seeds by pressure upon the cover-glass.

10. Examine genuine powdered lobelia, mounting it in the same reagents as were used for the sections and write out a list of the diagnostic characters.

11. Examine some asthma powders and report upon their composition.

NOTES ON HISTOLOGICAL SCHEDULE XVII

Characters of Powdered Lobelia—Leaves. 1. Cells of upper epidermis have straight walls, showing a more or less beaded appearance in surface view, owing to the pitting of the radial walls.

2. Upper epidermal cells papillose.

3. Palisade of one row; small globules of oil in all the cells of the mesophyll.

4. Lower epidermis, wavy walls. Stomata without special subsidiary cells, *i.e.*, the ranunculaceous type.

5. Trichomes conical, up to 600 microns long and 50 to 60 microns wide at the base; sometimes twisted and flattened; occasionally two-celled.

6. Teeth with numerous water pores on the upper surface.

Stem. 1. Epidermis of rectangular cells with beaded walls; cuticle striated; stomata with the pore parallel to the stem axis.

2. Anastomosing laticiferous vessels from the phloem.

3. Spiral and scalariform vessels; narrow wood-fibres.

4. Occasional solitary pericyclic fibres.

5. Lignified and pitted thin-walled parenchyma from the pith.

Corolla. The upper epidermis is papillose. The anthocyanin becomes red in solution of chloral hydrate.

Stamens. The anthers are syngenesious and at the apex of each connective is a tuft of unicellular linear trichomes about 300μ long. The pollen grains are spherical with three pores and a warty surface; 20 to 30 microns in diameter.

Fruit. The pericarp and dissepiment contain lignified sclereid idioblasts.

Seeds. 1. Dimensions about 0·64 to 0·7 mm. long and 0·25 to 0·30 mm. wide.

2. Reticulations are elongated polygonal in shape and have lignified anticlinal walls.

HISTOLOGICAL SCHEDULE XVIII

SQUILL BULB, COLCHICUM CORM, CALUMBA ROOT

Squill Bulb. The bulb of *Urginea Scilla* Steinh., family Liliaceæ.

1. Cut a transverse section of prepared material (see notes) ; mount in chloral and make sketches of the epidermis, the mesophyll and the bundles of acicular calcium oxalate, embedded in mucilage. Determine the composition of the crystals and measure their size.
2. Cut a transverse section of a piece of bulb softened by exposure to a moist atmosphere, and mount in corallin soda. Note the stained mucilage cells ; sketch.
3. Mount a transverse section of softened bulb in Fehling's reagent and warm ; note the formation of any red precipitate.
4. Cut surface preparations from both the concave and convex surfaces of a slice. Mount in chloral hydrate solution and sketch the epidermis. Are any stomata present, if so, where ?
5. Examine the powdered squill mounted in chloral hydrate solution and also in corallin soda.

Colchicum Corm. The corm of *Colchicum autumnale* Linn., family Liliaceæ, sliced transversely and dried.

1. Scrape a little powder from the flat surface of a slice, mount it in lacto-phenol and examine it microscopically. Sketch the starch and record its characteristics.
2. By means of transverse and longitudinal sections of a softened slice, examine the nature of the vascular bundles and make illustrative sketches.
3. From the edge of a softened slice, cut a surface section, Mount it in chloral hydrate solution and sketch the brown epidermis.
4. Examine powdered colchicum corm and identify the structures seen in the dissections.

Calumba Root. The dried transverse slices of the root of *Jateorhiza palmata* (Lamarck) Miers, family Menispermaceæ.

1. From a softened slice (see notes) cut out small pieces about 2 mm. square to include (*a*) the cork and outer layers, and (*b*) the cambium line together with some phloem and xylem. Support the pieces in pith and cut transverse sections from each and mount in chloral hydrate solution.

   Sketch them to show the cork cells, the sclerenchyma and its crystals, the details of phloem and xylem.
2. Scrape a little powder from the surface of a slice, mount it in lacto-phenol and sketch the starch. Measure the size of the starch grains and note their other characters.
3. Cut a radial longitudinal section, mount in chloral hydrate and sketch a vessel in detail.
4. Cut a longitudinal piece about 2 mm. wide quite across the diameter of a slice of calumba. Cut it up into small pieces longitudinally and macerate them, on a water-bath, in 5 per cent. caustic alkali for fifteen minutes. Tease out with needles, remove the woody strands and place them in a mixture of chromic and nitric acids (10 per cent. of each) for about thirty minutes. Thoroughly tease out both

the potash material and the woody strands and examine and sketch the isolated elements.

5. Examine powdered calumba root mounted in chloral hydrate solution, in lacto-phenol and in 66 per cent., by volume, sulphuric acid.

NOTES ON HISTOLOGICAL SCHEDULE XVIII

Squill Bulb. For making sections to study the structure of the tissues, squill may be prepared by exposing it to a moist atmosphere.

Characters of Powdered Squill. 1. Acicular raphides of calcium oxalate 50 to 900 microns, mostly 250 to 500 microns long and 5 to 8 microns wide.

2. Mounted in corallin soda, the mucilage stains red.

3. Stomata on the upper surface very rare ; on the lower surface few ; circular in outline with wide guard cells.

4. Epidermis of sub-rectangular cells.

5. Very occasional small starch grains.

Colchicum Corm. To prepare the slices of corm for section cutting, soak them in cold water for about eighteen hours.

Characters of Powdered Colchicum Corm. 1. Starch of simple and compound grains ; the compound grains predominate and usually consist of two to three components, more rarely four to seven ; the components are frequently muller-shaped. Hilum central, often a radiate split. Individual grains mostly about 10 to 16 microns in diameter.

2. Epidermis of isodiametric cells 40 to 95 microns, mostly about 60 microns, in width ; radial walls indistinctly pitted ; very occasional, nearly circular, stomata.

3. A few small spiral and annular vessels, up to 30 microns in width.

Calumba Root. Prepare this root for section-cutting by soaking in water till fully swollen (this requires two or three days) and then store in 30 per cent. alcohol mixed with one-fifth its volume of glycerin.

Characters of Powdered Calumba Root. 1. Starch grains, mostly simple, some compound with two to six components. Diameter of individual grains from 10 to 80 microns.

2. Abundant cellulose parenchyma.

3. Vessels with transversely elongated bordered pits and some reticulate vessels ; 80 to 150 microns in diameter. Walls yellow, changing to green with 66 per cent. *v/v* sulphuric acid.

4. Yellow, sub-rectangular, moderately thickened stone-cells containing small prisms of calcium oxalate. The walls become green with sulphuric acid 66 per cent. by volume).

5. Thin-walled, tabular, cork cells in several layers.

6. No true fibres ; small numbers of fibrous tracheids near the vessels.

HISTOLOGICAL SCHEDULE XIX

Ginger Rhizome (*Zingiber officinale*)

1. For the external characters and general appearance of a transverse section as seen with a lens, see Schedule XXXIV., p. 94.

2. From the cut surface of the dry rhizome scrape a little powder, moisten with alcohol and mount in water or in lactophenol and sketch the starch grains. Make the grains roll by irrigation or by pushing the cover-glass, and note their shape. Measure the length, breadth

and thickness of the grains. Are there any compound grains ? Write a description of the starch.

3. From a rhizome, softened by exposure to a moist atmosphere (see p. 38), cut several transverse sections. Mount them separately in iodine water, chloral hydrate solution, solution of caustic potash, phloroglucin and hydrochloric acid. Sections mounted in chloral hydrate and in caustic potash should be boiled to remove the starch. Make notes of the staining effects produced. Sketch in detail a piece of a section in the region of the endodermis and also a vascular bundle ; mark the oil-cells, endodermis, vessels, brown pigment cells, fibres, etc. Record the width of the fibres.

4. Cut longitudinal sections of the prepared rhizome, mount one in chloral hydrate solution, a second in phloroglucin and hydrochloric acid, and a third in aniline chloride solution. Sketch a vascular bundle to show the structure of the vessels, fibres and pigment cells. Sketch some of the oil-cells to show their shape and arrangement.

5. Make a crude fibre from some genuine powder, using the Dutch method (see notes below). Examine the fibre and identify the elements present.

6. Examine the genuine powder mounted in water, in iodine water, in chloral hydrate solution, and in phloroglucin and hydrochloric acid. Write out a statement of its diagnostic characters.

NOTES ON HISTOLOGICAL SCHEDULE XIX

Crude Fibre. For the examination of many kinds of starchy materials, such as flour, pepper, ginger and many drugs, as also for dark-coloured substances like coffee and chicory, the preparation of a crude fibre concentrates the resistant tissues into a small bulk and also separates and clears the constituent elements, so that they are in a good condition for microscopical examination. From all points of view the "Dutch Process" is to be preferred ; it is as follows :—Weigh out a quantity of the powdered drug, which may vary from 1 to 2 gm. according to circumstances, put it into a 100 ml. porcelain dish, add 50 ml. of nitric acid, 10 per cent., bring it to the boil and maintain ebullition with constant stirring during thirty seconds. Immediately strain out the residue by filtration at the pump through a piece of fine-meshed cotton cloth having about 92 threads to the linear inch (such as some forms of "tarantulle" or "longcloth") and wash the residue on the cloth by pouring through it about 100 ml. of boiling water. Remove the material from the cloth by stretching it tightly, like the membrane of a drum, over the rim of a watch-glass and scraping off the fibre with a flexible spatula ; return the fibre to the porcelain dish, add 50 ml. of caustic soda solution, 2·5 per cent., and boil for thirty seconds. Strain the liquid through the cloth and wash with 100 ml. of boiling water as before and remove the fibre from the cloth. The fibre may be transferred to a small corked tube, a little water added and also, if desired, a small amount of formaldehyde to act as a preservative. This fibre is now in an excellent condition for microscopical examination and a small quantity is removed with a dipping-tube and mounted on a slide in water, glycerin or chloral hydrate solution. A fibre prepared in this way will not give reactions for lignin, because the lignin is destroyed by oxidation with the nitric acid.

Note.—When preparing a crude fibre of oily materials, such as linseed or mustard, the greater part of the oil must be removed by preliminary treatment with a suitable solvent.

Characters of Powdered Ginger. 1. Abundant starch grains of the Scitaminaceous type.

2. Free-lying oleo-resin lumps, mostly broken up and staining with iodine water. Walls of oleo-resin cells cuticularised.

3. Abundant thin-walled parenchyma.

4. Thin-walled, septate fibres with elongated pits. Only the middle lamella shows a reaction for lignin. Fibres up to 60µ wide.

5. Portions of vessels with reticulate thickening, sometimes accompanied by narrow, brown pigment cells. The vessels give no reaction for lignin.

6. Absence of hairs, stone-cells and calcium oxalate crystals. Jamaica ginger also shows an absence of cork cells.

N.B.—The cells of the endodermis and pericycle contain no starch and, being thin-walled, collapse during drying of the rhizome. These cells are expanded by warming the sections in caustic potash solution, which also changes the yellow colour of the oleo-resin to a deep orange.

Starch of Ginger. Shape, sack-shaped, *i.e.*, flat and oval-oblong with a slight terminal protuberance.

Hilum. Eccentric ; situated in the terminal protuberance.

Striations. Not clearly marked. They are almost straight and at right angles to the long axis of the grain.

Size. 12 to 50 microns long, up to 30 microns wide and about 7 microns thick.

Compound Grains. Almost absent.

Polarised Light. Faint cross.

HISTOLOGICAL SCHEDULE XX

Rhubarb (*Rheum palmatum*)

1. Cut a transverse section of a root, softened by exposure to a moist atmosphere, and mount it in dilute glycerin. If the section passed through the outer ring of secondary wood, the medullary rays appear as fairly straight and parallel yellow bands. If the section traverses a star-spot, the medullary rays appear as curved radiating lines. Measure, sketch and describe the starch.

2. Mount a transverse section in chloral hydrate solution and boil it. The yellow matter disappears. Note the conspicuous calcium oxalate crystals ; sketch two or three and find their average diameter.

3. Find and sketch a transverse section of a star-spot, with its internal phloem and surrounding xylem, separated by cambium.

4. Mount other sections in alcohol and in phloroglucin and hydrochloric acid respectively.

5. Tease out a small piece of rhubarb which has been digested in 5 per cent. caustic alkali on a water-bath until thoroughly softened. Examine it and sketch vessels, parenchyma and crystals ; measure the diameter of the vessels.

6. Mount some powdered East Indian rhubarb in alcohol and irrigate with solution of caustic alkali ; record the result. Mount a further quantity in alcohol and irrigate with water. Clear some powder in chloral hydrate solution and identify all the elements seen

in the sections. Write out the diagnostic characters of powdered rhubarb.

7. Determine the nature of the vegetable structures present in the compressed tablet of rhubarb, soda and ginger, examining it as explained in the notes below. Indicate in your report, by diagrams and descriptions or both, the nature of the structures upon which your conclusions as to its composition are based.

NOTES ON HISTOLOGICAL SCHEDULE XX

Characters of Powdered Rhubarb. 1. Abundance of thin-walled parenchyma.

2. Large amount of starch, partly in single grains (mostly 12 to 20 microns) and partly in compound grains with two to five components (individual grains up to about 20 microns). The hilum is frequently in the form of a radiate split.

3. Calcium oxalate cluster crystals, from 20 to 200 microns in diameter, often over 100 microns; in the powder often broken up, and can be picked out by means of the polariscope.

4. Yellow-coloured masses from the medullary rays, insoluble in alcohol, soluble in water. They are dissolved to a reddish-pink colour by solution of ammonia, and a deep red by solution of caustic alkali.

5. Fragments of reticulate vessels (often about 80 microns in diameter), also some spiral and annular vessels, and some tracheids. These elements do not react for lignin, but stain blue with iodine and 80 per cent. (by volume) sulphuric acid.

6. Cork, sclerenchymatous cells and fibres are absent.

See also pp. 216 and 217.

Lozenges and tablets, when soaked in water, become disintegrated, and yield their sugar and other soluble constituents to the solvent, while vegetable powders and insoluble ingredients form a sediment suitable for immediate examination, and, if further treatment with other reagents, such as acids, chloral hydrate, acid and alkali, in succession, etc., as may seem desirable. To clear such a sediment with chloral hydrate some of the thick deposit is removed to a second clean test-tube by means of a dipping tube, and boiled with two or three times its volume of chloral hydrate solution. The deposit from the chloral is obtained either by sedimentation or centrifugation, and is examined in the usual way.

HISTOLOGICAL SCHEDULE XXI

Liquorice (*Glycyrrhiza glabra*)

1. Cut some transverse sections of a softened stolon; mount one in dilute glycerin or lacto-phenol, another in chloral hydrate solution, a third in iodine water and a fourth in phloroglucin and hydrochloric acid. Make a diagrammatic sketch and mark the cork, phellogen, cortex (if any), keratenchyma, bast parenchyma and fibres, sieve tissue, medullary rays, cambium, wood parenchyma, fibres and vessels, pith and calcium oxalate crystals. (See Fig 56, p. 95.)

2. Sketch in detail some starch grains, a group of bast fibres, some vessels and wood fibres with the accompanying crystal cells.

3. Cut radial longitudinal sections and mount in reagents as for the transverse sections. Sketch bast fibres with the neighbouring crystal

cells and some vessels with numerous bordered pits or reticulate thickening.

4. If possible, find a piece of root and make transverse sections. Note the absence of a pith and determine the number of primary xylem bundles.

5. Take a piece of the drug about 5 mm. long, and cut it longitudinally into small pieces. Macerate the pieces in 5 per cent. caustic alkali upon a water-bath till thoroughly softened; wash by decantation with distilled water. Tease out a piece of the macerated material with needles; find and sketch the isolated vessels, fibres, files of crystal cells, etc.

6. Examine powdered liquorice after soaking it in diluted glycerin for at least an hour. Examine also preparations mounted in chloral hydrate solution and in phloroglucin and hydrochloric acid. Identify the structures seen in the sections and write out a list of the diagnostic characters of the powdered drug.

7. Examine Pulv. Sennæ Co. *U.S.P.*, and identify the vegetable ingredients.

NOTES ON HISTOLOGICAL SCHEDULE XXI

To prepare liquorice root for making sections, soak short lengths (about 3 cm.) of the commercial drug in water for a few days until thoroughly swollen out and penetrated by the water. If necessary, the material may now be hardened slightly by placing it in alcohol, and may be stored in a mixture of 50 per cent. alcohol containing one-fifth of its volume of glycerin.

Characters of Powdered Liquorice. 1. Thick-walled fibres from both phloem and xylem in bundles of ten to fifty. Diameter of the fibres up to 20 microns.

2. Files of small rectangular crystal cells accompanying the fibres and containing single prisms of calcium oxalate, 10 to **15** to **25** to 35μ.

3. Large vessels with numerous bordered pits, having slit-shaped openings. Vessels 80 to 200 microns wide.

4. Starch grains small, mostly about 10 microns, round to oval or very narrowly oval; no striations; they occasionally show a hilum.

5. Sulphuric acid, 80 per cent. by volume, gives a yellow coloration.

6. Sweet taste; buff colour.

Pulv. Sennæ Co. U.S.P. has the following composition: Senna in No. 80 powder, 18; liquorice in No. 80 powder, 23·6; washed sulphur, 8; oil of fennel (by weight), 0·4; sugar, in fine powder, 50.

HISTOLOGICAL SCHEDULE XXII

BELLADONNA ROOT AND GENTIAN ROOT

Belladonna Root (*Atropa belladonna*)

1. Cut transverse sections of a softened root and mount separate sections in lacto-phenol, chloral hydrate solution, iodine water and phloroglucin and hydrochloric acid. Make a diagrammatic sketch and mark the tissues present, viz., cortex (if present, outside the cork in small patches with thicker-walled cells), cork, phellogen, phelloderm

and pericycle, phloem, cambium, wood vessels, tracheids and fibres. idioblasts with microsphenoidal crystals of calcium oxalate, groups of interxylary phloem, the central diarch mass of primary xylem.

2. Sketch in detail some starch grains and an idioblast with its crystals. Measure the diameter of some starch granules.

3. Cut a radial longitudinal section and sketch a small portion to show the somewhat axially elongated parenchyma and the cells with sandy crystals.

4. Digest a piece of root with caustic potash on a water-bath until thoroughly softened. Tease out a small piece, examine with the microscope, and sketch typical vessels, tracheids, fibres and cork cells. Sketch part of a vessel to show the pitting.

5. Examine powdered belladonna root mounted in reagents as directed for transverse sections. Identify the elements seen in the sections and write out a list of the diagnostic characters of powdered belladonna root.

6. Compare powdered poke root (*Phytolacca decandra*) with powdered belladonna root and point out the main distinguishing features.

Gentian Root (*Gentiana lutea*)

1. Cut transverse sections of a prepared root, mount one in chloral hydrate solution and a second one in phloroglucin and hydrochloric acid. Make a diagram to show the limits of the cork, phellogen, bark (mainly secondary phloem), cambium and xylem ; search for small groups of sieve tissue amongst the xylem. Sketch typical portions of each region in detail and find the minute crystals of calcium oxalate in the parenchyma. Note also the highly refractive spherical droplets scattered throughout the preparation.

2. Cut radial longitudinal sections and mount in chloral hydrate solution. Sketch some of the vessels and parenchyma with minute calcium oxalate crystals.

3. Cut transverse sections from a root, softened by exposure to a moist atmosphere ; mount one in water and, after it has spread out, add a drop of tincture of alkanna ; mount a second section in iodine water. What conclusions do you draw from your observations ?

4. Digest a piece of root in caustic potash solution on a water-bath, until thoroughly softened. Tease out a portion with needles and identify the isolated elements.

5. Examine genuine powdered gentian mounted in lacto-phenol and in the reagents used for the dissections. Write out the diagnostic characters of the powder.

NOTES ON HISTOLOGICAL SCHEDULE XXII

Belladonna Root is softened for section cutting by soaking in cold water for eighteen hours.

Characters of Powdered Belladonna Root. 1. Large veessls with closely-arranged bordered pits ; thin-walled xylem fibres and tracheidal fibres.

2. Much parenchyma with idioblasts filled with microsphenoidal crystals of calcium oxalate, measuring 1·7 to 7·0μ.

3. Starch grains, mostly simple, occasionally compound; individual grains up to 30 microns, usually 15 to 20 microns in diameter.

4. Patches of cork cells.

5. Phloem fibres and stone-cells absent.

Characters of Powdered Poke Root (*Phytolacca*). 1. Large vessels with closely-arranged bordered pits.

2. Parenchyma containing idioblasts with bundles of acicular raphides of calcium oxalate.

3. Fibres having thicker walls than those of belladonna.

4. Starch in rather large oval grains with a distinct hilum; often compound; individual grains up to 40 microns in diameter.

5. Cells containing resin.

Gentian root is prepared by soaking some of the smaller roots till thoroughly swollen in water as for liquorice root (see p. 158). Some roots should also be softened by exposure to a moist atmosphere in a desiccator.

Characters of Powdered Gentian Root. 1. Abundant parenchyma, the cells being rather thick-walled and containing droplets of oil, which are often difficult to find in the powder.

2. Minute needles of calcium oxalate occur in some cells of the parenchyma and also lying loose in the powder. The crystals are about 3 to 6 microns long and 0·5 to 1 micron wide.

3. Small amounts of reticulate, and a very few spiral and annular vessels.

4. Yellowish-brown cork cells.

5. Starch almost absent; a very few small grains here and there.

6. Stone-cells and fibres absent.

HISTOLOGICAL SCHEDULE XXIII

Ipecacuanha Root (*Cephaëlis Ipecacuanha*)

1. Using a razor flooded with alcohol, cut transverse sections of a root, softened by soaking in water for eighteen hours. Mount one in chloral hydrate solution and clear it by boiling; mount a second section in iodine water. Make a diagram to show the distribution of the xylem, phloem, medullary rays, cork and other tissues. Mark also the position of the bundles of acicular raphides; measure the length of the crystals.

2. Sketch in detail a bundle of raphides and a few typical cells from the different regions.

3. Mount a fresh section in lacto-phenol and sketch some starch grains. Measure and record their size, especially noting the dimensions of the largest grains present. Note also the number of components of the compound grains.

4. Cut thin surface sections from a root, mount in chloral hydrate solution and sketch some of the cork cells in surface view.

5. Digest some of the separated woody cylinder with potassium chlorate and nitric acid, or with sulphuric acid and chromic anhydride. Mount some of the disintegrated material, thoroughly teased out, and sketch typical tracheids. Note the absence of large vessels and the presence of starch grains filling the interior of the wood parenchyma and the cells of the medullary rays.

6. Examine some of the powdered ipecacuanha root and identify the structures observed in the sections. Write a brief statement of the diagnostic characters of powdered ipecacuanha root.

7. Examine some powdered Carthagena ipecacuanha and measure the starch grains.

8. Cut a transverse section of ipecacuanha stem and compare it with the root. Make a diagrammatic drawing. Note the central pith and the sclereids of the pericycle.

9. Analyse some pills of ipecacuanha with squill, according to instructions; identify the vegetable ingredients, giving your reasons.

NOTES ON HISTOLOGICAL SCHEDULE XXIII

Characters of Powdered Ipecacuanha Root. 1. Abundant starch grains, mostly compound. Some of the isolated grains are muller-shaped, being components of compound grains. Individual grains not larger than 15 microns in diameter.

2. Lignified medullary ray cells and cells of the wood parenchyma, often filled with starch grains; all with pitted walls. Vessels small and difficult to distinguish from tracheids.

3. Acicular crystals of calcium oxalate; the groups mostly broken up, and the small needles (20 to 80 microns long) are strewn throughout the preparation.

4. Patches of cork cells with dark brown contents.

5. Absence of large vessels, sclerenchymatous cells and phloem fibres.

Pil. Ipecacuanhæ cum Scilla, B.P.C., has the following composition: Compound powder of ipecacuanha, 60: squill, in powder, 20; ammoniacum, in powder, 20; syrup of glucose, a sufficient quantity.

Pills should first be stripped of their coating by carefully paring it off with a sharp knife, and the remainder is dropped into water in a test-tube, and soaked until disintegrated. The sediment is examined in water, and a part is removed to another tube, and boiled with chloral hydrate or treated with other clearing reagents, after which the new sediment is removed for examination. If information is desired as to the nature of the *coating,* the parings should be soaked in water in a separate tube, and the deposit examined in the same way as the pill mass itself. Starch and talc are the most usual ingredients detectable by the microscope. Many trade pills are coated with talc only. For *Pil. Ipecac. cum Scilla* mount a little of the mass in corallin-soda and note the staining of the mucilage.

HISTOLOGICAL SCHEDULE XXIV

ACONITE ROOT AND JALAP ROOT

Aconite Root (*Aconitum Napellus*)

1. Cut transverse sections from the narrower end of a prepared tuberous root. Mount one in iodine water, a second in chloral hydrate solution and a third in phloroglucin and hydrochloric acid. Make a diagrammatic drawing and mark upon it the cortex, endodermis, primary xylem, cambium, pith and phloem strands.

2. Take a fresh transverse section and determine the nature of the cell walls of the outer cortical layers. Treat the sections separately with tincture of alkanna, solution of Soudan Red III. and of Scharlach R. Confirm your result by the sulphuric acid test.

3. Scrape the exposed surface of a transversely-broken, dry root and examine the powder mounted in water or in lacto-phenol. Measure the starch grains, sketch them and record essential particulars about them.

4. From a prepared root, cut a surface section, mount it in chloral hydrate solution and sketch the surface view of the outer layer.

5. Tease out material after digesting it upon a water-bath with 5 per cent. caustic alkali until soft; make drawings of characteristic elements.

6. Examine the genuine powder mounted in reagents as for the sections. Write out an account of the characters of the powder.

Jalap Root (*Ipomœa purga*)

1. Cut a tubercle transversely and examine the cut surface with a pocket lens. Make a sketch to show the position of the following structures: Cork, a narrow layer of secondary phloem, cambium line and the central region. Note the dark points (resin cells) scattered throughout the section, and in the central portion note the scattered groups of vessels and the irregularly curved cambia.

2. Make thin transverse sections to include parts of all the regions noted in (1). Mount one in lacto-phenol, another in chloral hydrate and a third in phloroglucin and hydrochloric acid. Sketch some starch grains and determine their size. Note that the pale brown contents of the cuticularised secretion cells dissolve in the chloral hydrate.

3. Make drawings to show the structures present in each region, viz., the cork cells, the secondary phloem with its sieve tissue and parenchyma containing calcium oxalate clusters (determine their size) and resin cells, the cambium, the xylem vessels and xylem parenchyma. In the central region find and sketch one of the groups of vessels (from one to several) surrounded by a cambium, which forms phloem on the outside and xylem on the inside.

4. Mount fresh sections (cut with a razor flooded with water) in tincture of alkanet, in iodine water and in 80 per cent. by volume sulphuric acid. Note and record the behaviour of the secretion cells and their contents.

5. Cut radial longitudinal sections and mount in iodine water and in chloral hydrate solution. Make sketches to show the arrangement of the secretion cells in vertical rows.

6. Digest some small pieces of a tubercle in 5 per cent. potash for fifteen minutes on a water-bath. Wash and tease out and sketch the cork in surface view, the parenchyma, the secretion cells and the vessels.

7. Examine genuine powdered jalap mounted in the same reagents as were used for the sections. Make a list of the characters which appear to be most useful for the identification of jalap in the form of powder.

NOTES ON HISTOLOGICAL SCHEDULE XXIV

Aconite Root. Select small roots and soak them in water till thoroughly swollen.

Characters of Powdered Aconite Root. 1. Patches of metaderm, composed of brown-walled cuticularised tabular cells.

2. Abundant parenchyma containing small starch grains, single or 2–5 compound. Individual grains up to 30 microns diameter.

3. Occasional stone-cells, which are quadratic and evenly thickened with large lumina and simple pits.

4. Fragments of vessels.
5. Fibres and crystals of calcium oxalate absent.

Jalap Root. Prepare jalap roots for dissection by soaking small tubercles in water till sufficiently soft to be cut easily; this takes about 48 hours.

Characters of Powdered Jalap. 1. Calcium oxalate in cluster crystals, 15 to 30 microns in diameter. Also some small prisms, about 6μ long, scattered here and there in the parenchyma.

2. Abundant parenchyma containing large starch grains, single or 2–4 compound. Individual grains up to 65 microns, mostly about 30 microns in diameter. Some starch grains are gelatinised.

3. Yellow resin cells or drops of resinous secretion, stain with iodine water or with alkanet.

4. Fragments of brown cork cells.

5. Scattered fragments of vessels and fibrous tracheids.

6. A few yellowish stone-cells, not very strongly thickened. Found in very small roots, hardly ever in larger roots.

7. Fibres absent.

HISTOLOGICAL SCHEDULE XXV

MARSHMALLOW ROOT, SENEGA AND MALE FERN RHIZOME

Marshmallow Root (*Althœa officinalis*)

1. From a prepared root, cut transverse sections, using a razor flooded with alcohol. Mount sections in chloral hydrate solution, iodine water; in phloroglucin and hydrochloric acid, in ruthenium red, in caustic potash and in oil of cloves.

2. Make sketches to show the characteristic structures present in the phloem, xylem, medullary rays and cambium region. Record your conclusions as to the contents of the various cells and as to the nature of the cell walls. Determine the number of fibres present in the groups of fibres.

3. Mount a section in alcohol and irrigate it with water or dilute glycerin and observe the swelling of the mucilage.

4. From the surface of a root scrape a little powder, mount in lactophenol. Note and sketch the sclerenchymatous fibres, starch, mucilage, vessels, calcium oxalate crystals, etc. Determine the size of the starch grains and of the calcium oxalate crystals, which are best seen in a chloral hydrate preparation.

5. Examine genuine powdered marshmallow root and compare the particles present with the structures observed in the dissections. Write out a list of the important features by which the powder may be recognised.

Senega (*Polygala senaga*)

1. For the external characters and the general appearance of a transverse section as seen with a lens, see Schedule XXXVI, p. 98.

2. From a prepared root cut several transverse sections about 1 cm. below the crown, using a razor flooded with alcohol. Mount separate sections in chloral hydrate solution, iodine water, tincture of alkanna, and phloroglucin and hydrochloric acid. Make notes of the staining effects produced and record your conclusions.

3. Make a diagrammatic drawing of a transverse section and prepare detailed sketches of the central woody mass to show the primary axlem

groups, a small portion from the region of the cambium to show details of xylem, phloem and medullary rays, also a small piece of the external region to show the cork, phellogen, phelloderm, etc. Sketch also a small piece of the wedge of parenchyma (an abnormally large medullary ray) in the neighbourhood of the cambium.

4. Cut radial longitudinal sections so as to pass through the parenchymatous wedge and mount as for the transverse sections. Make sketches to show details of the xylem elements, the parenchyma of the wedge and of the phelloderm, and the phloem.

5. Cut surface sections from the root and sketch a few typical cells of the cork.

6. Isolate a piece of the central woody core (see p. 99) and macerate longitudinal slices cut from it in a mixture of chromic and nitric acids until disintegrated. Sketch typical elements, and determine the dimensions of the tracheids and vessel elements.

7. Examine genuine powdered senega root and identify the elements and cell contents observed in the dissections.

Male Fern Rhizome (*Dryopteris Filix-mas*)

1. Cut transverse sections of the rhizome and mount them separately in chloral hydrate solution, in iodine water and in phloroglucin with hydrochloric acid. Make a diagram to show the general distribution of the meristeles, the hypodermal sclerenchyma, etc. Make a detailed drawing of a single meristele showing the endodermis, pericycle, phloem and xylem. Sketch also a portion of the fundamental parenchyma to show an intercellular space with an internal secreting hair and a few starch grains.

2. Measure and record the dimensions of the starch grains. Make a note of their other characters.

3. Cut a longitudinal section of the rhizome and sketch a vessel to show the scalariform thickening.

4. Cut a transverse section of a frond base. Mount as for the rhizome and make a diagrammatic sketch to show the arrangement and number of the meristeles and the sclerenchyma.

5. Remove a ramentum, mount it in chloral hydrate solution. Sketch an entire ramentum diagrammatically to show the general outline, and sketch in detail a piece of the margin to show the characteristic outgrowths and sketch also the base.

6. Digest a piece of rhizome in 5 per cent. potash on a water-bath. Tease out thoroughly and sketch the isolated tracheids, parenchyma, sclerenchyma of the hypodermis, ramenta, etc.

7. Examine the powdered male fern and identify all the structures noted in the dissections.

NOTES ON HISTOLOGICAL SCHEDULE XXV

Marshmallow Root is prepared for section cutting by exposure to a moist atmosphere for about eighteen hours.

Characters of Powdered Marshmallow Root. 1. Phloem fibres in bundles of three to twenty-five, unlignified. Xylem fibres similar, but with lignification of the middle lamella.

2. Abundant parenchyma with ovoid starch grains, almost all simple, a few 2-4 compound. Diameter up to 15 microns.

3. Cells containing sphæro-crystals of asparagine, visible in oil of cloves and giving a yellow colour in strong caustic potash.

4. Crystal cells with clusters of calcium oxalate, 17 to 34 microns in diameter.

5. Mucilage cells which stain with ruthenium red.

6. A few reticulate vessels which often show abundant thylosis.

7. Cork absent from the peeled root or only very small amount from the grooves.

Senega. Prepare senega root for making sections by soaking it in water. In a transverse section stained with phloroglucin and hydrochloric acid, the diarch structure of the primary xylem is easily seen. The cells of the parenchymatous wedge in the xylem are radially elongated. The disintegration of the woody core by chromic and nitric acids requires about forty-five minutes.

Characters of Powdered Senega. 1. Fragments of vessels and of the more numerous tracheids with transversely elongated bordered pits. The vessels show lateral as well as terminal openings.

2. Rounded parenchyma of the phelloderm and slightly elongated parenchyma of the wedges, all containing droplets of oil.

3. Numerous patches of pale brown sub-rectangular cork cells.

4. Absence of crystals, starch and sclerenchymatous fibres and cells.

5. Odour resembling that of wintergreen; taste sweetish and then acrid. The powder froths when shaken with water.

Characters of Powdered Male Fern Rhizome. 1. Abundant large-celled parenchyma, containing numerous starch grains, up to 18 microns in diameter.

2. Internal hairs, secreting oleo-resin.

3. Yellow-brown sclerenchyma (not lignified) from the hypodermis.

4. Scalariform tracheids.

5. Fragments of ramenta showing characteristic two-celled marginal teeth.

6. Absence of crystals.

HISTOLOGICAL SCHEDULE XXVI

LINSEED AND NUX VOMICA

Linseed (*Linum usitatissimum*)

1. Cut a small slit in the end of a dispensing cork, insert the end of a seed into the slit and cut transverse sections with a dry razor. Mount a section in chloral hydrate and sketch it to show the following parts: Epidermis with mucilage, parenchymatous layer, sclerenchymatous layer, obliterated parenchyma, pigment layer, endosperm and cotyledons.

2. Mount a section in alcohol and allow water to flow in by irrigation. Note and record the action upon the mucilaginous epidermis. Mount another section in ruthenium red and note the staining of the mucilage. Mount a third section in iodine water and note the absence of starch. Test a fourth section for fixed oil.

3. Cut a seed longitudinally and remove the endosperm and cotyledons. Soak the seed-coats in 5 per cent. solution of caustic alkali until they can be disintegrated upon a slide with needles; this will take an hour or more. Identify the layers seen in the sections and sketch a small piece of each in surface view.

4. Defat some sections of the cotyledons by soaking in ether. Mount one in glycerin and another in iodine water. Make sketches of the aleurone grains.

5. Examine powdered linseed both in the ordinary condition and after defatting. Identify the structures seen in the sections and surface preparations and write out a list of the diagnostic characters of the powder.

Nux Vomica (*Strychnos Nux-vomica*)

1. Cut a dry seed in half at right angles to the flat faces and from the exposed surface cut a section with a dry razor. Mount it in alcohol and observe the cell walls of the endosperm ; add water by irrigation and watch the swelling of the walls. Note also the middle lamella.

2. From a seed softened by soaking in water, cut radial sections, moving the razor parallel to the direction of the hairs. Mount a section in chloral hydrate solution and sketch it to show the structure of the seed-coat (including the epidermis with its pitted cell bases and ribbed hairs, and the brown, collapsed cells of the nutrient layer) and the endosperm, noting the difference between the cells of the endosperm epidermis and of the inner portion.

3. Mount a second section in phloroglucin and hydrochloric acid. What conclusions do you draw from the observed action ?

4. Warm a section in chloral hydrate solution, wash with water and mount in tincture of alkanna ; note the oil-globules stained red.

5. Put some sections into ether or into petroleum spirit to remove oil. Mount one in iodine water and observe the deep staining of the aleurone grains in the cells of the endosperm and the fine strands of protoplasm (plasmodesma) connecting the protoplasts through the cell walls. Remove the iodine water with blotting-paper and add 80 per cent. (by volume) sulphuric acid and state the conclusions you draw as to the cell walls of the endosperm and the seed-coat.

6. Cut some sections from a dry seed and defat them by soaking in light petroleum in a covered hollowed glass block. Place a defatted section on a slide and cover it with a cover-glass. Focus the section with the 16 mm. objective and place a drop of strong nitric acid against the edge of the cover-glass. When the acid reaches the section, note the deep yellow colour given to the cell contents (due to brucine). In a similar way treat a section with sulphovanadic acid.

7. Cut the seed-coat from a seed ; macerate it in a solution of 10 per cent. sulphuric acid and 10 per cent. chromic acid until the hairs can be separated, wash with water, shake violently in a tube to separate the hairs, and examine them microscopically.

8. Examine powdered nux vomica and make a statement of its characteristic features.

NOTES ON HISTOLOGICAL SCHEDULE XXVI

Characters of Powdered Linseed. 1. Quadrangular pigment cells in a single layer ; walls moderately and evenly thickened and pitted ; contents a red-brown amorphous mass filling the lumen of each cell and often dropping out entire.

2. Narrow, oblong, lignified, sclerenchymatous cells in a single layer with their long axes parallel and with a layer of delicate, colourless, elongated, narrow parenchyma crossing them at right angles.

3. Thick-walled, circular cells of the sub-epidermal layer, with triangular intercellular spaces.

4. Aleurone grains with crystalloid and globoid, up to 18 microns in diameter.

5. Mucilage of the epidermis ; stains red with ruthenium red and blue with iodine water.

6. Starch and calcium oxalate absent. A little starch may sometimes be fóund. It is present in the epidermis, not having been entirely used in the formation of mucilage.

Characters of Powdered Nux Vomica. 1. Numerous lignified, slender, rod-shaped fragments of the ribs of thickening from the broken hairs. Occasional unbroken tips of hairs may be found.

2. Lignified and pitted, thick-walled bases of the epidermal hairs.

3. Abundant fragments of endosperm, consisting of colourless, thick-walled, polygonal cells, containing small aleurone grains, granular matter and oil. No pits in the walls, which are composed mainly of a mucilaginous form of cellulose and are penetrated by plasmodesma, which is most clearly visible in mounts made in iodine water.

4. Starch and calcium oxalate absent.

5. The powder responds to colour tests for brucine and strychnine.

HISTOLOGICAL SCHEDULE XXVII

Strophanthus Seed (*Strophanthus kombé*)

1. Embed a dry seed in pith and cut transverse sections of the entire seed, using a razor flooded with alcohol. Sweep off the sections into a hollow glass block containing alcohol.

2. Mount sections in chloral hydrate and in phloroglucin and hydrochloric acid. Find and sketch the seed-coat to show the epidermis with cells showing a band-like thickening and unicellular hairs with a rod-like thickening. Look for calcium oxalate crystals in the underlying cells.

3. Examine a transverse section of the endosperm and make a sketch to show the clearly marked outer epidermis and the collapsed condition of the innermost layers.

4. Transfer some sections to ether and defat them. Mount defatted sections of all parts of the seed in iodine water and look for aleurone and starch. Sketch a part of a section of a cotyledon with its cell contents. Look for laticiferous tubes in the neighbourhood of the procambial strands.

5. Mount some sections of the endosperm and cotyledon in tincture of alkanna, Soudan Red III. and Scharlach R. Record your conclusions.

6. Remove the seed coat from a soaked seed, boil it in chloral hydrate solution until clear. Sketch the epidermis in surface view and look for crystals.

7. Dissect out the endosperm from a seed, lay it upon a slide and boil with chloral hydrate solution. Sketch in surface view a portion of the epidermis and of the inner parenchyma.

8. Make surface preparations from a cotyledon and sketch the small-celled epidermis.

9. Soak a piece of seed-coat in a mixture of chromic and nitric acids (10 per cent. of each) until it can be disintegrated by violent shaking with water in a tube. Sketch some of the isolated cells.

10. Examine powdered strophanthus both before and after defatting

with ether. Make the mounts in the same reagents as were used for the dissections, and write out a list of the diagnostic features of the powder.

NOTES ON HISTOLOGICAL SCHEDULE XXVII

Characters of Powdered Strophanthus Seeds. 1. Numerous fragments of the lignified ribs from the epidermal hairs, resembling fibres or the ribs from the hairs of *nux vomica*.

2. Bases of hairs with band-shaped, lignified thickening.

CHARACTERS OF THE SEEDS OF COMMON SPECIES OF STROPHANTHUS

Species of *Strophanthus*.	Testa.			Endosperm and Embryo.		
	Colour.	Trichomes.	Calcium Oxalate.	Calcium Oxalate.	Reaction with H_2SO_4 66% by volume.	
					Endosperm.	Embryo.
Strophanthus kombé Oliv.	Greyish-green to greenish-fawn.	Abundant	Occasional clusters and prisms.	None.	Green.	Green and/or reddish.
Strophanthus hispidus P.DC.	Brownish.	Abundant, mostly rubbed off.	Occasional clusters and prisms.	None.	Green.	Green and/or reddish.
Strophanthus Courmonti Sad.	Brownish.	Abundant.	Single prisms and twin crystals, a few clusters and conglomerate crystals.	None.	Red to violet.	Red to violet.
Strophanthus sarmentosus P.DC.	Reddish-brown to greenish.	Abundant, mostly rubbed off.	As *S. Courmonti*.	Numerous clusters in the cotyledons.	Pale rose-red.	Pale rose-red.
Strophanthus Nicholsoni Holmes.	Whitish-brown.	Abundant and woolly.	None.	None.	Bright red to violet.	Bright red to violet.
Strophanthus Emini Aschers et Pax.	Light yellowish-brown.	Abundant.	None.	None.	Red to violet.	Red to violet.
Strophanthus gratus (Wall. et Hook) Franch.	Brown.	Small papillæ; appear glabrous.	None.	None.	Rose-red.	Rose-red.

3. Epidermis of the testa in surface view, consisting of somewhat elongated polygonal cells, with evenly thickened, straight, lignified walls. The scars left by the fall of hairs appear as circles near the centres of the cells bearing them.

4. Fixed oil and aleurone grains from the endosperm and cotyledons.

5. Occasional cluster crystals and small prisms of calcium oxalate from the inner layers of the seed-coat.

6. A small amount of small ovoid starch grains.

7. Green coloration with sulphuric acid (66 per cent. by volume).

HISTOLOGICAL SCHEDULE XXVIII

FENNEL FRUIT, ANISE FRUIT, CORIANDER

Fennel Fruit (*Fœniculum vulgare*)

1. Cut transverse sections of a soaked fennel fruit ; mount one in chloral hydrate and boil. Mount a second section in phloroglucin and hydrochloric acid, and a third in a mixture of equal volumes of tincture of alkanna and water and warm it.

2. Make a diagram of a section to show the general arrangement of the parts and sketch a portion in detail, marking upon your drawing the outer epidermis of the pericarp, the parenchymatous mesocarp containing vittæ with a secreting epithelium lignified reticulated parenchyma, vascular bundles with phloem groups on either side of a central group of vessels and fibres, thin-walled parenchyma, inner epidermis of the pericarp, and the epidermis of the seed-coat.

3. In the section of the seed, note the drops of oil (alkanna preparation) and the minute rosettes of calcium oxalate contained in the aleurone grains (chloral preparation). Sketch these details.

4. Defat a section and stain with iodine water ; note the aleurone grains.

5. Digest some fruits in a 5 per cent. solution of caustic alkali upon a water-bath until soft enough to break up easily. Tease out the tissue with needles and sketch surface views of all the structures noted in the sections.

6. Examine powdered fennel fruit in the same reagents as were used for the sections. Write out a statement of the charcteristic features of the powder.

Anise Fruit (*Pimpinella Anisum*)

Proceed as for Fennel ; but under (5) carefully dissect out the vittæ and determine the manner of their branching.

Coriander (*Coriandrum sativium*)

Proceed as for Fennel. Under (5), in addition to treatment with caustic alkali, steep the pericarp in nitric and chromic acids (10 per cent. of each), for about thirty minutes, wash with water and disintegrate the fibrous mesocarp with needles on a slide. Sketch the isolated fusiform sclerenchymatous cells and also a piece to show their arrangement in the tissue.

NOTES ON HISTOLOGICAL SCHEDULE XXVIII

Characters of Powdered Fennel Fruit. 1. Fragments of epidermis of quadrangular cells, with very occasional stomata ; trichomes and cuticular striations absent.

2. Numerous parenchymatous cells of the mesocarp with characteristic, lignified, reticulate thickening.

3. Fragments of endosperm consisting of colourless, somewhat thick-walled, polyhedral cells, containing fixed oil and aleurone grains with minute rosettes of calcium oxalate.

4. Portions of the brown vittæ.

5. Pieces of the inner epidermis of the pericarp, composed of very narrow, thin-walled cells, arranged parallel to one another in groups of five to seven. Separate groups sometimes variously oriented.

6. Starch grains absent.

Characters of Powdered Anise Fruit. 1. Epidermis with trichomes, about 80 to 160 microns long, conical, warty and straight or curved at the tip, which is often nearly solid with secondary thickening and is rounded.

2. Brown fragments of the small branching vittæ.

3. Fragments of the endosperm resembling that of fennel.

4. Absence of starch grains and of reticulate, lignified parenchyma.

Characters of Powdered Coriander. 1. Masses of lignified, fusiform, sclerenchymatous cells in sinuous rows, often crossing one another at right angles.

2. Epidermis, when present, having small prisms of calcium oxalate in many of its cells. Anticlinal walls straight and pitted ; stomata present.

3. Cellulosic polyhedral cells from the endosperm, containing fixed oil and small aleurone grains with micro-rosettes of calcium oxalate.

4. Trichomes and reticulate lignified parenchyma absent.

5. Parquetry cells and large hexagonal rather thin-walled sclerenchyma from the endocarp.

UMBELLIFERROUS FRUITS

Characters common to all are :—Abundant endosperm of cellulosic, polyhedral, somewhat thick-walled parenchyma containing much fixed oil and numerous small aluerone grains, most of which include micro-rosette crystals of calcium oxalate ; starch absent.

A. Trichomes present ; vittæ present.

- i. Short conical unicellular warty trichomes on the epidermis of the pericarp ; apex rounded, length 20–100 μ ; breadth at base 15–40 μ. Vittæ narrow, branching, numerous.

  Anise (*Pimpinella Anisum*)

- ii. Branched, pluriseriate trichomes on the epidermis of the pericarp, apex rounded ; length up to 500 μ. Mesocarp contains sclerenchymatous cells. Vittæ 6 in each mericarp.

  Cummin (*Cuminum Cyminum*)

B. Trichomes absent ; vittæ present.

- i. Reticulate, lignified parenchyma in the mesocarp.
  - (*a*) Abundant reticulate, lignified parenchyma in the mesocarp ; cuticle of epidermis of pericarp without striations ; endocarp of parquetry cells.

    Fennel (*Fœniculum vulgare*)
  - (*b*) Small amount of reticulate, lignified parenchyma in the mesocarp ; cuticle of epidermis of pericarp striated.

    Dill (*Anethum graveolus*)

††. Reticulate lignified parenchyma absent.

(*a*) Cuticle of epidermis of pericarp striated; some rectangular finely-pitted sclereids in the mesocarp; parquetry cells absent.

Caraway (*Carum Carvi*)

(*b*) In the mesocarp, masses of fusiform, sclerenchymatous cells in sinuous rows, often crossing at right angles; epidermis, when present, shows small prisms of calcium oxalate in many cells; endocarp consists of a layer of somewhat thin-walled, large, flattened, hexagonal sclerenchyma and a layer of parquetry cells.

Coriander (*Coriandrum sativium*)

C. Trichomes absent; vittæ absent.

No parquetry cells in the endocarp, which is developed as the coniine layer. When the fruits are rubbed with solution of caustic alkali, a strong mouse-like odour is developed.

Hemlock (*Conium maculatum*)

HISTOLOGICAL SCHEDULE XXIX

Cubebs (*Piper Cubeba*)

1. Cut some fruits transversely and select one with a well-developed seed. Remove the seed and cut several transverse sections of the pericarp, supported in pith. Mount sections separately in chloral hydrate solution, in iodine water and in phloroglucin and hydrochloric acid. Make a diagrammatic sketch and sketches of details. Note the following particulars: Epidermis of small cells containing minute crystals of calcium oxalate and having a thick cuticle; hypodermal sclerenchyma in an interrupted layer, parenchyma with oil cells, collapsed parenchyma with calcium oxalate prisms, inner layer of sclerenchyma.

2. Make transverse sections of the seed and note the thin brown layer (the seed-coat) and the perisperm containing abundant starch and numerous oil cells. Sketch these details.

3. Cut transverse and longitudinal sections of the "tail," and make sketches to show the fibres, fibrous cells and small annular and spiral vessels.

4. Digest the pericarp in caustic alkali till soft and tease it out with needles. Find all the layers named above and sketch them as seen in surface view.

5. Digest a seed in caustic alkali and tease out its tissues. Sketch the three layers of the seed-coat and the parenchyma of the perisperm with its oil cells.

6. Mount powdered cubebs in various reagents, identify the tissues found in the dissections, and write out a list of the diagnostic characters.

Pepper (*Piper nigrum*)

Proceed as directed for cubebs and see characters given in Table, p. 220.

NOTES ON HISTOLOGICAL SCHEDULE XXIX

Characters of Powdered Cubebs. 1. Epidermis with cells containing small rectangular prisms.

2. Stone-cells, rectangular or polygonal with fairly large lumina, in groups, with intervening parenchyma, from the hypodermis.

3. Stone-cells, oblong with very thick walls, small lumina and light yellow colour, in a continuous layer, from the endocarp.
4. Pieces of the reddish-brown seed-coat, usually with the hyaline layer attached.
5. Starch in small angular grains, mostly in large polyhedral masses; individual grains about 6 to 7 microns in diameter.
6. Parenchyma with small prisms of calcium oxalate and small, rounded starch grains, from the mesocarp.
7. Groups of sclerenchymatous fibres from the "tail."
8. Oil cells present, from the perisperm and pericarp.
9. Beaker cells absent.
10. Deep crimson with sulphuric acid (80 per cent. by volume).

HISTOLOGICAL SCHEDULE XXX

Cardamom Seeds (*Elettaria Cardamomum var. minuscula*)

1. Soak fully developed but not quite ripe seeds in water for three or four days. Cut several transverse sections of a seed and mount separate sections in chloral hydrate solution, iodine water, phloroglucin with hydrochloric acid and dilute glycerin.
2. Make a diagrammatic drawing to show the arrangement of the parts of the seed and make detailed sketches to show the structure of the seed-coats. Mark the following layers: Epidermis, a single layer of collapsed parenchyma (often brown), large oil cells, collapsed parenchyma in several layers, sclerenchymatous layer with siliceous inclusions. Sketch the perisperm cells with starch and calcium oxalate.
3. Digest seeds in solution of caustic alkali for one hour on a water-bath and tease out the layers of the seed-coats. Identify and sketch a few cells of each as seen in surface view.
4. Cut transverse sections of the pericarp, softened by soaking in water. Mount them separately in lacto-phenol, in chloral hydrate solution and in phloroglucin and hydrochloric acid. Make a sketch, noting especially the vascular bundles and the supporting sclerenchyma.
5. Macerate a piece of pericarp in 5 per cent. aqueous caustic potash on a water-bath. Tease out the digested material, mount it and sketch a piece of the epidermis, some sclerenchymatous cells and fibres. Record the width of the epidermal cells.
6. Examine powdered cardamoms mounted in the same reagents as were used for the sections, and identify all the structures seen in the dissections. Write out a list of the diagnostic characters of the powder.

Nutmeg (*Myristica fragrans*)

1. Soak nutmegs in water until sufficiently soft to cut easily. Cut transverse sections and mount in chloral hydrate solution, in phloroglucin and hydrochloric acid and in tincture of alkanna. Make a diagrammatic sketch to show the perisperm and its ruminations, the endosperm, the vascular strands and cells containing volatile oil.
2. Mount a section in chloral hydrate, warm it, wash out the chloral with water and stain with tincture of alkanna. Note the abundant fatty oil in the endosperm.

3. Make sketches of details as seen with the 4 mm. objective, including the outer part of the perisperm with its prism-shaped crystals (see note); a rumination with its oil cells and small vascular strand; the endosperm cells with starch grains and aleurone grains, one of which in each cell is very large and is accompanied by a few small grains, the large grain including a crystalloid. Note that the fat is usually in the form of crystals and that there are scattered pigment cells, often described as tannin idioblasts, containing brown contents, and a little starch.

4. Defat some sections by soaking in ether, mount in iodine water, examine and sketch the aleurone grains.

NOTES ON HISTOLOGICAL SCHEDULE XXX

Cardamom Seeds. The endosperm contains no starch; the cells are filled with a hyaline or granular mass, which gives the reactions for proteins.

Caustic potash is quite satisfactory to disintegrate the unripe pericarp, which is completely destroyed by strong oxidising agents. Schulze's maceration fluid may, however, be used for the ripe pericarp.

Cardamom, Pericarp of. The vascular bundles of the pericarp consist of phloem and xylem, which latter is unlignified. Each bundle is accompanied by an arc of fibres which are strongly lignified excepting a few on the outer side of the arc.

Characters of Powdered Cardamom Seeds. 1. Polyhedral masses of adherent starch grains from the perisperm; individual grains up to 4 microns in diameter.

2. One or several small prisms of calcium oxalate are embedded in each starchy mass.

3. Dark-brown patches of sclerenchyma of the inner seed-coat, consisting of small polygonal cells each with a circular lumen filled by a spherical nodule of silica.

4. Elongated parenchyma of the epidermis; cells up to 25 μ wide.

5. Absence of fibres and fibrous sclerenchyma and of large vessels.

Nutmeg. The crystals in the outer part of the perisperm are stated not to be oxalate of calcium and it is suggested that they may be acid tartrate of potassium, but the evidence is not conclusive.

Characters of Powdered Nutmeg. 1. Abundant cells containing crystals of fat, starch grains and aleurone grains.

2. Scattered brown pigment cells (tannin idioblasts).

3. Large oil cells, isolated and in groups.

4. Starch granules simple and with 2 to 10 components, individual granules up to 25 microns.

5. Aleurone grains, many of them large and each then containing a well-formed crystalloid.

6. A few colourless prisms, in the perisperm cells, of uncertain composition.

HISTOLOGICAL SCHEDULE XXXI

Chillies and Capsicums

1. From a fruit of *Capsicum minimum*, remove the pericarp, embed it in pith and cut transverse sections. Mount separate sections in chloral hydrate, chlorzinciodine (or iodine and sulphuric acid), in

phloroglucin and hydrochloric acid, in tincture of alkanna and in Soudan Red III.

Make a drawing of a transverse section and mark the position of lignified, cellulose-walled and suberised cells; mark also any oily contents and calcium oxalate crystals.

2. Take a piece of pericarp and strip off the inner layer. Mount both the outer and the inner layers separately in chloral hydrate and boil till clear. Mount a second piece of each in phloroglucin and hydrochloric acid. Make a diagrammatic drawing of a large area of the inner epidermis to show the islets of sclerenchyma. Sketch also in detail a small portion of each epidermis.

3. Cut transverse sections of the seed and mount in chloral hydrate, phloroglucin and hydrochloric acid, in eosin and in Millon's reagent. Make a sketch to show the remarkably thickened epidermis, the other layers of the seed-coat and the cells of the endosperm; search for fixed oil in the endosperm. Defat some sections in ether and mount in glycerin and in iodine water; sketch the aleurone grains.

4. Remove the seed epidermis by a surface section and boil it in chloral hydrate solution; sketch the appearance in surface view of portions from the flat surface and from the edge of the seed.

5. Disintegrate a piece of seed epidermis by potassium chlorate or chromic and nitric acids; tease apart the cells and sketch some isolated cells.

6. Cut transverse sections and make surface preparations of the calyx and stalk, as for a leaf and stem. Sketch them to show all important features.

7. Mount powdered chillies in chloral hydrate solution and in the other reagents used for the sections and surface preparations; defat some powder and mount it in reagents to display the aleurone grains. Write out the chief characters of powdered chillies.

8. Make similar preparations of the pericarps of *Capsicum annuum* and of Japanese chillies. Compare their structure with that of the official chillies.

NOTES ON HISTOLOGICAL SCHEDULE XXXI

The pericarps of chillies and capsicums are best prepared for dissection by exposing them to a moist atmosphere for eighteen to twenty-four hours. The seeds should be soaked for a similar period in cold water.

Characters of Powdered Chillies (*Capsicum minimum*). 1. Fragments of the outer epidermis of the seed-coat, consisting of lignified cells with yellowish, thick and sinuous walls.

2. Fragments of the endosperm, composed of polyhedral cells with highly refractive colourless walls and containing fixed oil and aleurone.

3. Reddish oily drops scattered throughout the powder.

4. Pieces of the outer epidermis of the pericarp, composed of thick and straight-walled sub-rectangular cells with few pits, often arranged in groups of five to seven; cuticle uniformly striated.

5. Scattered sandy crystals of calcium oxalate and a few prisms.

6. Portions of the sclerenchymatous islets from the inner epidermis of the pericarp.

7. Absence of starch and the presence of only a few small vessels and fibres.

Powder of Capsicum annuum and of *Japanese chillies* is best recognised by the characters, in surface view, of the epidermis and hypodermis of the pericarp, as explained below.

COMMERCIAL CAPSICUMS

Capsicum minimum.

EPIDERMIS. Thick, straight-walled, rectangular cells with few pits, often arranged in groups of five to seven in a row and sometimes showing a uniformly striated cuticle. Cells 25 to 60 microns in either direction. Easily visible in surface preparations.

HYPODERMIS. Delicate, thin-walled, cellulosic parenchyma.

Capsicum annuum.

EPIDERMIS. Irregular, polygonal, tabular cells with evenly thickened walls, traversed by numerous well-marked simple pits. Occasionally the cuticle shows well-separated striated ridges. Cells 50 to 100 microns long and 25 to 50 microns wide. Walls very transparent, difficult to focus and not easily visible in surface preparations.

HYPODERMIS. Several layers of cuticularised collenchyma; cells rounded, with very few pits.

Capsicum sp. (Japanese Capsicums).

EPIDERMIS. Cells with strongly thickened walls and a radiate lumen; the pits only rarely appear to penetrate the whole thickness of the wall. No striations. Cells 30 to 80 microns long and 15 to 45 microns wide.

HYPODERMIS. A single layer of regular polygonal cells with cuticularised, fairly thick walls, traversed by numerous pits, which give them a beaded appearance.

HISTOLOGICAL SCHEDULE XXXII

Colocynth (*Citrullus Colocynthis*)

1. Cut thin sections of the pulp and mount them separately in chloral hydrate solution, in phloroglucin and hydrochloric acid, and in chlorzinciodine. Examine them microscopically and record your conclusions as to the chemical nature of the cell walls.

2. Sketch a portion of a section to show the rounded cells and abundant intercellular spaces. On the surface of the cells find the faintly marked oval or rounded areas containing simple pits.

3. Cut transverse sections of the hard outer part of the pericarp and mount in reagents as for the pulp. Sketch a portion to show the characters of the epidermis, the sub-epidermal parenchyma and the inner sclerenchyma. Record upon your drawing the reaction and character of the walls of the several layers.

4. Cut a surface section of the rind and mount it in chloral hydrate solution. Sketch the epidermis in surface view.

5. Cut transverse sections of a colocynth seed and mount as for the rind and pulp. Sketch and key a section and mark the epidermis, the sub-epidermal sclerenchyma and other layers.

6. With a dipping tube take a little of the disintegrated seed-coats (broken up by potassium chlorate and nitric acid) and mount in water or chloral hydrate solution. Examine and sketch typical cells from the various layers as seen in surface view. For the surface view of the seed epidermis, cut surface sections with a razor and mount in chloral hydrate solution.

7. Cut a transverse section of the cotyledons of the seed and test for oil and aleurone.

8. Examine the genuine powdered colocynth and record the diagnostic features.

NOTES ON HISTOLOGICAL SCHEDULE XXXII

Sections of colocynth pulp can be made without any special preparation. The outer part of the pericarp and the seeds should be soaked in cold water for twenty-four hours before use ; it is wise to choose unripe seeds for the purpose.

Characters of Powdered Colocynth Pulp. 1. Consists mainly of rounded parenchyma with cellulose walls, which are thin and show oval or circular, flat, pitted areas where contiguous cells touch.

2. Only a very few small spiral and annular vessels are present.

3. Absence of starch and of calcium oxalate.

4. Almost complete absence of sclerenchymatous cells and of oil (very small amounts of these may be present, corresponding to the small percentage of seeds that is permitted).

5. Intensely bitter taste ; very pale buff colour.

PART IV

QUANTITATIVE ANALYSIS

QUANTITATIVE SCHEDULE I

To Determine the Percentage of Foreign Leaf in a Drug Composed of Leaves or the Composition of a Mixture of Leaves, more or less Broken

1. Divide the sample into two parts. Use one part for the general examination (2 to 4 below) and the other for the quantitative work.

2. Carefully examine the part reserved for general examination and note and record the following details :—

(*a*) Size and prominence of the veins.
(*b*) Distinctness and straightness of the veinlets.
(*c*) Colour of the veins and veinlets.
(*d*) Distinctness and shape of the vein-islets.
(*e*) Presence or absence of trichomes.
(*f*) Surface characters, *e.g.*, shining, matt, rugose, etc.
(*g*) Flatness of the lamina, *e.g.*, undulated, flat, etc.
(*h*) Compare the upper and under surfaces.
(*i*) Odour an tasted.
(*k*) Chemical tests.

3. From the results of the above observations, pick out as many differnt types of leaf as are present.

4. Confirm the difference between the selected portions by microscopical examination.

(*a*) Cut a transverse section of the main vein of each component leaf. Make diagrams.
(*b*) Clear a piece of each component and make drawings of any crystals and trichomes present.

5. Take the portion reserved for quantitative work, sort it into its components and weigh the separate portions. Calculate the percentages of the component leaves.

NOTES ON QUANTITATIVE SCHEDULE I

Good mixtures for this exercise can be made by mixing 1. Hamamelis leaf with sweet chestnut leaf. 2. Senna leaf with Ailanthus. 3. Belladonna leaf with Ailanthus or Phytolacca.

The mixtures should consist of broken leaves which have passed a No. 6 sieve and have been retained by a No. 10 sieve.

QUANTITATIVE SCHEDULE II

To Determine the Percentage Composition of Mixtures of Broken Roots, Rhizomes or Barks

1. Divide the specimen into two parts ; use one for a qualitative examination of the ingredients (see 2 below) and reserve the other for quantitative work (see 3 and 4 below).

2. By observing the following characters of the fragments present, determine the number of ingredients.

(*a*) Colour of the various surfaces.

(*b*) Presence or absence of starch in the fragments.

(*c*) Fibrous structure or brittle nature, including behaviour when broken longitudinally.

(*d*) Examine a smoothed transverse surface, noting especially (i) occurrence, size and distribution of the vessels, (ii) occurrence and distribution of fibres and other sclerenchyma, (iii) occurrence of bundles and their arrangement in a single ring, in concentric rings or scattered irregularly.

(*e*) Odour and taste.

(*f*) Make selected chemical tests, such as tests for alkaloids, cyanophoric glycosides, anthraquinone derivatives, tannin and mucilage.

(*g*) Determine the occurrence and nature of any crystals of calcium oxalate.

3. Take the second reserved portion and sort it into the ingredients which have been identified by the work carried out under 2, above.

4. Weigh the separated ingredients and calculate the percentage amounts present.

NOTES ON QUANTITATIVE SCHEDULE II

Useful mixtures for this exercise are 1. Belladonna root with Phytolacca root, 2. Gentian with Dock root, 3. Gentian with Veratrum rhizome, 4. Cinnamon with Sassafras bark.

The mixtures should consist of broken pieces which have passed a No. 6 sieve and have been retained by a No. 10 sieve.

QUANTITATIVE SCHEDULE III

To Determine the Purity of a Sample of Strophanthus

1. Take a sample weighing about 100 g., prepared so as to represent the whole consignment to be tested.

2. From the sample take a seed at random. Cut a rather thick section and put it at the top left-hand corner of a glass plate, measuring about 25 by 16 cm. and placed on a sheet of white paper. Put the remainder of the cut seed in a similar position on a second sheet of white paper placed beside the first sheet. Continue in this way until ten seeds have been cut and their sections form a row extending across the glass plate near its upper edge.

3. With a glass rod put a drop of sulphuric acid, 80 per cent. *v/v*, on to each section and observe the colour produced. If the seed is going green, it does so rapidly, if red, it usually colours slowly. On the paper make a circle round each seed the section of which fails to become green.

4. Make a second line of ten sections and test them. Continue until five lines are completed. Test similarly a second fifty seeds.

5. Each seed surrounded by a circle is examined according to the table in Histological Schedule XXVII., p. 168, and its species determined.

6. Count the genuine and false seeds and calculate the percentage of genuine seed.

NOTES ON QUANTITATIVE SCHEDULE III

When several cases of seed are to be examined, a representative sample of the consignment may be obtained as follows: take a handful of seed from various parts of each case, mix them well and make a sample of about 500 g. representing each case. From each sample remove a small handful and mix all thoroughly together. Use about 100 g. of this final mixture, representing the entire consignment, for the actual test. If the result shows a percentage of false seed, it will be necessary to make a separate test for each case to discover which contains adulterated and which pure seed.

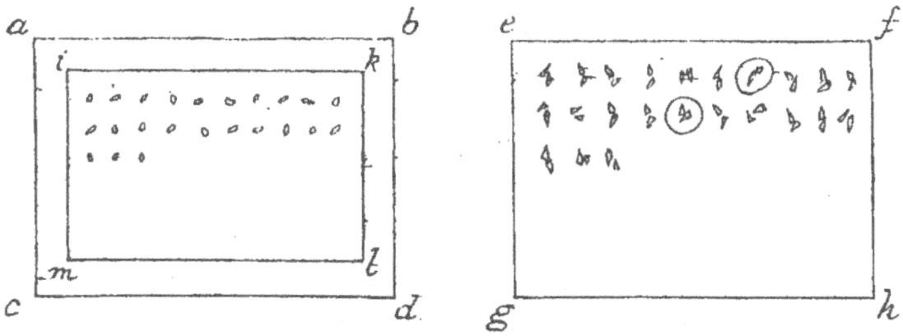

FIG. 70.—Diagram to illustrate the testing of strophanthus seed. *abcd* and *efgh* are two sheets of white paper; *iklm* is a sheet of glass 25 × 16 cm. On the glass are arranged the sections and the seeds from which they were made are on *efgh*, each foreign seed being surrounded by a circle.

QUANTITATIVE SCHEDULE IV

Determination of Ash

A. *Total Ash*

1. Weigh an ignited flat, thin, porcelain dish.
2. Weigh about 2 g. of the powdered drug into the dish.
3. Support the dish on a pipe-clay triangle placed on a ring of a retort-stand. Heat with a ring-shaped solid-flame burner. Using a flame about 2 cm. high and supporting the dish about 7 cm. above the flame, heat till vapours almost cease to be evolved; then lower the dish and heat more strongly until all the carbon is burnt off.
4. Cool in a desiccator and weigh.

B. *Acid-insoluble Ash*

1. Using 25 ml. of dilute hydrochloric acid, wash the ash from the dish, used for total ash, in a 100-ml. beaker. Place on a wire gauze over a Bunsen burner and boil for 5 minutes.
2. Filter through an "ashless" filter-paper, wash the residue twice with hot water and dry the filter-paper and residue in the oven at 100° C. (This drying requires about 15 minutes.)
3. Meanwhile ignite a crucible in the flame, cool and weigh.
4. Put the dried filter-paper and residue together into the crucible;

heat gently until vapours cease to be evolved and then more strongly until all carbon has been removed. Cool and weigh.

C. *Moisture Determination*

1. Weigh about 1·5 g. of the powdered drug into a weighed flat and thin porcelain dish. Dry in the oven at 100° C. Cool in a desiccator and weigh.

D. *Calculation*

Calculate the percentages of total ash and of acid insoluble ash with reference to the drug dried at 100° C.

E. *Water-soluble Ash*

This is determined in a similar way to acid-insoluble ash, using 25 ml. of water in place of dilute hydrochloric acid.

NOTES ON QUANTITATIVE SCHEDULE IV

A very useful form of dish for the determination of moisture and of ash is a thin flat porcelain dish such as is used for total solids of milk. If a platinum dish is available it may be used. The burning of the powder should proceed slowly and the material must not be allowed to catch fire or to give off smoke as dense fumes.

QUANTITATIVE SCHEDULE V

Determination of Extractive yielded to Specified Solvents

1. Weigh out 5 g. of the powdered drug in a weighing bottle and transfer it to a dry 250-ml. conical flask.
2. Fill a 100-ml. graduated flask to the delivery mark with the solvent. Wash out the weighing bottle and pour the washings, together with the remainder of the solvent, into the conical flask.
3. Cork the flask and set aside for 24 hours, shaking frequently.
4. Filter into a 50-ml. cylinder. When sufficient filtrate has collected, transfer from 10 to 25 ml. with a pipette to a weighed, flat, thin porcelain dish, as used for the ash determinations.
5. Evaporate to dryness on a water-bath and complete the drying in an oven at 100° C. Cool in a desiccator and weigh.
6. Calculate the percentage of extractive.

NOTES ON QUANTITATIVE SCHEDULE V

Use a weighing-bottle because it is easier of manipulation than a watch-glass when transferring the powder to the flask and the bottle can be more easily washed out. For water-soluble extractive, use chloroform water; for alcohol-soluble extractive use the particular strength of alcohol prescribed for each drug.

QUANTITATIVE SCHEDULE VI

Determination of the Percentage of Volatile Oil in Drugs

1. Set up the apparatus represented in the figure, consisting of a round-bottomed 1-litre boiling-flask to which is attached a special still-head consisting of condenser, receiver and return-tube combined in

one unit. The still-head must be thoroughly clean and, if necessary, should be cleaned by washing successively with water, acetone and chromic acid mixture, which last should be left in the inverted tube for about 18 hours.

2. Put 300 ml. of water in the flask and bring it nearly to the boil; then add 10 to 20 g. of drug, together with some fragments of porous pot, and attach the still-head. An Argand burner is recommended for heating the flask, but a Bunsen burner and asbestos-filled wire gauze may be used.

3. Until the liquid is boiling steadily, lift the flask at intervals and shake the contents. Finally adjust the flame so that the distillate in the graduated tube remains cold. Continue till no more oil collects. This requires two hours or more.

4. Turn out the gas and allow the liquid in the condenser to drain for 5 or 10 minutes; then read off the volume of oil. Express the result as a volume in weight percentage.

N.B.—(1) When the oil is heavier than water, a known volume of xylene is added to the graduated tube by a pipette which is passed through the side-tube of the still head. The increase in volume of the xylene gives the volume of oil distilled.

(2) Better results are obtained with some drugs by using 150 ml. each of glycerin and water in place of pure water in the boiling flask. This modification should be used for dill, coriander, cloves, fennel and dried orange peel.

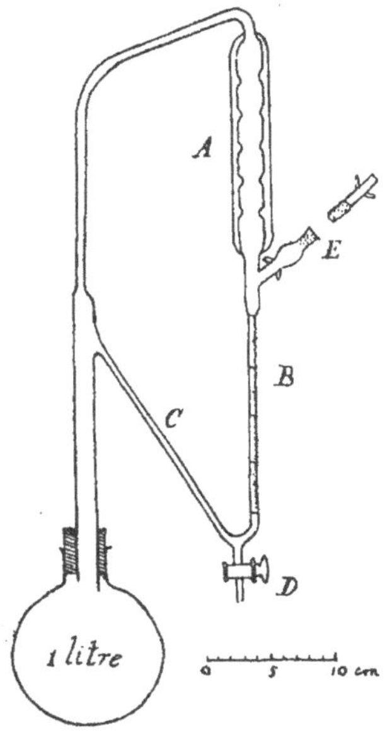

FIG. 71.—Apparatus for the determination of volatile oil in drugs; after Cocking and Middleton (1935). *A*, condenser; *B*, receiver, graduated to 0·05 ml.; *C*, return tube; *D*, tap to remove distillate; *E*, side-tube to introduce xylene.

NOTES ON QUANTITATIVE SCHEDULE VI

Use 10 g. of whole cardamom seeds or 10 g. of powdered ginger and proceed as directed above. Use 10 g. of powdered buchu and put 1 ml. of xylene in the graduated tube. For cloves, take 5 g., use glycerin and water in the flask and put 1 ml. of xylene in the graduated tube.

QUANTITATIVE SCHEDULE VII

To Determine the Number of Granules per Milligram of Commercial Potato Starch

1. Weigh accurately 0·04 gm. of potato starch and 0·04 gm. of lycopodium. Put 5 ml. of olive oil into a small conical measure. Transfer the powders to a glass plate about 15 cm. square, mix them

thoroughly with a few drops of olive oil by means of a flexible spatula and gradually incorporate more oil to produce a thin smooth paste.

2. When sufficiently fluid, drain off the suspension from a corner of the plate into a clean and dry corked specimen tube (about 6·5 × 1·5 cm.). Rub the residue on the plate with a little fresh oil and drain it into the specimen tube and repeat the operation until the whole of the powder has been transferred to the tube. Add the remainder of the 5 ml. of oil and mix the contents of the tube by gentle oscillation.

3. With a glass rod place a drop of the suspension in the centre of a microscope slide and apply a cover-glass. Into the eyepiece of the microscope drop a net-ruled scale (usually one sq. cm. divided into

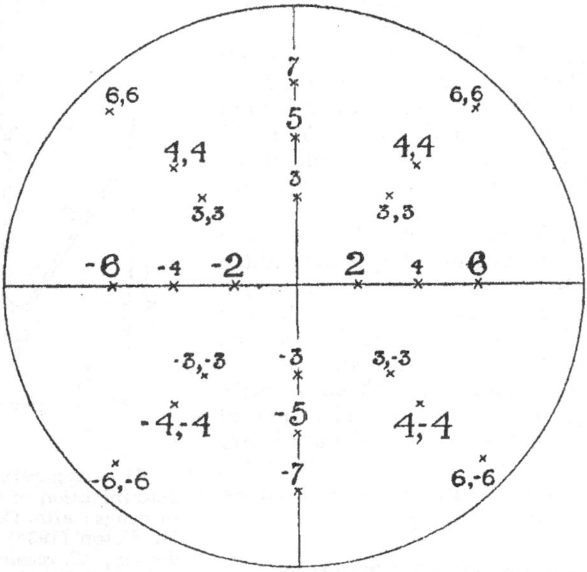

FIG. 72.—Diagram to show the position of ten selected fields, indicated by the larger figures, and of fifteen other selected fields, indicated by the smaller figures and the centre of the circle. The figures in all cases represent distances in millimetres from the two intersecting axes.

sq. mm.) so that it rests upon the diaphragm. Fasten a counting-field finder (see below), to the stage of the microscope and place the slide on it so that its edges coincide with the central rectangle. Now, using the 4 mm. objective, count the number of spores and of starch granules seen within the rulings of the eyepiece; these will be the counts for the first field.

4. Move the slide successively to each of the centre lines ruled on the "finder" and for each field count and record the numbers of potato granules and of lycopodium spores. From the total of the results for ten fields determine the number of starch granules corresponding to 94,000 lycopodium spores. Since 94,000 spores weigh one milligram and the starch and lycopodium were present in equal

amounts by weight, it follows that the number of granules found represents one milligram of air-dry commercial potato starch.

NOTES ON QUANTITATIVE SCHEDULE VII

Suspending Agent. In place of oil, one may use a mixture of 1 vol. of glycerine and 2 vols. of N/50 iodine; this will stain the starch granules and tends to make the counting easier.

Fields to be Counted. These must be evenly distributed throughout the mount and the positions shown in the diagram, Fig. 72, are convenient for the purpose. The numerals indicating each field give the distances in millimetres above and below or to the right and left of the two diameters crossing at right angles.

Counting-field Finder. This consists of a piece of stiff paper or of thin cardboard upon which is drawn a rectangle 3 in. by 1 in. Parallel to the sides of the rectangle and outside it, lines are drawn at distances in millimetres corresponding to the positions of the fields marked in the diagram,

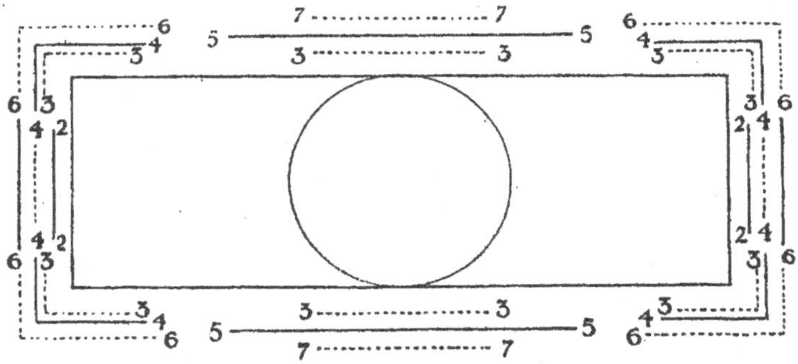

FIG. 73.—Counting-field Finder. The arrangement represented corresponds to the selection of fields marked in Fig. 72.

Fig. 72. The distances of the lines from the sides of the rectangle are indicated by the figures against them and the ten unbroken lines correspond to the fields marked by the larger figures while the fourteen broken lines correspond to the fourteen positions marked by smaller figures. The finder can be attached to the plain stage of the microscope by piercing it with the pins of the clips on the stage or by the use of an adhesive or by some kind of clip.

For certain work ten fields are sufficient for the purpose of making a count and then the unbroken lines only are used; but when a larger number of fields is necessary the positions marked by the broken lines should be used in addition, making a total of twenty-five fields.

The *number of granules per mg.* of commercial potato starch may vary very considerably because this starch is graded into qualities which differ according to the size of the granules present. They are known by such names as Finest Quality, Superior *Prima*, Second Product *Prima*, *Secunda* and *Tertia*, the size of the granules decreasing in the order given from about 36 microns in the best to about 12 microns in the lowest. It is therefore impossible to give a number of granules per mg. which will represent potato starch generally. In one sample examined, the number was 78,000 granules per mgr. of air-dry starch, the moisture present being 20·76 per cent.

QUANTITATIVE SCHEDULE VIII

To Determine the Proportions by Weight of the Constituents of a Mixture of Powdered Drugs

1. Examine the gentian powder A for the presence of extraneous matter. Use a starchy adulterant for this exercise.
2. Prepare a mixture of genuine powdered gentian with an equal weight of the extraneous matter found, weighing out about 0·5 gm. of each constituent.
3. Examine the 50 per cent. mixture microscopically and note how it compares with the sample A. If it appears to differ widely in the amount of the extraneous substance, form a mental estimate of the quantity present in A and prepare a fresh standard mixture of the strength you decide upon.
4. Weigh out an exact amount, about 0·02 gm., of lycopodium and also an exact amount, about 0·5 gm., of the mixture of known composition. Put 3 ml. of a mixture of 1 vol. of glycerin and 2 vols, of N/50 iodine into a measure. Transfer the powders to a glass plate and incorporate them with the suspending agent as directed for potato starch in the preceding schedule, p. 181.
5. Remove a drop of the suspension with a glass rod and mount it for microscopical examination. Using a net-ruled micrometer eye-piece, count the number of lycopodium spores and of starch grains in ten fields selected by moving the slide successively to each of the entire lines ruled on the counting-field finder. Record the counts.
6. Repeat the whole set of operations 4 and 5, using the powder A and record the counts.
7. Calculate the percentage of extraneous matter present in A.

NOTES ON QUANTITATIVE SCHEDULE VIII

An example will help to make the method and calculation clear :—

Gentian mixed with ginger was used and after examining the specimen and a 50 per cent. mixture it was decided to take an accurately prepared 5 per cent. admixture of ginger with gentian as the standard. Using this standard mixture *the number of starch granules per mg. of ginger* was determined as follows :—

Weight of lycopodium 0·0221 g. *i.e.*, 22·1 mg.
„ „ 5% mixture 0·5020 g. *i.e.*, 502 mg.

After mixing with the suspending medium and counting the particles in ten fields, the following numbers were obtained :—

Lycopodium spores	9, 10, 13, 8, 6, 7, 11, 12, 10, 9 = 95
Ginger starch granules	25, 28, 40, 32, 22, 26, 31, 34, 36, 26 = 300

Now 22·1 mg. of lycopodium = 22·1 × 94,000 spores and since 95 lycopodium spores occur with 300 ginger starch granules

∴ 22·1 × 94,000 lycopodium spores occur with $\frac{300 \times 22{\cdot}1 \times 94{,}000}{95}$

= 6,560,000 ginger starch granules.

∴ 502 mg. of the 5 per cent. mixture contains 6,560,000 ginger starch granules.

∴ 1 mg. „ „ „ „ „ 6,560,000 ÷ 502
= 13,070 ginger starch granules

and 1 mg. of the ginger contains 13,070 × 20
= 261.400 ginger starch granules.

The *percentage of ginger in the mixture of unknown composition* was then determined as follows :—

Weight of lycopodium 0·0215 gm. *i.e.*, 21·5 mg.
„ „ mixture A 0·5383 gm. *i.e.*, 538·3 mg.

After mixing with the suspending medium and counting the particles in ten fields, the following numbers were obtained :

Lycopodium spores	7, 18, 8, 16, 12, 9, 10, 14, 11, 12 = 117
Ginger starch granules	25, 41, 25, 37, 31, 26, 27, 36, 28, 29 = 305

Now 21·5 mg. of lycopodium = 21·5 × 94,000 spores and since 117 lycopodium spores occur with 305 ginger starch granules,

∴ 21·5 × 94,000 „ „ „ $\frac{305 \times 21{\cdot}5 \times 94{,}000}{117}$

= 5,267,000 ginger starch granules
= 5,267,000 ÷ 261,400
= 20·15 mg. of ginger

∴ 538·3 mg. of the mixture A contain 20·15 mg. of ginger
= 3·75 per cent.

This result may be obtained by using the following formula :

$$\frac{n \times w \times 94{,}000 \times 100}{s \times p \times m}$$

where n = number of starch granules in the ten fields.
s = „ „ spores in the same ten fields.
w = weight in milligrams of the lycopodium taken.
m = „ „ milligrams of the sample.
p = number of starch granules per mg. of the pure ginger.
94,000 „ „ spores per mg. of lycopodium.

QUANTITATIVE SCHEDULE IX

To Determine the Epidermal Area per Gram of Powdered Senna Leaf

1. Weigh accurately about 0·1 gm. of senna leaf in No. 90 powder and 0·05 gm. of lycopodium. Put 3 ml. of solution of chloral hydrate (5 in 2) into a measure. Mix the powders on a glass plate and, using a flexible steel spatula, rub them to a smooth paste with a few drops of the chloral hydrate and transfer the suspension to a corked glass tube as described for potato starch in Quantitative Schedule VII, p. 182.

2. Lower the corked tube into a boiling tube, having first attached a string by which it can be lifted out of the boiling-tube for shaking.

Immerse the lower part of the boiling-tube in boiling water and occasionally shake it during five minutes or until the particles of powder are nearly colourless. To the suspension add 6 ml. of a mixture of 4 vols. of glycerin, 2 vols. of mucilage of tragacanth and 4 vols. of water; shake the tube for about three minutes by gentle oscillation.

3. Quickly remove a drop of the suspension to a slide by means of a glass rod or by a clean dry glass tube having a bore of 2 or 3 mm. Spread the drop by means of a needle or thin glass rod over an area slightly less than that of the cover-glass and apply the cover. Set aside for a few minutes in a level place.

4. Place the slide on the counting-field-finder on the stage of the microscope and count the spores present in twenty-five fields, and also trace the outlines of all the epidermal particles present in the same twenty-five fields by means of a camera lucida arranged to give a magnification of 400 diameters.

5. Cut out the tracings from the paper and weigh them; determine their area by weighing a piece of the same paper of known area, say 10 in. square, and calculating from the weight of the tracings.

6. Divide the area found by 160,000 (400^2) and one has the actual area of the particles of epidermis present in the twenty-five fields in which the lycopodium spores have been counted.

7. From the number of spores calculate the weight of the senna present, using the fact that 94,000 spores weigh 1 mg., and finally calculate the area of epidermis per gram of air-dry drug.

8. If the result obtained is to be used as a standard for future work, it should be corrected for the moisture present in the drug.

NOTES ON QUANTITATIVE SCHEDULE IX

The following is an example of the calculation:—

Weight of air-dry senna 0·1128 gm.
Weight of lycopodium 0·0528 gm.
Moisture in the senna = 7·63 per cent.

Number of lycopodium spores in twenty-five fields = 307·5.

Epidermal area of particles in the same twenty-five fields at a magnification of 400 diameters = 254·12 sq. cm.

Actual epidermal area of the particles

$$= \frac{254{\cdot}12}{160{,}000} \times 100 \text{ sq. mm.}$$
$$= 0{\cdot}15883 \text{ sq. mm.}$$

∴ 307·5 spores correspond to 0·15883 sq. mm. of epidermis

$$\therefore\ 52{\cdot}8 \times 94{,}000 \text{ spores correspond to } \frac{0{\cdot}15883 \times 52{\cdot}8 \times 94{,}000}{307{\cdot}5 \times 100}$$
$$= 25{\cdot}64 \text{ sq. cm. of epidermis.}$$

∴ 0·1128 gm. of air-dry senna powder has 25·64 sq. cm. and 1 gm. air dry powder has $\frac{25{\cdot}64}{0{\cdot}1128} = 227{\cdot}5$ sq. cm.

Correcting for moisture,

$$1 \text{ gm. of powdered senna dried at } 100^\circ \text{ C. has } \frac{227{\cdot}5 \times 100}{92{\cdot}37}$$
$$= 246 \text{ sq. cm. of epidermis.}$$

Using these figures it is a simple matter to *determine the percentage of senna in a compound powder*, such as Pulv, Sennæ Co. U.S.P. For example: The epidermal area present in 1 gm. of air-dry compound powder was found, by the method explained above, to be 41·2 sq. cm. Hence the amount of senna present is $\frac{41{\cdot}2 \times 100}{227{\cdot}5} = 18{\cdot}2$ per cent. (the amount actually present is 18 per cent.).

The composition of Pulv. Sennæ Co. U.S.P. is

Senna, very fine powder	180
Glycyrrhiza, very fine powder	236
Washed sulphur	80
Oil of fennel	4
Sucrose, finely powdered	500

QUANTITATIVE SCHEDULE X

To Determine the Number of Pollen Grains in Powdered Pyrethrum

1. Weigh out accurately about 1·0 gm. of powdered pyrethrum (*Chrysanthemum cinerariæfolium*) and about 0·05 gm. of lycopodium. Mix the two powders, and from the mixture prepare a crude fibre by the process described on p. 155, being careful that nothing is lost during the operation.

2. Mix the moist crude fibre with the suspending fluid (2 vols. of glycerin, 1 vol. of mucilage of tragacanth and 2 vols. of water) until the volume is about 20 ml. Shake by gentle oscillation for a few minutes in the corked tube until thoroughly mixed. Quickly remove a drop of the suspension by means of a glass tube and mount it for examination (as described in Quantitative Schedule IX., **3**, p. 186).

3. Count the number of pollen grains in a strip across one diameter of the cover-glass, having a width equal to that of the field of view. Count also the number of lycopodium spores in twenty or twenty-five fields evenly distributed along the strip and determine the average number per field.

4. Measure the diameter of the field of view and calculate the area of one field, and also of the entire strip in which the pollen grains were counted. From the results, find the number of fields in the strip and, from the average number of spores per field, find the total number of spores in the strip.

5. From the number of spores and the weights of pyrethrum and lycopodium used, calculate the wight of pyrethrum in the strip and then calculate the number of pollen grains per milligram.

NOTES ON QUANTITATIVE SCHEDULE X

Example of the Method

Weight of pyrethrum powder . .	= 1·0311 gm.
Weight of lycopodium spores . . .	= 0·0510 gm.
No. of compositous pollen grains in one diameter	= 20
No. of lycopodium spores in twenty fields of view	= 87, *i.e.*, 4·35 spores per field
Diameter of the field of view . . .	= 0·51 mm.
∴ Area of the field of view . . .	= 0·2041 sq. mm.
Diameter of the cover-glass . . .	= 19 mm.
∴ Area of strip along one diameter .	= 19 × 0·51 = 9·69 sq. mm.
No. of fields in the strip . . .	= 9·69 ÷ 0·204
	= 47·5 fields
No. of spores in the strip . . .	= 47·5 × 4·35
	= 206·6 spores
∴ there are 20 pollen grains for . .	206·6 spores
0·051 mg. of lycopodium . . .	= ·051 × 94,000
	= 4,794 spores.
The corresponding number of pollen grains	= 4794 × 20 ÷ 206·6
	= 462·1
∴ 1·0311 mg. pyrethrum contains .	462·1 pollen grains
and 1·0 mg. of pyrethrum contains .	448 pollen grains.

Good samples of pyrethrum flowers contain between 1,000 and 2,000 pollen grains per mg., and samples with less than 500 per mg. are considered to be of inferior quality. Hence the above sample is not of good quality.

The quality of pyrethrum flowers is now commonly assessed by determination of the pyrethrins present; but the question sometimes arises as to the type of flower-head supplied—buds, half-open or fully open, when the count of pollen-grains is the only method of finding an answer, when dealing with powder. It is also still a good method of judging quality. The method described is useful in other instances, and is a good example of the utilisation of crude fibre in connection with microscopical counts.

PART V

THE EXAMINATION OF POWDERED DRUGS

THE first necessity for the microscopical examination and analysis of powdered drugs is a practical knowledge of the histology of those plant members and animal organs occurring as drugs and a wide acquaintance with the types of cell and cell contents which provide the diagnostic characters of individual drugs. The organs of animals and plants are recognised by histological information gained by observing the arrangement of the constituent elements as they occur in those particles of powder which are composed of several cell types. The size and form of the cell types and the nature of their contents then enable the worker to form an opinion as to the identity of the plant or animal of which some particular member is present.

In addition to this, something further is needed for two purposes :— First, to provide in outline a scheme for the systematic handling of these examinations and analyses ; and, secondly, to provide a method for finding out rapidly what materials are characterised by the diagnostic features observed during the systematic search. Any suggested scheme need not be followed too rigidly, but it should be adopted as far as possible to avoid the omission of some essential test, and so save much trouble at a later stage, or even to identify a substance that otherwise would have been overlooked. For this reason certain preliminary observations must be carried out before making the preparations for the actual microscopical studies. The method of procedure should be as follows :—

Preliminary Observations

1. Observe the physical and sensory characteristics :—(*a*) Colour ; (*b*) taste and odour ; (*c*) fineness and degree of uniformity of the particles ; (*d*) sensation of smoothness or grittiness when the powder is gently rubbed on the hand, and crepitation when pressed ; (*e*) surface appearance by reflected light, shining particles, such as hairs, fibres, and calcium oxalate crystals.

2. If the powder is not uniform, sift it through a series of sieves (*e.g.*, Nos. 30, 60 and 90) and examine the fractions separately. The bulk of the loose starch will be found in the fraction passing the No. 90 sieve. The material retained by the coarsest sieve should be examined with a pocket lens.

3. To a little of the powder on a tile or slide add a drop or two of water and mix ; note the effect—*e.g.*, a mucilaginous mass may result, as with slippery elm bark, althæa root, and tragacanth ; or an emulsion may be formed as with myrrh or asafetida. Shake a little of the powder with a few cubic centimetres of water in a test-tube and note the extent to which solution takes place, as with aloes,

gambier, and gum acacia, or the production of a froth, as with quillaia and senega.

4. Press the powder between the folds of a piece of paper and look for any oily stain, as produced by almond meal, linseed meal, powdered umbelliferous fruits, etc.

5. Add a few drops of 5 per cent. caustic alkali to some of the powder on a white tile. Note any colour changes—*e.g.*, red with rhubarb, purple with cascara and frangula.

6. Add a few drops of 60 per cent. (by volume) sulphuric acid to some of the powder and observe any colour change—*e.g.*, crimson with cubebs, yellow with colchicum and liquorice; or any effervescence as with chalk.

7. Add a little of a 5 per cent. solution of ferric chloride and observe any colour changes as shown by drugs containing tannin.

Preparation of Microscopical Mounts

1. Make mounts to determine the types of cells and the nature of the cell walls present. Measure the sizes of fibres, stone cells, epidermal cells, and other important cell forms. Observe: (*a*) Any well-marked cell types which are absent; (*b*) the grouping of the cells, as seen in the larger particles.

The most useful clearing reagents for this purpose are solution of chloral hydrate (75 per cent.), lactophenol, dilute glycerin, solution of chlorinated soda, and, for certain powders (*e.g.*, oily powders and galls), clove oil. The most important staining reagent is phloroglucin followed by hydrochloric acid.

2. Make mounts to determine the nature of the cell contents. Measure the sizes of starch grains, crystals of calcium oxalate, and other contents having a definite form. Observe the relationship of the contents to the cells or groups of cells.

The most generally useful reagents, in addition to the clearing reagents named above, are water, iodine water, corallin soda, tincture of alkanet, and ruthenium red.

3. If necessary, make a crude fibre, using the Dutch process (see p. 155). This operation is, in practice, useful for a large proportion of the powders presented for analysis or examination; it concentrates the more highly resistant elements and frequently reveals the presence of materials occurring in small proportions only.

The Removal of Air Bubbles

One of the chief difficulties experienced in making microscopical mounts is to free the preparations from air bubbles. This may be accomplished in different ways, the simplest and most commonly useful being to boil the powder with the mountant until the particles are clear and air is completely removed. The boiling may be carried out on the slide, but care must be taken to replace the fluid which evaporates, so that the space beneath the cover-glass is completely filled with mountant at the conclusion of the operation. Another method is to boil a little of the powder with a cubic centimetre or two of the mountant in a test-tube, and, when clear, transfer to a slide. When boiling is impracticable, because of its possible destructive action, the powder may be soaked in the cold reagent for several hours, or even for a day or two, until clear. In a few instances, as for starches, it is sufficient to moisten the powder with alcohol and then add the reagent.

Dark-coloured powders which have been bleached by maceration in solution of chlorinated soda frequently become filled with bubbles of gas. These can be removed by transferring the bleached powder to some recently boiled and cooled distilled water, which rapidly dissolves the bubbles of gas. *Oily powders* are best prepared for mounting by extracting a large proportion of the oil with some solvent such as chloroform. Shake the powder with the solvent in a small flask, pour on to a filter paper, and, after draining, displace the remaining solution of fat or oil by pouring on fresh quantities of solvent. The powder will then be sufficiently defatted for mounting in the ordinary reagents.

This, in brief outline, is the sequence of the operations which must be carried out in the investigation of a powdered drug. At each stage of the process systematic notes and sketches must be made.

Next, the analyst must determine the nature of the plant or animal organs present in the powder by considering the way in which the tissues and cells are grouped together in the complex particles of the powder. The decision is reached by using information of the kind given in the following scheme. By this classification the drug is referred to a morphological group, and its identification then becomes relatively more simple.

Morphological Groups

Each of the following twelve groups forms a distinct section of the scheme of analysis, and should be considered separately from the remainder.

STARCHES AND ARROWROOTS. The powder consists of starch grains only. *Flours and meals* are recognised by the presence of protein matter accompanying the starch, and the identity of the flour is confirmed by an examination of the structures present in the crude fibre.

WOODS. *Structures present;* Vessels, fibres, wood parenchyma, and medullary rays which often cross the fibres and vessels. The powder is usually entirely lignified.

Structures absent; Cork, sieve tubes, ordinary cellulose parenchyma. Vessels are absent from the wood of most gymnosperms, *e.g.*, pine and juniper.

Nut-Shells and Fruit-Stones, in powder, consist almost entirely of lignified stone-cells, with a few pieces of spiral vessels and cellulose parenchyma.

BARKS AND GALLS. *Structures present;* Sieve tubes and cellulose parenchyma. Frequently also cork, pericyclic and phloem fibres, stone cells, calcium oxalate crystals, starch grains, and occasionally secretory tissue, *e.g.*, oil cells and laticiferous cells or tubes.

Structures absent; Epidermal tissues, palisade cells, xylem vessels, tracheids, and aleurone grains.

LEAVES. *Structures present*; Epidermis with stomata, cellulose parenchyma, not very abundant small-sized vascular elements. Frequently also trichomes, glands, palisade cells, and crystals of calcium oxalate. Foliage leaves contain chlorophyll. Leaves from bulbs contain no chlorophyll.

FLOWERS. *Structures present*; Pollen grains, fibrous layer of the anther wall, papillose surface of the stigma. Frequently also delicate yellow, red, or blue fragments of leaf-like structures showing a slightly papillose epidermis.

HERBS. *Structures prseent*; All structures characteristic of both leaves and flowers. Also epidermis, vessels, fibres, and parenchyma characteristic of herbaceous stems, frequently particles of small seeds, especially the diagnostic epidermis.

RHIZOMES AND ROOTS. *Structures present*; Cork and vascular tissues in varying amount, usually abundant parenchyma, which often contains starch in large amount.

Structures absent; Chlorenchyma, palisade tissue, and aleurone grains.

SEEDS. *Structures present*; Aleurone grains are always present. A little vascular tissue, consisting of small sized-elements only. Some form of carbohydrate reserve, *e.g.*, starch, hemicellulose, or oil.

FRUITS. *Structures present*; The same structures as for seeds and also more highly developed vascular tissues and other lignified and strongly built elements from the pericarp, often including a well-marked epidermis and a sclerenchymatous endocarp.

FIBRES USED FOR SURGICAL DRESSINGS. *Structures present*; Interlacing filaments, which may be either lignified or unlignified. In some instances structures characteristic of woods, but usually failing to give the lignin reaction.

ANIMAL SUBSTANCES. *Structures present*; Muscle fibres.

MISCELLANEOUS SUBSTANCES. *Structures present*; Unicellular organisms, trichomes, glands, etc.

If the drug shows no definite structure, it is probably one of the *unorganised drugs*, *e.g.*, aloes, gambier, etc. These may be sorted by first observing the solubility towards alcohol and then applying other tests, thus :—

A. Insoluble in alcohol :

1. Triturate with water—white emulsion, *Asafetida*.
   yellowish emulsion, *Myrrh*
2. Mount in alcohol and irrigate with water—
   (*a*) particles dissolve without swelling, *Acacia*.
   (*b*) particles swell and ultimately dissolve or become diffused, *Tragacanth*.
   Sterculia Gum.
   Gelatin.
   Agar.
3. Mount in ruthenium red—
   stains pink, *Agar* or *Sterculia gum*.

4. Heat with soda-lime in a dry tube—
   ammoniacal vapours evolved, *Albumen, Gelatin.*
5. Boil about 1 part with 100 parts of water—
   stiff jelly forms on cooling, *Agar.*
   the liquid coagulates, *Albumen.*
6. Warm with solution of caustic soda, 5 per cent.—
   a canary yellow colour indicates *Agar*.

B. Soluble in alcohol :

1. Add alcoholic ferric chloride to a dilute solution—
   green colour, *Gambier, Tolu.*
2. Apply the test for hydroxymethylanthraquinone derivatives—
   rose-pink colour, *Aloes*, except *Zanzibar Aloes.*
3. Test with potassium permanganate—
   odour of benzaldehyde, *Balsams.*

The presence of the individual drugs must be confirmed by applying the various special tests for each.

Having decided that a drug belongs to a particular morphological group, turn to the relevant table amongst those which follow and search for the drug which shows the cell forms and contents exhibited by the specimen under examination and so complete the identification.

TABLES OF HISTOLOGICAL CHARACTERS

The tables give the diagnostic characters of the more important members of each of the following morphological groups :—starches, woods, barks (including galls), leaves, inflorescences and floral members, rhizomes and roots, seeds and fruits. In other parts of the book there are supplementary tables for

Nut-shells and fruit-stones, p. 138.
Species of Strophanthus, p. 168.
Umbelliferous fruits, p. 170.
Varieties of capsicums, p. 175.

Each of the following tables has the names of the drugs in the first column and the other columns of the table are headed with the names of the more important structures which are generally diagnostic of the group. So far as possible, each column is completed for every drug, so that a ready means of comparison is provided and details of a diagnostic structure of any particular type can be quickly found, even when it has no specific significance for the drug concerned. The last column of each table gives a note of any special peculiarities and of chemical tests. It is therefore possible, with the aid of these tables, very rapidly to identify any powdered drug which is mentioned in them. After coming to a decision as to the identity of a powder, one should obtain a genuine specimen for comparison before making a final report.

In the tables, a number of the commoner adulterants are included so as to aid in their detection by affording a ready comparison between their characters and those of the drugs for which they are commonly substituted.

N.B.—The numerals used to state the dimensions of starch granules, fibres, etc., are printed in two kinds of type. The usual limits of size are given in ordinary type and the commoner sizes are printed in heavy type.

Types of Stomata, based upon the arrangement of the surrounding cells :—

Ranunculaceous type. The cells surrounding the stoma resemble the other epidermal cells, *i.e.*, there are no special subsidiary cells.

Cruciferous type. The stoma is usually surrounded by three or more subsidiary cells, one of which is markedly smaller than the others.

Rubiaceous type. The stoma has usually two subsidiary cells having their long axes parallel to the pore.

Caryophyllaceous type. The stoma has usually two subsidiary cells having their axes at right angles to the axis of the pore, *i.e.*, lying round the ends of the guard-cells.

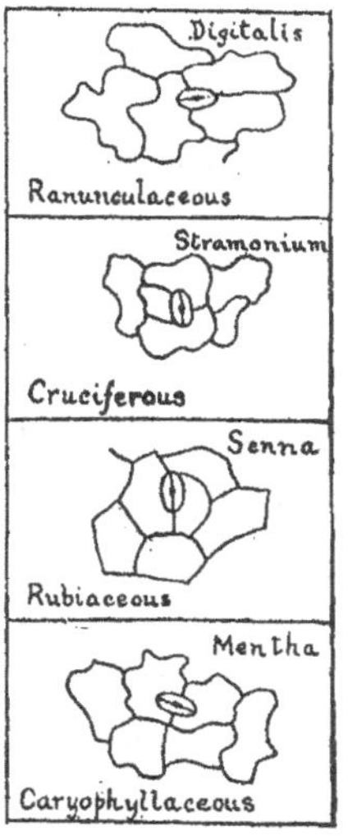

Drawings all × 100.

Name and Source.	Shape.	Hilum.	Striations.
[1] Wheat. *Triticum sativum.*	Lenticular. Outline circular, oval or sub-reniform.	A central point appearing as a line when a grain is on its edge.	Concentric. Faintly marked in commercial starch.
Maize or Corn. *Zea Mays.*	Polyhedral or sub-spherical.	A central triangular or 2 to 5-stellate split.	None.
[2] Rice. *Oryza sativa.*	Polyhedral.	A central point.	None.
Potato. *Solanum tuberosum.*	Ovoid ; irregularly ovoid or sub-spherical. Somewhat flattened.	A point at the narrower end. Usually eccentric $\frac{1}{3}$ to $\frac{1}{4}$.	Concentric. Well marked ; some rings darker than others.
Arrowroot. West Indian. *Maranta arundinacea.*	Ovoid to ellipsoid, with tuberosities.	A cleft, resembling wings of a bird in flight, at the broader end.	Faintly marked.
Arrowroot. East Indian. *Curcuma angustifolia* and *C. leucorrhiza.*	Flattened rectangular ovoid, with a terminal projection.	A point in the terminal projection.	Numerous, faint and transverse.
Sago. *Metroxylon Rumphii, M. Sagu* and *M. læve.*	Simple grains, mostly ovoid, some sub-spherical. Components of compound grains, muller-shaped.	A 2 to 5-rayed split. Central or eccentric $\frac{1}{2}$ to $\frac{1}{5}$.	Concentric.
Tapioca. *Manihot utilissima* and other species.	Mostly sub-spherical. Separated components, muller-shaped.	Round, linear or stellate. Central or up to $\frac{1}{2}$ eccentric.	Concentric.
Sweet Potato. *Ipomœa Batatas.*	Rounded, polyhedral and muller-shaped.	Fissured or stellate. Central or $\frac{1}{2}$ to $\frac{1}{5}$ eccentric.	Concentric.
Florida Arrowroot. *Zamia floridana.*	Ovoid, muller-shaped or irregularly triangular or quadrilateral.	A point or a split. Central or eccentric.	Concentric.

[1] Barley. *Hordeum sativum.* Resembles wheat starch, but is rather
Rye. *Secale cereale.* Resembles wheat starch, but is slightly
[2] Oat. *Avena sativa.* Resembles rice, but always shows some

Size.	Aggregation.	Polariscope, etc.	Drawings all × 150.
Smaller grains 0 to **5** to 10 microns. Larger grains 16 to **20** to **25** to 50 microns. More than 400 grains per milligram over 40 microns.	Mostly simple. Very few compound grains of 2 to 4 components.	Faint Maltese cross. Grains on their edges show a clearly defined "cross" thus >——<.	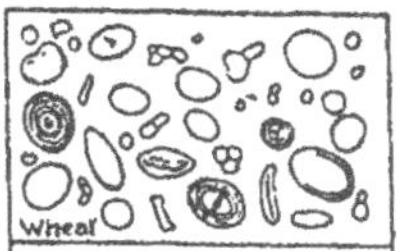 Wheat
5 to **10** to **15** to 25 microns.	In commercial starch, all simple.	Well-marked cross.	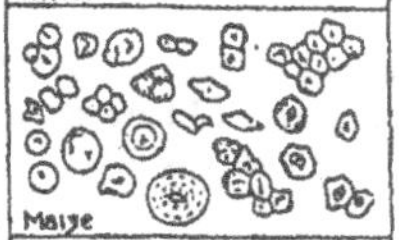 Maize
3 to **5** to **8** to 12 microns.	Ovate compound grains, 2 to 150 components. Size 7 to 20 microns × 12 to 30 microns.	Well-marked cross.	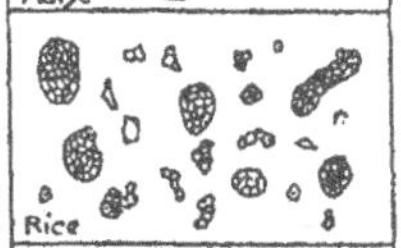 Rice
Rounded 10 to 35 microns. Ovoid 30 to 100 microns.	Small number of compound grains of 2 to 3 components.	Well-marked cross.	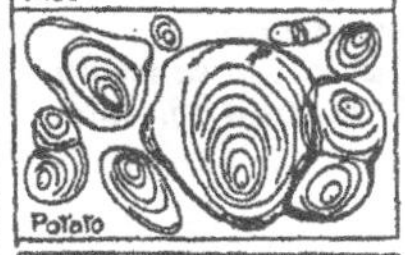 Potato
7 to **30** to **45** to 75 microns.	All simple.	Well-marked cross.	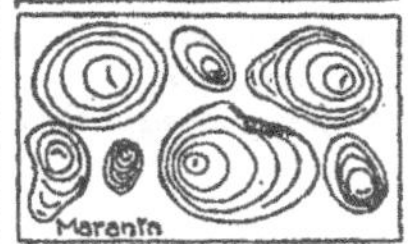 Maranta
Length 15 to **30** to **60** to 140 microns. Breadth 25 to 35 microns. Thickness 7 to 8 microns.	All simple.	Well-marked cross.	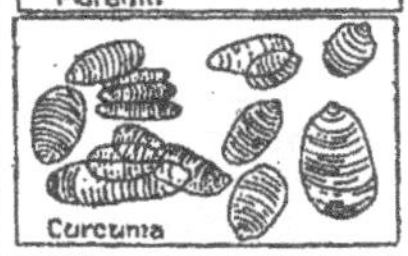 Curcuma
Large components 50 to **65** to 80 microns. Small components 10 to 20 microns.	Mostly compound with 2 to 4 components. Usually one large and 1 to 3 small.	Well-marked cross. Some grains are gelatinised.	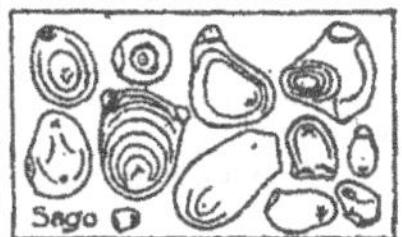 Sago
Large components 25 to 35 microns. Small components **5** to 12 or 25 microns.	Mostly compound, 2 to 8 components, mostly 2, 3 or 4.	Well-marked cross. Some grains are gelatinised.	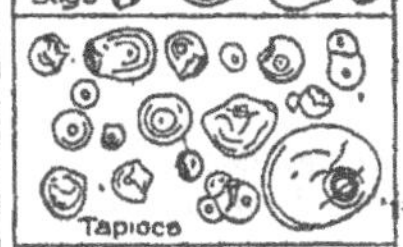 Tapioca
Large **25** to **50** to 55 microns. Small 15 to 22 microns.	Compound grains 2 to 3 or up to 6 components.	Well-marked cross.	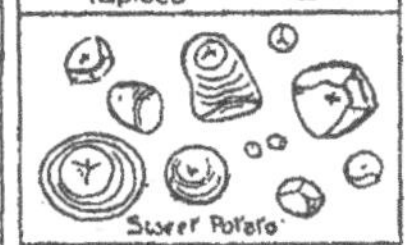 Sweet Potato
5 to **15** to **40** to 75 microns.	Mostly compound of 3 to 8 components.	Well-marked cross. The starch contains a few clusters of calcium oxalate 14 to **35** to 60 microns. Also some grains of sand.	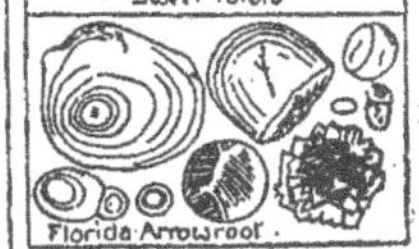 Florida Arrowroot.

more irregular in outline and slightly smaller. No grains over 40 microns.
larger and the hilum is a split with 3 to 5 rays.
spindle-shaped or lemon-shaped forms.

Name and Source.	Annual Rings, etc.	Medullary Rays.	Vessels.
[1] Pine. *Pinus sylvestris.*	Well marked.	Heterogeneous and uniseriate. A few multiseriate and including a resin duct.	None, except of the primary xylem.
[2] Quassia (Jamaica). *Picræna excelsa.*	None. Shows storied arrangement.	About 80 per cent. are 2 to 5 cells wide; 20 per cent. are uniseriate. 10 to 25 cells high. A few prisms of calcium oxalate are present.	Isolated or 2 to 11 in a group; up to 200 microns wide. Thickly covered with minute bordered pits.
Guaiacum. *Guaiacum sanctum. Guaiacum officinale.*	Fairly well marked. Shows storied arrangement.	Uniseriate. 3 to 6 cells high.	Isolated or 2 to 3 in a group; up to 150 microns wide. Closely covered with small bordered pits.
Red Sanders. *Pterocarpus santalinus.*	None. Shows storied arrangement.	Mostly uniseriate; some 2 to 3 cells wide. About 2 to 12 cells high.	Isolated or 2 to 5 in a group; up to 300 microns wide, mostly 100–250 microns; closely pitted walls.
Logwood. *Hæmatoxylon campechianum.*	None.	Up to 7 (mostly 3–4) cells wide. A few uniseriate.	Mostly isolated. A few in pairs.
Sappan. *Cæsalpinia Sappan.*	Clearly marked.	Usually 2 to 3 cells wide.	Mostly in pairs or in radial groups; up to about 250 microns wide.
Sandal Wood. *Santalum album.*	Not clearly marked. There are alternating darker and lighter concentric bands.	Usually 2 to 4 cells wide.	Mostly isolated and showing oil-containing thyloses. Up to 150 microns wide, mostly 50–90 microns.
Sassafras Wood. *Sassafras officinale.*	Clearly marked.	One to 4 cells wide. They contain small starch grains.	Usually in groups; up to about 110 microns wide. Numerous bordered pits. Thyloses often present.

[1] Juniper. *Juniperus communis.* Wood similar to that of *Pinus sylvestris*, but
Yew. *Taxus baccata.* Wood similar to that of *Pinus sylvestris*, but no resin
[2] Surinam Quassia. *Quassia amara.* Wood similar to that of *Picræna excelsa.*

Fibres.	Parenchyma.	Contents.	Peculiarities and Tests.
None.	Few thin-walled cells near the resin ducts.	Resin in the ducts. Occasional starch grains in the medullary rays.	Consists mainly of rectangular prismatic tracheids with tapering ends. Circular bordered pits in a single row on the radial walls.
Thin-walled. Pits slit-like.	Abundant, chiefly metatracheal. In files. Longer cells without calcium oxalate prisms.	Calcium oxalate prisms in the files of short-celled parenchyma. Usually one crystal in each cell. A few starch grains.	Bitter taste.
Thick-walled.	Scanty; contains occasional single prisms of calcium oxalate.	Resin in all the elements, yellow-brown or red in colour.	Gives a bluish-green colour with ferric chloride.
Rather thin-walled in the middle; tips more thickened.	Abundant, chiefly metatracheal. Calcium oxalate prisms in the files of cells.	Red resin in all elements. All walls coloured brownish-red.	Colour soluble in alcohol; insoluble in water.
Strongly thickened walls.	Abundant in wide metatracheal bands. Many cells contain prisms of calcium oxalate.	Gummy matter and a whitish substance in the vessels.	Colour soluble in water. Coloured purple by lime-water and blackish-violet by ferric chloride.
Thick-walled.	Abundant, mostly around the vessels. Prisms of calcium oxalate in many of the cells.	Coloured cell-walls and contents.	Colour soluble in water. Coloured crimson by lime-water; no change with ferric chloride.
Thick-walled.	Encircling the vessels. A few files of cells contain prisms of calcium oxalate.	Oil in all the elements. Oil soluble in alcohol.	Characteristic odour.
Thick-walled.	Cells contain numerous small starch grains.	Calcium oxalate absent. Oil in cells embedded in the wood and the medullary rays.	Characteristic odour.

resin ducts are absent and the medullary rays are homogeneous.
ducts and the tracheids have a spiral thickening as well as circular bordered pits.
but the medullary rays are mostly uniseriate and calcium oxalate is absent.

Name and Source.	Fibres.	Calcium Oxalate.	Stone Cells.
Pomegranate Root. *Punica granatum.*	None.	Abundant clusters in longitudinal rows. Prisms very few indeed.	Very few, but characteristic.
Canella. *Canella alba.*	None, except an occasional pericyclic fibre.	Clusters only, about 20 to 35 microns in diameter.	Cells of the phelloderm thickened on the inner walls.
Black Haw. *Viburnum prunifolium.*	None.	Clusters, 10 to 40 microns in diameter. Some prisms.	Very numerous in large ovoid groups.
Wahoo. *Euonymus atropurpureus.*	None.	Numerous cluster crystals 30 to 40 microns in diameter.	None.
Wild Cherry. *Prunus serotina.*	No typical fibres.	Prisms near the sclerenchyma ; few clusters in the inner layers.	Abundant in ellipsoidal groups of up to 250 cells. Smallest groups of 3 or 4 cells often fibrous.
Cinchona. *Cinchona succirubra* and other spp.	Isolated or in short radial rows, 25 to 90 microns wide, often over 70 microns.	Microcrystals in idioblasts in the parenchymatous elements. Crystals 2 to 6μ long.	None.
Cassia. *Cinnamomum Cassia.*	Isolated or in short tangential rows, often 30 to 40 microns wide.	Very small needles scattered in the parenchyma.	Numerous. Thickened on the inner and radial walls.
Cinnamon. *Cinnamomum zeylanicum.*	Isolated or in short tangential rows, rarely exceeding 30 microns in width.	Very small needles scattered in the parenchyma.	Numerous. Thickened on the inner and radial walls.
Sassafras. *Sassafras variifolium.*	Isolated. About 25 microns wide and 150 to 500 microns long.	Very small needles in the phloem parenchyma and in the medullary rays.	Few.
Cascarilla. *Croton Eluteria.*	Isolated.	Cluster crystals and also some prisms. See also under Cork.	No ordinary stone cells ; see under Cork.

Cork.	Starch.	Special Features and Tests.
Most of the cells strongly thickened on the inner walls, which are also lignified.	Abundant rounded grains, mostly simple, up to 8 microns in diameter, rarely up to 25 microns.	Coloured blue-black with solution of ferric chloride.
None or only very small amount.	Abundant. Simple grains and compound with up to 4 components, 6–10 microns or up to 20 microns.	Oil cells present. Aromatic odour.
Abundant, large-celled, yellowish-brown.	Scanty.	Slight valerian-like odour.
Thin-walled and mostly lignified.	Numerous spheroidal grains 3–12 microns	Rectangular parenchyma with brown contents from the cortex and medullary rays. Thin- and cellulose-walled fibre shaped cells with granular nearly colourless contents, very numerous.
Thin-walled cells.	Small grains, simple and 2 to 5 compound.	When moistened with cold water, the odour of bitter almonds is developed and the vapour turns picrate paper brick-red.
Thin-walled.	Small amount in very small grains.	Bitter taste. Heated in a dry tube evolves a red vapour which condenses to red droplets.
Thin-walled cells in fairly large amount.	Abundant ; rarely under 10 microns wide.	Aromatic odour. Oil and mucilage cells present.
A very small amount usually present.	Abundant ; rarely over 8 microns in diameter.	Aromatic odour. Oil cells present.
Small amount, cells with red contents.	Abundant rounded grains about 3 to 20 microns diameter.	Odour of safrol. Oil cells present.
Lignified; outer walls strongly thickened ; small calcium oxalate prisms on the inner walls.	Abundant very small rounded grains.	Latex tubes present. Oil cells present. Resin cells in the phloem parenchyma. Gives a deep blue with solution of ferric chloride.

Name and Source.	Fibres.	Calcium Oxalate.	Stone Cells.
Alstonia. *Alstonia scholaris.*	Isolated.	Prismatic crystals only.	Groups of rather thin-walled rectangular cells and groups of heavily thickened irregularly shaped cells Yellow in colour.
Angustura. *Cusparia trifoliata.*	Isolated and in small groups.	Bundles of acicular raphides and also large prisms.	Present in the phelloderm, see also Cork
Soap Bark. *Quillaia Saponaria.*	In bundles, tortuous and irregularly enlarged at intervals.	Large prisms, 50 to 170 microns long and up to 30 microns wide.	Few, sub-rectangular singly or in small groups.
Slippery Elm. *Ulmus fulva.*	In bundles of 6 to 30; about 20 microns in diameter; rather thin walls; only slightly lignified.	Prisms 10 to 25 to 60 microns long, in files of crystal cells surrounding the bundles of fibres.	None.
Witch Hazel. *Hamamelis virginiana.*	In bundles of 20 to 100 arranged in tangential bands. Fibres 15 to 30 microns in diameter.	Prisms in endodermis and scattered in the parenchyma and in crystal sheaths to the bundles of fibres.	Abundant Heavily and evenly thickened walls
[1] Cascara Sagrada. *Rhamnus Purshiana.*	In bundles of up to 30 fibres. Fibres about 8 to 15 microns in diameter.	Clusters in the cortex and parenchyma; prisms in sheaths surrounding the groups of stone cells and fibres.	In ovoid groups.

GALLS

Name and Source.	Fibres.	Calcium Oxalate.	Stone Cells.
Oak Galls. *Quercus infectoria.*	None.	Clusters and prisms in fairly thick-walled and pitted parenchyma.	Abundant; also "*lignin bodies*" and a few small vessels.

[1] Alder Buckthorn. *Rhamnus Frangula.* Resembles

Cork.	Starch.	Special Features and Tests.
Thin-walled.	In the medullary rays. Rounded grains 7 to 15 microns.	Latex tubes present.
Thick-walled, lignified and yellow in part and the remainder thin-walled.	Small rounded grains.	Drops of oily secretion. Gives a red colour with ferric chloride.
Very little.	Abundant grains about 6 to 10 microns in diameter.	Powder is sternutatory. Froths when shaken with water.
None.	Abundant, spheroidal or polygonal 10 to 15 to 25 microns in diameter.	Very large mucilage cells about 200 microns in diameter. Mucilage stains with ruthenium red. Odour recalling that of fenugreek. Make a thick mucilage with water.
Thin-walled tabular cells.	Very little in small grains.	Taste astringent. Ferric chloride solution colours the parenchyma bluish black.
Thin-walled ; with yellow-brown contents.	Scanty. In very small grains found in the chloroplastids.	Yellow cell contents are coloured purple by solution of caustic alkali. Both these barks give the characteristic rose-pink colour to solution of ammonia when subjected to the test for hydroxymethylanthraquinones (see p. 24).

GALLS

No cork ; but the outer layers are suberised (metaderm).	Few grains about 20 microns in diameter.	Tannin flakes in all the parenchyma. Solution of ferric chloride gives a bluish-black colour. Occasional insect fragments. Astringent taste.

Cascara Sagrada, but stone cells are absent.

Name and Source.	Calcium Oxalate.	Stomata.		Trichomes.
		Upper Surface.	Lower Surface.	Covering.
Foxglove. *Digitalis purpurea.*	None.	Ranunculaceous. Few.	Numerous.	3 to 5 cells long, uniseriate, finely warty. 230 to 280μ long; 8 to 15 to 35 to 45μ wide.
Xanthium. *Xanthium strumarium.*	None.	Ranunculaceous.		Large and conical, 2 to 3 cells long; the 1 or 2 basal cells filled with a mass of $CaCO_3$. Also slender uniseriate trichomes of 6 to 7 cells.
Savin. *Juniperus Sabina.*	In the cuticle, minute prisms (2 to 3 microns). In some cells of the mesophyll small prisms, 2 to 6 microns.	Deeply sunken and in longitudinal rows, with the pores parallel to the axis of the leaf. Walls of guard cells lignified.		None.
Buchu. *Barosma betulina.*	Cluster crystals only.	None.	Ranunculaceous. Some over 38 microns long.	Few, unicellular, on the midrib and petiole, on the upper surface only.
Tea. *Camellia sinensis.*	Cluster crystals in the spongy parenchyma.	None.	Ranunculaceous. Each surrounded by 3 or 4 narrow cells.	Few, unicellular, on the under surface only. Up to 700 microns long.
Maté. *Ilex paraguensis.*	Cluster crystals.	None.	Ranunculaceous. Each surrounded by 4 or 5 apparently narrow cells.	Few, unicellular, conical-linear.
Henna. *Lawsonia inermis.*	Cluster crystals abundant in the spongy parenchyma up to about 40 microns	Ranunculaceous.		None.
Ailanthus. *Ailanthus glandulosa.*	Cluster crystals along the veins.	None.	Ranunculaceous.	Unicellular (rarely 2-celled) sharply conical, slightly curved, lignified.
Bearberry. *Arctostaphylos Uva-ursi.*	Irregular single crystals (prisms) in the collenchyma.	None.	Ranunculaceous, grouped in patches over the vein islets.	Very few, mostly unicellular, conical and thick-walled. On the petiole and margin.

Trichomes.	Epidermis.		Mesophyll.	Special Features.
Glandular.	Upper	Lower.		
Few ; mostly with a unicellular stalk and head of 2 cells.	Walls slightly wavy.	Walls markedly wavy.	One row of palisade ; sometimes not differentiated.	One large water pore, rarely 2, on each tooth.
Few ; composed of 2 or 3 tiers of 2 cells each.	Walls straight.	Walls straight.	Palisade of 2 or 3 rows.	Effervescence with acid.
None.	Walls straight and beaded ; cells somewhat elongated longitudinally except where the stomata are numerous.		No palisade layer. Contains lignified transfusion cells.	The hypodermis in parts of the leaf is fibrous and lignified.
None.	Walls straight.	Walls straight. Patches of thin-walled, modified cells over the glands.	One row of palisade, rarely 2.	Numerous schizolysigenous oil-glands. Mucilage and diosmin in the epidermis.
None.	Walls, nearly straight; slightly undulating.	Somewhat wavy walls.	One row of palisade ; 2 rows here and there.	Needle-shaped crystals of caffein obtained by microsublimation.
None.	Straight walls. Cells rather small. Cuticle striated.		One row of palisade.	Small globules of oil in many of the cells. Yields needle - shaped crystals of caffeine by microsublimation.
None.	Walls straight or slightly wavy.	Walls straight or very slightly wavy.	Two rows, sometime three, of palisade on each side.	Epidermis over the veins is strongly striated.
On teeth at the base of the laminæ. Very rare and not easy to find.	Walls straight ; cuticle strongly striated ; also the cuticle of the trichomes.		One row of palisade.	
Very few with a short 2 - celled stalk and multicellular secreting head.	Walls straight.	Walls straight.	Palisade 3 to 5 rows, usually 3. Small droplets of oil in most of the cells.	Ferric chloride give a bluish-black colour.

Name and Source	Calcium Oxalate.	Stomata		Trichomes.
		Upper Surface.	Lower Surface.	Covering.
Phytolacca. *Phytolacca decandra.*	Bundles of needles in idioblasts.	Ranunculaceous.	Ranunculaceous.	None.
Belladonna. *Atropa Belladonna.*	Microsphenoids in idioblasts (sandy crystals).	Cruciferous few.	Cruciferous many.	Uniseriate 4 to 5 cells long.
Coca. *Erythroxylum Coca.*	Prisms and a few cluster crystals.	None.	Rubiaceous.	None.
Witch-hazel. *Hamamelis virginiana.*	Prisms near the fibres ; a few clusters.	None.	Rubiaceous numerous.	Stellate clusters, 4 to 12 branches, rarely single trichomes.
Eucalyptus. *Eucalyptus globulus.*	Prisms near the fibres. Clusters in the palisade.	Ranunculaceous.	Ranunculaceous.	None.
Senna. *Cassia acutifolia. Cassia angustifolia.*	Prisms near the fibres. Clusters in palisade and spongy tissue.	Rubiaceous numerous.	Rubiaceous numerous.	Unicellular. Thick walls, strong cuticular warts, often appressed.
Lily of the Valley. *Convallaria majalis.*	Prisms and bundles of acicular raphides.	In lines ; small, each between 2 large elongated rectangular cells.	In lines ; small, between 2 large elongated rectangular cells.	None.
[1] Stramonium. *Datura Stramonium.*	Clusters in a crystal layer. Few prisms and microsphenoids near the veins.	Cruciferous few.	Cruciferous many.	Conical and uniseriate ; usually 3 cells.
Datura. *Datura innoxia.*	Similar to stramonium.	Cruciferous numerous.	Cruciferous numerous, about equal numbers on both surfaces.	Conical and slender ; 1 to 3 cells.
Datura. *Datura Metel* and *D. fastuosa.*	Similar to stramonium.	Cruciferous few. Collapsed guard cells fairly numerous.	Cruciferous many. Collapsed guard cells fairly numerous.	As stramonium but basal cell is shorter and narrower (under 75 microns in length).
Henbane. *Hyoscyamus niger.*	Prisms or twins or clusters of few components. A few microsphenoids near veins.	Cruciferous few.	Cruciferous many.	Uniseriate of 3 to 4 cells ; conical.

[1] *Datura Tatula.* Similar to stramonium. The uniseriate covering hairs are usually

Trichomes.	Epidermis.		Mesophyll.	Special Features.
Glandular.	Upper.	Lower.		
None.	Straight walls.	Straight walls.	One row of palisade.	
Club-shaped solanceous and also with a long uniseriate stalk and a glandular head.	Slightly sinuous walls, striated cuticle.	More sinuous walls, striated cuticle.	One row of palisade.	
None.	Straight walls.	Straight walls. Papillose.	One row of palisade.	Numbing taste.
None.	Somewhat sinuous walls.	Somewhat sinuous walls.	One row of palisade. Occasional lignified idioblasts.	Green colour with ferric chloride.
None.	Straight walls. Patches of cells over the glands.	Straight walls. Patches of cells over the glands.	Isobilateral. Palisade 3 or 4 rows.	Corky spots due to emptied glands. Large ovoid oil-glands.
None.	Straight walls. Mucilage in lower part of many cells.	Straight walls. Mucilage in lower part of many cells.	Isobilateral. Palisade of one row.	Give the hydroxy-methylanthra-quinone reaction (see p. 24).
None.	Straight walls. Cells axially elongated and in rows.	Straight walls. Cells axially elongated and in rows.	Homogeneous.	Groups of well-developed peri-cyclic fibres ex-tend the bundles from one epider-mis to the other.
Club-shaped solanaceous.	Slightly sinuous walls.	More sinuous walls.	Palisade of one row of cells. Well marked crys-tal layer.	
Uniseriate, usually 4 cells, with a 1-celled terminal gland (numerous). Also club-shaped solanaceous type.	As stra-monium.	As stra-monium.	One row of palisade.	
Similar to stra-monium.	Similar to stramonium.	Similar to stramonium.	One row of palisade.	Large crystalline masses in the epidermis and mesophyll.
Large ovoid pluri-cellular glands at ends of uni-seriate stalks.	Sinuous walls.	Sinuous walls.	One row of palisade. Well marked crystal layer	

4-celled. Petioles and stems give a pink with hydrochloric acid or chloral hydrate

Name and Source.	Bracts, Receptacle, etc.	Calyx.	Corolla.
Saffron. *Crocus sativus.*			Very occasional fragments present.
Red Rose Petals. *Rosa gallica.*			Papillose on the upper surface. Cells of lower epidermis with inward projections. Outer surface with few stomata and narrow unicellular trichomes.
Poppy Petals. *Papaver Rhœas.*			Stomata in small numbers on both surfaces. Laticiferous vessels in the veins.
Cloves. *Eugenia aromatica.*	Bracts resemble the calyx teeth. *Stalks* or pedicels contain numerous stone-cells, fibres and prisms of calcium oxalate.	Glabrous. Epidermis of straight-walled cells ; many stomata on outer surface. Ovoid glands in mesophyll.	Glabrous. Contains ovoid oil-glands and small cluster crystals of calcium oxalate. No papillæ. Stomata absent.
Kousso. *Brayera anthelmintica.*	Bracts carry glandular trichomes with a uniseriate stalk of 2 to 5 cells and a large unicellular secreting head ; also some with pluricellular heads.	Calyx tube carries numerous unicellular, thick-walled, conical trichomes. Prisms of calcium oxalate in the parenchyma.	Often absent. Quite small. Mesophyll parenchyma of branching cells.
Lily of the Valley. *Convallaria majalis.*			Stomata on the outer surface. Acicular raphides in small bundles in the cells of the mesophyll.
Lavender. *Lavandula officinalis.*		Long, unicellular, conical trichomes on the margin. Labiate glandular trichomes in the grooves. On the ridges branching purple trichomes, both unicellular and pluricellular.	Labiate glandular trichomes on outer surface. On the inner surface, at the throat and where the stamens are attached, long, uniseriate glandular trichomes with a small spherical unicellular head and a stalk consisting mainly of one long, knotted, narrow cell.

Stamens, Anthers and Pollen.	Ovary and Fruit.	Style and Stigma.	Special Features.
Few pollen grains, 80 to 150 microns, finely granular and spherical. Occasional piece of anther wall with fibrous cells.	Cells of style epidermis are narrow and axially elongated, each with a small conical papilla.	Hollow; open one side. Finger-like marginal papillæ 50 to 150 microns long and 25 to 40 microns wide. Small spiral vessels.	Gives a deep blue with 80 per cent. v/v sulphuric acid. Strong characteristic odour. Slightly bitter taste. Starch absent.
Pollen grains spherical, smooth, with 3 pores, 36 to 43 microns in diameter.			Red with acid, green with alkali; deep blue with iron salts. A few cluster crystals of calcium oxalate in the mesophyll near the base.
Pollen grains spherical, with 3 pores, 23 to 30 microns in diameter.			Ultimate veinlets anastomose by small arches forming a line 150 to 250 microns within the margin.
Oil-gland in apex of connective. Anther walls with fibrous layer and minute clusters of calcium oxalate along the lines of dehiscence. Pollen grains rounded triangular, 15 to 20 microns in diameter.	Spongy parenchyma, ovoid oil-glands and cluster crystals of calcium oxalate in the hypanthium. No prisms of calcium oxalate.	No papillæ.	Few small pericyclic fibres. No stone-cells; no starch. 50 per cent. caustic potash gives needles of potassium eugenate. Ferric chloride gives a blue-black. Aromatic, spicy odour, pungent taste.
Pollen spherical with 3 indefinite slit-shaped pores, 30 to 36 microns in diameter. Less than 200 pollen grains per mgr.	Wall of three layers, the innermost developed as a parquetry layer of thick-walled and pitted cells.	Stigma papillose. Thick-walled conical, sharply-pointed trichomes on the style.	Large cluster crystals of calcium oxalate in the axis; small ones in the floral parts.
Anther walls with fibrous layer. Pollen grains, ellipsoidal, almost smooth, 33 to 37 microns in diameter.		Short club-shaped papillæ on the stigma.	
Anther wall with long trichomes. Pollen spherical, with 6 slit-shaped pores, 26 to 30 microns in diameter	Epidermis of ovary small-celled and glabrous.	Fine rounded papillæ on the stigma. Sharply conical unicellular and forked bi-cellular trichomes on the style	Oxalate almost absent. Occasional small prisms in the inner epidermis of the calyx. Characteristic odour.

Name and Source.	Bracts, Receptacle, etc.	Calyx.	Corolla.
Marigold. *Calendula officinalis.*			On the tube, trichomes formed of 2 rows of cells, up to 120 microns long. Glandular trichomes with long stalks. Yellow plastids in the corolla.
Santonica. *Artemisia Cina.*	Bract margin scarious, no marginal trichomes ; few T-shaped cottony hairs over midrib ; numerous compositous glandular trichomes.	None present.	Tubular only. Compositous glandular trichomes at the base and on the free lobes.
Arnica. *Arnica montana.*	Large conical uniseriate trichomes on the involucral bracts. No paleæ.	Pappus bristles 5 to 6 cells wide and covered thickly with projecting points.	Ligulate and tubular corollas yellow. Compositous glandular trichomes on the strap and on the tube.
Chamomile. *Anthemis nobilis.*	Paleæ with scarious margin and thick-walled, narrow, conical trichomes on the outer surface of the thicker central region, up to 600 microns long, each composed of a very long apical cell and a row of 3 to 5 small basal cells.	None present.	Mostly ligulate with a few tubular. Ligule with a slightly papillose upper epidermis : compositous glandular trichomes on the tube. Few calcium oxalate clusters, about 5 microns diameter, at base of corolla tube.
Matricaria. *Matricaria Chamomilla.*	Involucral bracts glabrous. No paleæ.	None present.	12 to 21 ligulate florets, about 200 tubular florets. Ligulate corolla white ; tubular corolla yellow. Compositous glandular trichomes on both.
Insect Flowers. *Chrysanthemum cinerariæfolium.*	Outer epidermis of involucral bracts bears T-shaped balance hairs and numerous stomata. The bracts contain small prisms of calcium oxalate. No paleæ.	Membranous and about 0·8 to 1·0 millimetre long, with small prisms of calcium oxalate in the epidermis.	Ligulate corolla with papillose upper epidermis. Compositous glandular trichomes on outer epidermis of the corollas of both ligulate and tubular florets. Small cluster crystals of calcium oxalate in the corolla of tubular florets.
Dandelion. *Taraxacum officinale.*	No paleæ.	Pappus bristles 2 to 3 cells wide, with distant alternate points.	All ligulate and yellow.

Stamens, Anthers and Pollen.	Ovary and Fruit.	Style and Stigma.	Special Features.
Spherical with 3 pores ; spiny, 30 to 45 microns in diameter.			
Small cluster crystals of calcium oxalate in the connectives. Pollen grains, spherical, smooth, 3 pores, 14 to 18 to 25 microns in diameter.	Immature.	Unexpanded, bifid, with papillæ.	Small fibre-tracheids from the bracts. Odour resembling that of eucalyptus
Pollen grains spherical, rather long spines, 3 pores, about 36 microns in diameter.	On the wall, appressed twin hairs each of 2 cells separated longitudinally by a pitted wall ; also compositous glandular trichomes.	Bifid stigma, that of the ligulate florets having long papillæ. Phytomelan in the fruit wall.	
Pollen grains spherical and with short spines, 3 pores, 30 to 45 microns in diameter.	Compositous glandular trichomes on ovary wall in vertical lines.	Bifid stigma with slightly papillose tips. Numerous small calcium oxalate clusters, about 5 microns diameter, where base of style joins ovary.	Aromatic odour. Taste aromatic and very bitter.
Pollen grains similar to *Anthemis* ; 25 to 30 microns in diameter. A few small calcium oxalate cluster crystals in the connective.	Compositous glandular trichomes on ovary wall in vertical rows and between the rows oblong-fusiform groups of about 20 to 40 small cells containing mucilage, each about 5 microns long and 25 microns wide.	Similar to *Anthemis*.	Strong, characteristic aromatic odour. Aromatic and bitter taste.
Pollen grains spherical, with 3 pores and shortly spiny ; about 28 microns in diameter.	Compositous glandular trichomes on the ovary wall and prisms of calcium oxalate in the epidermis of the ovary and in the cells of the much lignified and thickened hypodermis.	Bifid style with slightly papillose tips.	There should be at least 2,000 pollen grains per milligramme of the powder.
Pollen grains spherical and spiny, 35 to 40 microns in diameter.	Large spines on summit of the ovary. No glands or trichomes on the epidermis.	Bifid style with sharply pointed papillæ on the tips.	

Name and Source.	Starch.	Calcium Oxalate.	Fibres.	Vessels.
Dandelion. *Taraxacum officinale.*	None.	None.	None.	Reticulate with elongated pits; numerous and usually isolated; up to 80 microns in width.
Chicory. *Cichorium Intybus.*	None.	None.	Thin-walled fibres of the xylem.	Numerous, 20 to 50 microns wide; in small groups. Reticulate with transverse oval pits rarely more than half across the vessel width.
Pellitory. *Anacyclus Pyrethrum.*	None.	None.	Some xylem fibres.	10 to 15 microns wide; in groups; pits circular.
Couch Grass. *Agropyrum repens.*	None.	None.	Strongly thickened fibrous sclerenchyma of the hypoderma and pericycle.	Mostly spiral and annular.
Senega. *Polygala senega.*	None.	None.	Short xylem fibres.	Small vessels, often with lateral openings.
Gentian. *Gentiana lutea.*	Occasional simple grains.	Needles up to 0·1 by 8·0 microns, scattered in the parenchyma.	None.	Large reticulate.
Ginger. *Zingiber officinale.*	Abundant; granules sack-shaped, mostly simple, up to 50×30×7 microns.	None.	Non-lignified, thin-walled, septate, surrounding the vascular bundles.	Non-lignified, reticulate, accompanied by narrow pigment cells. Vessels 50 to 75µ wide.
Hydrastis. *Hydrastis canadensis.*	Sub-spherical; 2 to 15 microns in diameter. Few 2 to 6 compound.	None.	Bundles of thin-walled yellow xylem fibres.	Numerous; in groups; 8 to 25 microns wide. Slit-like bordered pits.
Male fern. *Dryopteris Filix-mas.*	Abundant, mostly simple rounded granules up to 18 to 25 microns.	None.	No true fibres. *See under* Stone-Cells.	Numerous, scalariform, 10 to 60 microns wide. A few spiral.
Colchicum. *Colchicum autumnale.*	Simple granules, spherical or polygonal, 3 to 16 to 28 microns. Mostly 2 to 3 compound or up to 7 compound.	None.	None.	Small spiral and annular.

Stone-Cells.	Cork.	Parenchyma.	Special Features and Tests.
None.	Thin-walled tabular cells.	Abundant, thin-walled, pitted, containing amorphous masses of inulin.	Lacticiferous vessels abundant. Bitter taste.
None.	Thin-walled poly-gonal, tabular cells.	Abundant, thin-walled, pitted, containing inulin in amorphous masses.	Laticiferous vessels. Sweetish taste. Characteristic odour.
Rectangular and polygonal from the cork.	Thin-walled layers alternating with layers of stone-cells.	Fairly abundant; contains inulin in amorphous masses.	Schizogenous glands and canals.
Endodermal cells, elongated axially, thickened on three walls.	None.	Abundant rounded and polygonal cells of pith and cortex.	Epidermis of rows of alternating long and short rectangular cells with wavy walls. Stomata characteristic.
Cells of the lignified medullary rays.	Thin-walled; yellow to brown.	Moderately thick-walled cells containing droplets of oil.	Numerous tracheids. Froths with water. Irritating odour.
None.	Thin-walled, polygonal, tabular cells; walls slightly waved.	Abundant; rather thick-walled; cells contain droplets of oil and calcium oxalate needles.	Very bitter taste. Characteristic odour.
None.	Thin-walled; absent from scraped Jamaica ginger.	Abundant; thin-walled, slightly elongated polygonal prisms; filled with starch.	Secretion cells, like the parenchyma, thin suberised walls, containing oleo-resin.
None.	Thin-walled, yellow, lignified, tabular, polygonal cells.	Abundant, thin-walled, filled with starch; cells often contain amorphous yellow masses.	Yellow powder, yields a micro-sublimate of yellow needles. Gives bunches of yellow crystals with hydrochloric or 2 per cent. sulphuric acid.
Brown, thick-walled, fibre-like from the hypoderma.	None.	Abundant, somewhat thickened walls. Intercellular spaces lined by thin cuticle and with internal unicellular glandular hairs.	Ramenta 1 cell thick, with 2-celled marginal teeth; no marginal glands.
None.	None.	Abundant, large polyhedral cells filled with starch.	Epidermis of slightly wavy brown-walled, rectangular to polygonal cells, pitted, with an occasional stoma. Gives a yellow colour with hydrochloric acid.

Name and Source.	Starch.	Calcium Oxalate.	Fibres.	Vessels.
Valerian. *Valeriana officinalis.*	Fairly abundant, granules, 3 to 12 to 20 microns ; simple and 2 to 6 compound.	None.	Thin-walled, narrow fibres from the xylem.	Not numerous. Pitted, spiral and annular.
Serpentary. *Aristolochia reticulata.*	Simple and compound granules, 3 to 15 microns.	None.	Few phloem fibres and also xylem fibres.	Pitted ; up to 40 microns wide.
Aconite *Aconitum Napellus.*	Abundant simple spherical granules ; also 2 to 4 compound, 8 to 13 and up to 15 microns.	None.	None.	Few ; reticulate and pitted. 20 to 30 microns wide.
Black Hellebore. *Helleborus niger.*	Abundant single and 2 to 4 compound. Individual granules 4 to 8 microns.	None.	None.	Spiral and reticulate.
Belladonna. *Atropa Belladonna.*	Simple and 2 to 4 compound. Granules 15 to 30 microns diameter.	Sphenoidal microcrystals in parenchymatous idioblasts.	Few, thin-walled and irregularly thickened, from the xylem.	Fairly numerous, pitted, with rounded bordered pits.
Orris. *Iris florentina.*	Simple granules 20 to 50 by 10 to 25 microns. Hilum stellate.	Large prisms 100 to 200 to 500 by 20 to 30 microns.	None.	Few spiral and reticulate.
Calumba. *Jateorhiza palmata.*	Mostly simple granules, some 2 to 3 compound ; 20 up to 85 microns wide ; hilum eccentric, radiate or cleft.	Small prisms in the stone-cells and also scattered throughout the parenchymatous ground tissue.	No true fibres. A small amount of fibrous tracheids near the vessels.	Pitted with transversely elongated bordered pits ; also reticulate vessels. Up to 150 microns wide.
Liquorice. *Glycyrrhiza glabra.*	Mostly simple granules 2 to 10 to 20 microns wide ; a few compound granules.	Prisms in files of small cells accompanying the fibres, also a few in the outer parenchyma.	Abundant in groups of 10 to 50. Individual fibres 10 to 15 to 20 microns wide.	Pitted with numerous oval bordered pits and a slit-shaped opening. Up to 200 microns wide.
Sweet Flag. *Acorus Calamus.*	Mostly simple granules, 2 to 4 to 8 microns wide. Few 2 to 4 compound.	Prisms in a few files accompanying the fibres.	Scanty, thick-walled, accompanying the bundles in the cortex.	Annular, spiral and reticulate, 10 to 30 microns wide.
Ipecacuanha. *Cephaëlis Ipecacuanha.*	Mostly compound with 2 to 4 components. Rio 4 to 10, but less than 15 microns. Carthagena up to 22 microns.	Bundles of acicular raphides in idioblasts scattered in the parenchyma. Length of the crystals 30 to 80 microns.	No true fibres. Fibrous tracheids and substitute fibres from the xylem.	Small and tracheidal, 10 to 20 microns wide.

Stone-Cells.	Cork.	Parenchyma.	Special Features and Tests.
Square prismatic cells from the pith.	Lignified. The cells contain drops of oil.	Rounded oblong cells filled with starch; somewhat thick walls.	Oil drops in the endodermis Epiblema with root-hairs present. Characteristic odour. Oil drops in the hypodermis of the roots.
Lignified cells of the medullary rays.	Thin-walled.	Thin-walled, pitted and lignified from the pith; polyhedral cellulose cells from cortex, both contain starch.	Yellowish-brown powder; camphoraceous odour; acrid bitter taste.
Few from the cortex; polygonal prismatic cells.	None.	Abundant thin-walled, polyhedral cells from the large pith and medullary rays. All with starch.	Metaderm of brown, cuticularised, tabular cells. Numbing taste.
From the pith of some of the roots.	None.	Rounded polygonal cells with pitted walls, containing starch.	Sternutatory powder. Brown tegumentary tissue composed of metaderm. Oil droplets in the parenchyma.
None.	Thin-walled, polygonal, tabular cells.	Somewhat abundant, walls slightly thickened; filled with starch, a few cells with sandy calcium oxalate.	Interxylary phloem present.
None.	Thin-walled, absent from the scraped rhizome.	Moderately thick-walled polyhedral cells with slightly beaded walls from the well-marked rounded simple pits.	Characteristic aromatic odour, resembling violets. Oil cells present.
Few rectangular in the outer part of the root. Walls yellow. Contain calcium oxalate.	Thin-walled, brown, polygonal, tabular cells.	Abundant, large-celled, thin-walled, elongated-polyhedral cells filled with starch.	Colour of vessels and stone-cells changed to green by 66 per cent. v/v sulphuric acid.
None.	Brownish, thin-walled, polygonal, tabular cells. Absent from the peeled drug.	Fairly abundant thin-walled, rounded polyhedral cells, filled with starch.	Sweet taste. Powder is coloured yellow by 66 per cent. v/v sulphuric acid.
None.	From the root scars, otherwise the outer covering is epidermis.	Collenchyma in outer part of the cortex. Frames of aerenchyma of thin-walled cells filled with starch.	Oil cells, with cuticularised walls, in the parenchyma; also tannin cells. Characteristic odour.
None.	Thin-walled, polygonal, tabular cells with dark brown contents.	Thin-walled, polyhedral cells filled with starch.	Cells of the lignified medullary rays, of the xylem parenchyma and the substitute fibres filled with starch.

Name and Source.	Starch.	Calcium-Oxalate.	Fibres.	Vessels.
Poke Root. *Phytolacca decandra.*	Oval granules, hilum radiate, up to 40 microns. Some compound.	Bundles of acicular raphides in idioblasts of the parenchyma. Needles 30 to 80 microns long.	Fairly thick-walled fibres from the xylem.	Large reticulate vessels and pitted vessels with oval or diamond - shaped bordered pits.
White Hellebore. *Veratrum album.*	Simple rounded granules, a few 2 to 4 compound. Individual grains 4 to 16 microns and up to 25 microns.	Bundles of acicular raphides. Needles 15 to 150 microns long.	Fibrous cells from the centres of the roots.	Large pitted vessels; also reticulate.
Sarsaparilla. *Smilax ornata.*	Very little from the pith.	Bundles of acicular raphides.	None.	Small spiral vessels 15 to 20 microns wide. Pitted and reticulate vessels up to 110 microns wide.
Rhubarb. *Rheum palmatum* and other species.	Simple granules and compound ones with 2 to 5 components. 4 to 20 or even 30 microns wide.	Clusters 20 to 200 microns wide; often over 100 microns.	None.	Non - lignified and reticulate; some spiral and annular. Up to 100 microns wide.
Marshmallow. *Althæa officinalis.*	Mostly simple granules, some 2 to 4 compound. 10 to 15 to 20 microns.	Clusters about 15 microns in diameter.	Unlignified phloem fibres; xylem fibres unlignified except the middle lamella. Both in groups of 4 to 25.	Scalariform and reticulate, 25 to 30 microns wide. They often show thylosis.
Podophyllum *Podophyllum peltatum.*	Usually 2 to 4 (up to 40) compound. Some simple. Granules 2 to 15 to 30 microns.	Clusters 20 to 100 microns across; often over 60 microns.	Small groups outside some of the bundles; up to 4 mm. long.	Cylindrical, pitted and scalariform, 15 to 20 microns wide.
Indian Podophyllum. *Podophyllum emodi.*	Simple and 2 to 25 compound. Individual granules 2 to 7 to 35 microns.	Few clusters 30 to 40 microns wide. Rarely over 60 microns.	Very occasional; up to 0·9 mm. long. Almost absent.	Irregular in shape; pitted.
Jalap. *Ipomœa purga.*	Simple granules and 2 to 4 compound. About 30 microns wide and up to 65 microns.	Clusters, 15 to 25 microns wide; up to 30 microns.	Fibrous tracheids.	Pitted with numerous bordered pits, up to 50 microns wide.
Ipomœa. *Ipomœa orizabensis.*	Abundant; mostly muller-shaped components of 2 to 5 compound granules. Few rounded simple granules. Up to 35 microns wide.	Numerous clusters, 15 to 45 microns wide. A few prisms.	Numerous fibres from the xylem, rather thick-walled.	Pitted with bordered pits.

Stone-Cells.	Cork.	Parenchyma.	Special Features and Tests.
None.	Thin-walled cells.	Rounded - rectangular cells, thin - walled, filled with starch ; occasional idioblasts with raphides.	Resin in some of the cells.
Yellowish endodermal cells, clongated axially and with horseshoe thickening.	None.	Rounded polygonal cells, filled with starch. Idioblasts with bundles of acicular raphides.	Metaderm of axially elongated cells. Powder is sternutatory.
Cells of the endodermis; exodermis and the pericyclic region.	None.	Rounded - rectangular cells, from the pith, with pitted walls and containing starch ; thin-walled cells from cortex without starch, some with raphides.	Froths when shaken with water.
None.	Thin-walled, polygonal, tabular cells ; cut away in the commercial drug.	Abundant, thin-walled, polygonal cells containing starch ; some cells with calcium oxalate clusters.	Parenchyma of the medullary rays contains yellow masses, insoluble in alcohol ; coloured red by caustic alkali.
None.	Thin-walled, polygonal, tabular cells. Absent from decorticated root.	Abundant thin-walled, axially elongated polygonal cells. Many mucilage and calcium oxalate idioblasts ; the remaining cells contain starch.	Mucilage stains with ruthenium red. Powder is coloured yellow by caustic alkali.
Sub-cylindrical cells from the pith.	Thin-walled cells, about one row under the epidermis.	Thin-walled, polygonal, pitted parenchyma ; some collenchymatous in outer cortex. Contains starch. Some calcium oxalate idioblasts.	Epidermis of isodiametric or elongated rectangular cells with red-brown contents. Copper acetate gives a green colour with an alcoholic tincture.
From the pith of root and rhizome, abundant short, contorted cells.	Thin - walled, polygonal, tabular cells.	Thin-walled, polygonal, pitted parenchyma filled with starch.	Epidermis absent. Copper acetate solution gives a brown precipitate with an alcoholic tincture.
Rare, yellowish in colour.	Brown-walled, polygonal, tabular cells.	Thin-walled, rounded rectangular cells filled with starch. Some calcium oxalate idioblasts. Secretion idioblasts in longitudinal rows.	Masses of resin stain brown with iodine and red with tincture of alkanna.
Few rectangular tables from the outer layers.	Thin-walled, somewhat scanty, much of it lignified.	Thin-walled cells ; in the outer part thick-walled. Numerous secretion idioblasts containing a resinous latex.	Grey-brown resin cells stain yellow with iodine water, scattered thickly in the parenchyma.

Name and Source.	Starch.	Aleurone.	Calcium Oxalate.	Pericarp.	
				Epicarp.	Mesocarp.
Almond. *Prunus communis.*	None.	Large grains, each with a small cluster crystal of calcium oxalate	Cluster crystals in the testa.	None.	None.
Kaladana. *Ipomœa hederacea.*	None.	Small, in the cotyledons with fixed oil.	Cluster crystals in the cotyledons, 10 to 15 microns.	None.	None.
Capsicum. *Capsicum minimum,* see p. 175.	None.	Grains, 3 to 6 microns, with fixed oil.	Microcrystals in idioblasts in the mesocarp.	Sub-rectangular cells in rows of 5 to 7. Striated.	Thin-walled parenchyma, many cells with red oily drops. Innermost layer composed of giant cells.
Strophanthus. *Strophanthus kombé.* see p. 168.	None.	Well-formed grains.	Few prisms and clusters in the testa.	None.	None.
Mustards. *Brassica spp.*	None.	Abundant grains of various shapes up to 16 or 25 microns. Each contains several globoids.	None.	None.	None.
Linseed. *Linum usitatissimum.*	None.	Well-formed grains, about 15 microns, with crystalloid and globoid.	None.	None.	None
Fenugreek. *Trigonella Fœnum-græcum.*	None.	Small in the epidermis of the endosperm and in the embryo.	None.	None.	None.
Soy. *Glycine hispida.*	None.	Well-formed grains, (3 to 10 microns), with crystalloid and globoid.	Prisms in many cells of the cotyledons, 24 × 4 microns.	None.	None.
Umbelliferous Fruits, see p. 170.	None.	Small grains, many containing a rosette of calcium oxalate.	Rosettes, about 4 microns in diameter, in aleurone grains.	Often diagnostic, see special table, p. 170.	Sometimes with reticulate parenchyma or sclerenchyma.
Coffee. *Caffea arabica.*	None.	Small grains embedded in an oil-plasma.	None.	None.	None.

	Testa			
Endocarp	Epidermis	Other Layers.	Stone-Cells	Special Features and Tests.
None.	Contains stone-cells, isolated and in small groups. Remainder is thin-walled parenchyma.	Parenchyma.	See epidermis. Rather thin-walled with simple pits; 60 to 400 microns, usually over 100 microns.	Fixed oil in the cotyledons
None.	Wavy, thin-walled cells with scattered unicellular conical trichomes.	The third layer is developed as a thick-walled palisade.		Mucilage in the endosperm. Large resin cells in the cotyledons.
Islands of sclerenchyma in a thin-walled parenchyma.	Heavily thickened and lignified with wavy anticlinal walls.	Collapsed parenchyma.	See endocarp and testa: both lignified.	Very pungent taste, due to crystals of capsaicin in the dissepiment. Pungency not destroyed by 2 per cent. caustic potash.
None.	Elongated polygonal cells, with thick, evenly lignified anticlinal walls; extended into trichomes with one lignified rib.	Contain occasional calcium oxalate crystals.	None.	Fixed oil in the endosperm and cotyledons. Endosperm gives a bright green colour with sulphuric acid 80 per cent. *v/v.*
None.	Thin-walled, filled with mucilage which stains with ruthenium red.	The inner coat is a hyaline layer in white mustard, but is brown in black mustard.	Inner epidermis of the outer coat consists of beaker-shaped sclerenchymatous cells.	Fixed oil in the embryo.
None.	Thin-walled, filled with mucilage, which stains with ruthenium red.	Hypodermis of collenchyma. Inner epidermis of inner coat of very flat, quadrangular cells with brown pigment.	Outer epidermis of the inner coat formed of small longitudinally elongated stone-cells, lignified	Thin-walled narrow-celled parenchyma crossing the sclerenchyma at right angles. Fixed oil in endosperm and cotyledons.
None.	Thick-walled palisade, cellulose cells about 65 × 15 microns.	Basket-like bearer cells.	None.	Mucilaginous endosperm.
None.	Thick-walled palisade; cells about 45 × 14 microns.	Hour-glass bearer cells.	None.	Fixed oil in the cotyledons.
Usually developed as a parquetry layer.	Adherent to the pericarp.		See pericarp.	Fixed oil in the endosperm, which consists of moderately thick-walled, polygonal, cellulose parenchyma.
None.	Thin-walled parenchyma with groups of 2 to 3 or more stone-cells.		From testa, lignified, 100 to 250 to 750 microns long, about 30 microns wide.	Endosperm cells with beaded cellulosic walls and large oval simple pits.

Name and Source.	Starch.	Aleurone.	Calcium Oxalate.	Pericarp.	
				Epicarp.	Mesocarp.
Nux Vomica. *Strychnos Nux vomica.*	None.	Grains of irregular shapes.	None.	None.	None.
Colocynth. *Citrullus Colocynthis.*	None.	In the cotyledons with fixed oil.	None.	Outer layers of lignified stone-cells. Occasional stomata in the epidermis.	Slightly lignified, thin - walled, rounded parenchyma with oval pitted areas.
Colchicum. *Colchicum autumnale.*	In the strophiole only. Simple and 2 to 8 compound. 4 to 10 to 20 microns.	Up to 5 microns in the endosperm with oil in a protoplasmic network.	None.	None.	None.
Nutmeg. *Myristica fragrans.*	Simple and 5 to 8 compound in cells of endosperm. Up to 20 microns.	One large grain with a crystalloid in each endosperm cell.	Prisms in the perisperm, but not oxalate, probably acid potassium tartrate.	None.	None.
Pepper. *Piper nigrum.*	Small polyhedral grains in large polyhedral masses.	Very small amorphous grains chiefly in the outer layers of the perisperm.	Small prisms in epidermis of pericarp.	Straight - walled cells. Occasional stoma. See stone-cells.	Thin-walled parenchyma with vascular bundles and oil cells.
Cubeb. *Piper cubeba.*	As pepper.	As pepper.	As pepper.	As pepper.	As pepper.
Cardamom. *Elettaria Cardamomum* var. *minuscula.*	Small polyhedral grains in masses from the cells of the perisperm.	Very small grains in the endosperm and embryo.	Prisms, one embedded in the starch of each perisperm cell.	Small polygonal tabular cells.	Radiating calcium oxalate needles in the parenchyma. Sclerenchymatous fibres surround the vascular bundles.
Pimento. *Pimenta officinalis.*	In the cotyledons mostly compound.		Small clusters and some prisms in the dissepiment and in the seed-coat.	Polygonal cells, with stomata and thick-walled unicellular trichomes.	Parenchyma with numerous groups of stone-cells.
Peas and Beans.	Ellipsoidal up to 60 to 70 microns, with an irregular slit-shaped hilum.	Small grains with the starch.	Usually absent, but see Soy and Haricot Bean.	None.	None.

Endocarp.	Testa.		Stone-Cells.	Special Features and Tests.
	Epidermis.	Other Layers.		
None.	Thick-walled lignified and pitted cells, each prolonged into a trichome with many lignified ribs.	Collapsed cells.	See epidermis.	Endosperm of thick, hemi-cellulosic walls and showing plasmodesma. Intensely bitter taste.
	Thick-walled, unlignified palisade. Vertical strips of thickening on the anticlinal walls.	Composed of thick-walled lignified sclerenchyma.	See testa and epicarp.	Intensely bitter taste.
None.	Slightly wavy, somewhat thickened, brown walls.	Innermost region of 2 layers of flattened thick-walled cells; next region of 2 layers of thick-walled polygonal cells.	None.	Endosperm of polygonal, thick-walled cellulose cells with simple pits.
None.	Removed.	Removed.	None.	Brown patches of perisperm with oil cells. Characteristic odour and taste. Much solid fat in the cells of the endosperm.
Single layer of beaker cells, lignified.	Brown pigment layer.	Hyaline layer.	In hypodermis of pericarp; in groups, mostly 1 layer only.	Oil cells in pericarp and in perisperm. Pungent odour and taste.
One or two layers of yellowish thick-walled sclerenchyma, lignified.	As pepper.	As pepper.	See endocarp. Also in the hypodermis of pericarp.	As pepper. Sprinkled on strong sulphuric acid, a crimson coloration develops.
	Fibre-like cells up to 350 microns long and 25 wide. Somewhat thickened walls.	Outer epidermis of the inner coat is composed of beaker cells, each with a silica nodule; dark brown.	See pericarp and testa.	Large rectangular cells of the middle layer of the outer seed coat are filled with oil globules. In the pericarp are occasional cells with brown resin.
Band of tissue composed of flattened cells.	Flattened cells, mostly polygonal in surface view.	Collapsed cells with red-brown contents.	See pericarp.	Spherical glands with oil in the outer part of the pericarp. Characteristic odour and taste.
None.	Epidermis of thick, cellulosic-walled palisade cells.	Often branched cells of a loose parenchyma	None.	Hour-glass bearer cells in the hypodermis of the testa, except in haricot bean.

APPENDIX I

SOME NUMERICAL DATA

Seeds	Weight of 100 seeds in grams.
Atropa Belladonna	0·107
Brassica alba	0·60
,, nigra	0·14 to 0·17
,, Rapa	0·50
Colchicum autumnale	0·36 to 0·55
Digitalis purpurea	0·004 to 0·007
Hyoscyamus niger	0·04 to 0·07
Ipomœa hederacea	2·6 to 3·9
,, muricata	14·0 to 18·4
Linum usitatissimum *var.* macrospermum	0·54 to 1·5
,, ,, *var.* microspermum	0·34 to 0·54
Myristica fragrans	350·0 to 760·0
Plantago arenaria	0·12 to 0·14
,, lanceolata	0·15 to 0·16
,, Psyllium	0·09 to 0·10
,, ovata	0·15 to 0·19
Strophanthus kombe	3·0 to 4·0
Strychnos Nux-vomica	120·0 to 208·0

Leaves. Vein-Islet Numbers, see p. 148.

Barosma Bathii	15 to 20
,, betulina	10 to 15
,, crenulata	10 to 16·5
,, ovata	15 to 20
,, serratifolia	9 to 24
,, venusta	5 to 7
Cassia acutifolia	25 to 30
,, augustifolia	19 to 23
Digitalis lanata	2 to 8
,, lutea	1 to 1·5, rarely 2
,, purpurea	2 to 5·5
,, Thapsi	8·5 to 16
Erythroxylum Coca	8 to 12
,, truxillense	15 to 26

Leaves. Palisade Ratio, see p. 148.

Ailanthus glandulosa	7 to 13
Atropa Belladonna	6 to 10
Barosma Bathii	8 to 24
,, betulina	10 to 26
,, ovata	5 to 14
,, serratifolia	8·5 to 18·5

Leaves. Palisade Ratio—*continued.*

Datura Stramonium	4 to 6, rarely 7
,, tatula	4 to 6, rarely 7
Digitalis lanata	2·5 to 6·5
,, lutea	2·5 to 6
,, purpurea	3·7 to 4·2
,, Thapsi	3 to 5
Hamamelis virginiana	5 to 8
Mentha viridis	5 to 7
Scopolia carniolica	3 to 5, rarely 6
Solanum nigrum	2 to 4
Xanthium Strumarium	3 to 4

Leaves. Stomatal Numbers, see p. 148.

	Upper surface.	Lower surface.
Arctostaphylos Uva-ursi	0	about 120
Atropa Belladonna	about 60	about 150
Barosma betulina	0	about 45
Cassia augustifolia	180 to **200** to 223	195 to **220** to 257
Datura innoxia	82 to **141** to 172	105 to **165** to 223
,, Stramonium	59 to **87** to 140	145 to **200** to 254
,, tatula	93 to **126** to 175	155 to **208** to 331
Digitalis purpurea	8 to 100	160 to 200

Crude Fibre

Dutch process, see p. 155.

	Per cent.
Cassia bark, Chinese	15·5 to 17
Cinnamon, Ceylon	25 to 28
Podophyllum, American	5·35 on drug dry at 100° C.
,, Indian	7·1 ,, ,, ,,
Senna leaves, Alexandrian	7·1
,, ,, Indian	8·2
Senna stalk, Alexandrian	25·3
,, ,, Indian	22·2

Ministry of Agriculture process.

Cassia bark, Chinese	18 to 24·5
Cinnamon bark, Ceylon	26 to 36
Chillies, Zanzibar	17 to 18
Clove stalks	13·6 to 18·7
Cloves	6 to **8** to 10·5
Ginger rhizome	1·7 to **4** to 9
Pepper, black	11 to 16
,, white	0·6 to 3·8
Pimento	13 to 22·4
Podophyllum, American	7·5
,, Indian	10·5

Microscopical Particles per Milligram of Certain Drugs

Starch Granules

Commercial starch.	Number of granules per mg. of the air-dry starch.	Moisture per cent.	Number of granules per mg. of the starch dry at 100° C.
Maize	846,000	13·4	977,000
	728,700	12·74	835,090
Maranta	172,700	14·24	201,375
	252,250	no record	
Potato	78,000	20·76	98,600
	67,120	17·04	80,900
Rice	10,381,360	15·96	12,360,000
	10,511,300	12·61	12,028,035
Wheat	1,827,360	17·2	2,207,000
Ginger rhizome . . .	286,000	13·9	332,172
Calumba root	51,200	no Record	—

Stone cells

Ipecacuanha stem contains 33 stone cells per mg.

Pollen grains

Insect Flowers (*Chrysanthemum cinerariæfolium*) contain from 1,000 to 2,000 pollen grains per mg. The number should not be less than 500.

Cousso (female inflorescence of *Brayera anthelmintica*) contains from 45 to 150 pollen grains per mg. ; the powdered drug should not contain more than 200 pollen grains per mg.

Spores

Lycopodium (the spores of *Lycopodium clavotum*) contains from 89,300 to 101,600 spores per mg. or an average of 94,000 spores.

Microscopical Measurement of Length, using powders of No. 90 fineness.

Length of rib of the epidermal trichomes per mg. of air-dry Nux Vomica seed, 167 to 206 cm., with a mean of 184 cm. per mg.

The moisture in these samples varied from 11·2 to 12·6 per cent., the average moisture being 11·6 per cent.

Microscopical Measurements of Area, using powders of No. 90 fineness.

	Sq. cm. per gm. of air-dry drug.	Moisture per cent.	Sq. cm. per gm. of drug dry at 100° C.
Area of Epidermis			
Ailanthus leaf . . .	295	7·27	318
Senna, Indian . . .	214	9·0	235
Senna, Alexandrian . .	202	9·0	222
Senna stalk, Indian . .	—	—	100
Senna, Indian; epidermis resembling that of the stalk	—	—	12
Area of Sclerenchymatous Layer			
Linseed . . .	32	8	34·8
Linseed, defatted . .	52	10	58
Area of Phloem Fibres			
Cassia bark . . .	11·3 to 12·5 mean 11·75	10·6	12·5 to 13·8 mean 13
Cinnamon bark . . .	80 to 90·5 mean 85	8·25	87 to 98 mean 92·5

APPENDIX II

REAGENTS

referred to in the Schedules

Acacia, Mucilage of

Quickly rinse 40 parts of gum acacia, in small tears, with a little distilled water, then dissolve in 60 parts of water and strain.

Alkanna, Tincture of

Macerate 1 part of bruised alkanet root in 5 volumes of 90 per cent. alcohol for one week and filter. This tincture will not keep in good condition for longer than about six months.

Aniline Chloride, Solution of

Dissolve 2 gm. of aniline hydrochloride in a mixture of 65 ml. of 90 per cent. alcohol and 35 ml. of distilled water and add 2 ml. of hydrochloric acid (sp. gr. 1·16).

Berlese Mountant

Distilled water	10 mils.
Dextrose	5 g.
Gum acacia	8 g.
Chloral hydrate	74 g.
Glacial acetic acid	3 mils.

Dissolve the dextrose in the water ; dissolve the gum acacia in the solution of dextrose and then add the chloral hydrate ; finally add the acetic acid.

Bleaching Solution (Solution of Sodium Hypochlorite)

Dissolve 75 gm. of crystalline sodium carbonate in 125 ml. of distilled water ; rub down 50 gm. of chlorinated lime in a mortar with 375 ml. of distilled water, added a little at a time. Mix the two fluids and shake occasionally during three or four hours ; filter.

Braemer's Reagent

Dissolve 1 gm. of sodium tungstate and 2 gm. of crystalline sodium acetate in sufficient distilled water to make 10 ml.

Canada Balsam Mountant

Heat Canada balsam on a water-bath until the volatile matter is removed and the residue sets to a hard mass on cooling. Dissolve the residue in xylene or in benzene to form a thin syrupy liquid.

Chloral Hydrate, Solution of

Dissolve 50 gm. of chloral hydrate in 20 ml. of distilled water.

Chlorzinciodine

Evaporate 100 ml. of Liquor Zinci Chloridi B.P. to 70 ml. or until it has lost a weight of 30 gm., dissolve in the residue 10 gm. of potassium iodide ; add 0·2 gm. of iodine and shake in a stoppered bottle at intervals until saturated with iodine.

Corallin Soda

Dissolve 5 gm. of corallin in 100 ml. of 90 per cent. alcohol. Dissolve 25 gm. of crystalline sodium carbonate in 100 ml. of water. Keep the two solutions in separate bottles and mix them, when required for use, in the following proportions : add 1 ml. of the 5 per cent. alcoholic corallin solution to 20 ml. of the 25 per cent. aqueous sodium carbonate. The mixed reagent will not keep in good condition for more than a few weeks.

Cuoxam or Ammoniacal Solution of Copper Oxide

Rub down 0·5 gm. of copper carbonate in a mortar with 10 ml. of distilled water and gradually add 10 ml. of strong solution of ammonia (sp. gr. 0·880) with continued stirring.

Eosin

Use a 1 per cent. solution of eosin in 90 per cent. alcohol.

Ether Alcohol

Mix equal volumes of ether and 90 per cent. alcohol.

Fehling's Reagent

Crystalline copper sulphate	34·6 gm.
Distilled water to	500 ml.

Dissolve and, if not quite clear, add a drop or two of sulphuric acid.

Sodium potassium tartrate	175 gm.
Sodium hydroxide	77 ,,
Distilled water to	500 ml.

Dissolve.

Mix equal volumes of the two solutions when required for use.

Ferric Chloride Solution

A 5 per cent. solution of ferric chloride in distilled water.

Glycerin, Dilute

One volume of glycerin mixed with 2 volumes of distilled water.

Hæmatoxylin, Delafield's

Prepare a saturated solution of ammonia alum, which is soluble 1 in 11 of water.

To 100 ml. of the saturated solution of ammonia alum add a solution of 1 gm. of hæmatoxylin in 6 ml. of alcohol (97 per cent.). Leave the mixed solution exposed to air and light in a stoppered bottle for 3 or 4 days ; filter and add to the filtrate 25 ml. of glycerin and 25 ml. of methyl alcohol. Allow the solution to stand in the light until it has acquired a dark colour—this requires about two months ; refilter and preserve in a stoppered bottle. For use the stock solution needs diluting to 3 or 4 times its volume with distilled water.

Hydrochloric Acid

The strong acid of the British Pharmacopœia ; sp. gr. 1·16, containing about 31 per cent. of real hydrogen chloride.

Iodine Water

Mix 1 volume of decinormal iodine with 4 volumes of distilled water or mix 1 volume of weak solution of iodine of the British Pharmacopœia with 9 volumes of water.

Indicator, Universal

The universal indicator made by the British Drug Houses, Graham Street, City Road, London, N.

Lactophenol (Amann's)

Phenol 20 gm., lactic acid 20 gm., glycerin 40 gm., distilled water 20 ml. Dissolve.

Millon's Reagent

Dissolve 1 volume of mercury in 9 volumes of fuming nitric acid (sp. gr. 1·52), keeping the mixture well cooled during the reaction. When the action is complete, add an equal volume of distilled water.

Phloroglucin

Dissolve 1 gm. of phloroglucin in 100 ml. of 90 per cent. alcohol.

Picric Acid

A saturated aqueous solution, made by dissolving 1 gm. of picric acid in 95 ml. of distilled water.

For staining aleurone grains use a solution in alcohol.

Potash, Caustic

For most purposes use a 5 per cent. solution in distilled water. Caustic soda may be substituted for caustic potash.

Ruthenium Red

Make a 10 per cent. solution of lead acetate. In 10 ml. of the lead acetate solution dissolve 0·008 gm. of ruthenium red. This reagent must be freshly prepared.

Safranin

Make a saturated solution of safranin in alcohol, 70 per cent.

Sandarac Mountant

Sandarac resin	32 gm.
Castor oil	5 ml.
Amylic alcohol	60 ,,

Dissolve and filter through paper.

Scharlach R. (Scarlet R.)

Alcohol, 90 per cent.	70 ml.
Distilled water	10 ,,
Ten per cent. aqueous solution of caustic potash	20 ,,

Mix and add Scharlach R. to saturation.

Soudan Red III

Soudan Red III	0·01 gm.
Alcohol, 90 per cent.	5·0 ml.
Glycerin	5·0 ,,

Dissolve.

Sulphovanadic Acid (Mandelin's Reagent)

Rub down 1 gm. of ammonium vanadate with 100 ml. of strong sulphuric acid (sp. gr. 1·843). Allow the deposit to subside and use the clear liquid. This reagent must be freshly prepared.

Sulphuric Acid

Various dilutions of the strong acid (sp. gr. 1·843) are used. The strongest acid suitable for chemomicroscopical testing is 80 per cent. by volume of the commercial strong acid, a strength of acid which will not char the cell walls, while it is sufficiently strong to give the necessary reactions.

Tannic Acid

Dissolve 5 gm. of tannic acid in distilled water and adjust the volume to 100 ml.

INDEX

PRINTED IN GREAT BRITAIN BY THE WHITEFRIARS PRESS LTD.
LONDON AND TONBRIDGE